ATLAS
OF
GENERAL
SURGERY

ATLAS OF GENERAL SURGERY

David C. Sabiston, Jr., M.D.

James B. Duke Professor and Chairman
Department of Surgery
Duke University Medical Center
Durham, North Carolina

Illustrations by

Robert G. Gordon, M.F.A.

Duke University Medical Center

W.B. SAUNDERS COMPANY
A Division of Harcourt Brace & Company
Philadelphia   London   Toronto   Montreal   Sydney   Tokyo

W.B. SAUNDERS COMPANY
A Division of
Harcourt Brace & Company

The Curtis Center
Independence Square West
Philadelphia, Pennsylvania 19106

Library of Congress Cataloging-in-Publication Data

Sabiston, David C.
Atlas of general surgery / David C. Sabiston, Jr.; illustrated by
Robert G. Gordon.

     p.   cm.

ISBN 0–7216–7883–1

1. Surgery, Operative—Atlases.   I. Title.

[DNLM: 1. Surgery, Operative—atlases. WO 517 S113a]

RD41.S23 1994

DNLM/DLC   92-48756

Atlas of General Surgery   ISBN 0–7216–7883–1

Printed in the United States of America.

Last digit is the print number: 9   8   7   6   5   4   3   2

CONTRIBUTORS

ONYE E. AKWARI, MD Associate Professor of Surgery and Associate Professor of Cell Biology and Physiology, Duke University Medical Center, Durham, North Carolina *Midline Incision Opening and Closing; Subtotal Left Colectomy; Pylorus-Saving Pancreaticoduodenectomy; Excision of Pilonidal Cysts and Sinuses; Splenectomy, Including Elective and Traumatic*

R. RANDAL BOLLINGER, MD, PHD Professor of Surgery and Associate Professor of Immunology; Chief of Surgical Transplant Service, Duke University Medical Center, Durham, North Carolina. *Kock Pouch; Ileoanal Anastomosis; Correction of Rectal Polapse*

DANIEL CLARKE-PEARSON, MD Professor of Gynecology and Obstetrics and Oncology, Duke University Medical Center, Durham, North Carolina *Abdominal Hysterectomy; Salpingectomy-Oophorectomy*

HOWARD C. FILSTON, MD Professor of Surgery and Chief, Division of Pediatric Surgery, The University of Tennessee Medical Center at Knoxville, College of Medicine-Knoxville, Knoxville, Tennessee *Inguinal Herniorrhaphy in Infants and Children*

SAMUEL R. FISHER, MD Associate Professor of Otolaryngology-Head and Neck Surgery, Duke University Medical Center, Durham, North Carolina *Radical Neck Dissection with Spinal Accessory Nerve Preservation Technique; Parotidectomy*

RICHARD D. GOLDNER, MD Associate Professor of Orthopaedic Surgery, Duke University Medical Center, Durham, North Carolina *Suture of Nerve; Suture of Tendon; Drainage of Hand Infections*

JOHN P. GRANT, MD Associate Professor of Surgery; Director, Nutritional Support Service, Duke University Medical Center, Durham, North Carolina *Insertion of Right Atrial Catheters for Chemotherapy, Antibiotics, and Hyperalimentation; Repair of Incisional Hernia; Repair of Petit's Hernia; Stamm Gastrostomy; Witzel Gastrostomy; Percutaneous Endoscopic Gastrostomy; Witzel Jejunostomy; Feeding (Needle Tube) Jejunostomy; Laparoscopic Jejunostomy; Appendectomy; Left Colectomy; Surgical Procedures for Morbid Obesity*

ROBERT C. HARLAND, MD Assistant Professor of Surgery; Duke University Medical Center, Durham, North Carolina *Insertion of Peritoneal Shunts*

J. DIRK IGLEHART, MD Associate Professor of Surgery and Cell Biology, Duke University Medical Center, Durham, North Carolina *Excision of Benign Tumor; Wide Local Excision Breast Biopsy—Segmentectomy, Tylectomy, or Lumpectomy; Breast Biopsy After Needle Localization; Splenectomy, Including Elective and Traumatic*

R. SCOTT JONES, MD Stephen H. Watts Professor and Chairman, Department of Surgery, University of Virginia Health Sciences Center, Charlottesville, Virginia; Attending Staff, University of Virginia Hospital, Charlottesville, Virginia *Gastric Resection: Billroth I Anastomosis; Gastric Resection: Billroth II*

LOWELL R. KING, MD Professor of Urology and Associate Professor of Pediatrics; Head, Section of Pediatric Urology, Duke University Medical Center, Durham, North Carolina *Hydrocelectomy: Bottle Procedure*

GEORGE S. LEIGHT, JR., MD Associate Professor of Surgery, Duke University Medical Center, Durham, North Carolina *Subtotal and Total Thyroidectomy and Thyroid Lobectomy; Parathyroidectomy for Hyperplasia and Adenoma; Excision of Benign Adrenal Neoplasm (Posterior Adrenalectomy, Right); Total Adrenalectomy (Anterior)*

H. KIM LYERLY, MD Assistant Professor of Surgery and Pathology, Duke University Medical Center, Durham, North Carolina *Modified Radical Mastectomy; Laparoscopic Colostomy*

RICHARD L. McCANN, MD Professor of Surgery; Chief, Vascular Surgical Service, Duke University Medical Center, Durham, North Carolina *Excision of Iliac Arterial Aneurysm; Excision of Thoracoabdominal Aneurysms; Carotid Endarterectomy (with Internal Shunt); Femoropopliteal Bypass; Femoropopliteal Bypass (In Situ); Femorotibial and Peroneal Bypass; Hepatorenal Bypass; Aortorenal Revascularization; Splenorenal Anastomosis; Portocaval Shunt; Ligation and Stripping of Varicose Veins; Below Knee Amputation; Supracondylar Amputation; Transmetatarsal Amputation*

WILLIAM C. MEYERS, MD Professor of Surgery; Chief, Gastrointestinal Surgical Service; Co-Director, Duke/U.S. Surgical Endosurgical Center, Duke University Medical Center, Durham, North Carolina *Heineke-Mikulicz Pyloroplasty; Finney Pyloroplasty; Jaboulay Pyloroplasty; Repair of Hiatal Hernia (Nissen); Total Gastrectomy; Enterotomy for Gallstone Ileus; Roux-en-Y Gastrojejunostomy; Right Colectomy; Transverse Colostomy; Miles Abdominoperitoneal Resection; Excision of Ampulla of Vater and Bile Duct; Segmental Hepatic Resection; Right Hepatic Lobectomy; Left Hepatic Lobectomy; Liver Transplantation*

JOSEPH A. MOYLAN, MD Professor of Surgery, Director of the Trauma Center, Duke University Medical Center, Durham, North Carolina *Inguinal Herniorrhaphy: Bassini (Inguinal Ligament); Laparoscopic Inguinal Hernia; Umbilical Hernia (Adult); Preperitoneal Herniorrhaphy; Repair of Spigelian Hernia; Sigmoid Colectomy; Hemorrhoidectomy; Drainage of Rectal Abscess; Excision of Fissure-in-Ano; Incision of Fistula-in-Ano*

THEODORE N. PAPPAS, MD Associate Professor of Surgery; Co-Director, Duke/U.S. Surgical Endosurgical Center, Duke University Medical Center, Chief of Surgical Service, Durham VA Medical Center, Durham, North Carolina *Laparoscopic Inguinal Hernia; Laparoscopic Nissen Fundoplication; Closure of Perforated Peptic Ulcer; Truncal Vagotomy; Laparoscopic Truncal Vagotomy and Gastrojejunostomy; Highly Selective Vagotomy; Meckel's Diverticulectomy; Laparoscopic Appendectomy; Laparoscopically Assisted Ileocolectomy; Laparoscopic Cholecystectomy; Cholecystectomy and Exploration of Common Duct; Partial Pancreatectomy (Distal); Drainage of Pancreatic Pseudocyst: Cystogastrostomy; Pancreaticojejunostomy (Puestow); Pancreaticoduodenectomy: Whipple Procedure*

WILLIAM P. J. PEETE, MD Professor of Surgery, Emeritus, Duke University Medical Center, Durham, North Carolina *Hernia Repair: General Principles; Inguinal Herniorrhaphy: McVay (Cooper's Ligament); Inguinal Herniorrhaphy: Shouldice; Gastrojejunostomy*

R. LAWRENCE REED, II, MD Associate Professor of Surgery and Associate Professor of Anesthesiology; Director, Surgical Intensive Care Unit, Duke University Medical Center, Durham, North Carolina *Surgical Management of Hepatic Trauma*

ARTHUR J. ROSS, III, MD Associate Professor of Pediatric Surgery, Division of Pediatric Surgery, University of Pennsylvania School of Medicine and Children's Hospital of Philadelphia, Philadelphia, Pennsylvania *Fundoplication for Gastroesophageal Reflux in Infants and Children; Correction of Malrotation with Midgut Volvulus; Splenic Repair (Pediatric)*

DAVID C. SABISTON, JR., MD James B. Duke Professor and Chairman, Department of Surgery, Duke University Medical Center, Durham, North Carolina *Excision of Femoral Arterial Aneurysm; Resection of Abdominal Aortic Aneurysm; Aortofemoral Bypass Graft for Occlusive Disease (Leriche's Syndrome); Distal Splenorenal Shunt (Distal and Proximal)*

HILLIARD F. SEIGLER, MD Professor of Surgery and Professor of Microbiology and Immunology, Duke University Medical Center, Durham, North Carolina *Heineke-Mikulicz Pyloroplasty (Stapler); Gastric Resection: Billroth I Anastomosis (Stapler); Total Gastrectomy (Stapler); Gastrojejunostomy (Stapler); Roux-en-Y Gastrojejunostomy (Stapler); Right Colectomy (Stapler); Low Anterior Resection; Axillary Node Dissection; Inguinal Node Dissection*

DONALD SERAFIN, MD Professor of Plastic, Reconstructive, Maxillofacial, and Oral Surgery; Chief, Division of Plastic, Reconstructive, Maxillofacial, and Oral Surgery, Duke University Medical Center, Durham, North Carolina *Insertion of Breast Prosthesis*

NICHOLAS A. SHORTER, MD Assistant Professor of Surgery and Pediatrics; Director, Pediatric Surgical Service, Dartmouth-Hitchcock Medical Center, The Hitchcock Clinic, Lebanon, New Hampshire *Umbilical Hernia (Child); Hydrocelectomy; Pyloromyotomy for Congenital Hypertrophic Pyloric Stenosis; Reduction of Intussusception*

DELFORD L. STICKEL, MD Professor of Surgery; Associate Director for Medical Affairs, Duke University Medical Center, Durham, North Carolina *Renal Dialysis Access Procedures; Insertion of Tenckhoff Catheter*

WALTER B. VERNON, MD Director, Pancreas Transplant Program, Porter Transplant Service, Porter Memorial Hospital, Denver, Colorado *Pancreas Transplantation*

JOHN L. WEINERTH, MD Professor of Surgery and Urology; Associate Dean, Graduate Medical Education, School of Medicine, Duke University Medical Center, Durham, North Carolina *Kidney Transplantation*

W. GLENN YOUNG, JR., MD Professor of Surgery, Duke University Medical Center, Durham, North Carolina *Excision of Carotid Body Tumor*

FOREWORD

"A work on surgery. . . .without principles, may be compared to a vessel at sea without helm or rudder to guide it to its place of destination."

SAMUEL D. GROSS, 1839

Medical textbooks are educational tools that describe mechanisms of disease and therapeutic intervention. Diseases treated by surgery require translation of the details of therapy—the operation—from a three-dimensional description to a two-dimensional illustration. The challenge of preparing an atlas is blending two-dimensional illustrations with descriptive and complementary text.

Atlas of General Surgery is a superb contribution to the surgical literature. The volume reflects the advance of laparoscopic technique and its appropriate inclusion in the lexicon of operative surgery.

The illustrations, superbly done by Robert G. Gordon, M.F.A., are in the best tradition of the great schools of medical illustration, reflecting the background of the editor.

The 16 chapters that comprise 125 procedures or operations and 1010 illustrations encompass the spectrum and breadth of general surgery. The book is more like a highly illustrated textbook than a collection of illustrated procedures, as is the case with most atlases. In that dimension, *Atlas of General Surgery* is similar to its most distant American predecessor, the first textbook of surgery published in the United States in 1813, John Syng Dorsey's *Elements of Surgery*.

The authors who describe the illustrated procedures are part of the faculty of Duke University Medical Center, Durham, North Carolina. The editor, David C. Sabiston, Jr., M.D., James B. Duke Professor and Chairman at Duke since 1964, is the senior academic chair in surgery in the United States. He brings the perspective of acknowledged leadership and excellence in academic medicine of many years.

Dr. Sabiston's academic honors include presidencies of most of the academic surgical organizations, such as the American College of Surgeons, the American Surgical Association, the Society of University Surgeons, and the Southern Surgical Association, and chairmanship of the American Board of Surgery. His leadership outside of surgery includes posts as Chairman of the Surgery Study Section of the National Institutes of Health, Chairman of the Accreditation Council for Graduate Medical Education, Graduate Medical Education Committee of the Robert Wood Johnson Foundation, and others.

Pertinent to this publication, Dr. Sabiston is contemporary medicine's most skilled and prolific editor. He is editor of *Annals of Surgery* and serves on eight other editorial boards.

This *Atlas* joins 11 other textbook products of the Sabiston–W.B. Saunders collaboration. That editorial collaboration includes the venerable *Textbook of Surgery*, now entering its 15th edition. Although this Atlas was not specifically written as a companion volume to this work, it does complement it. The high quality of this book allows it to comfortably supplement any work in the surgical literature.

A surgical atlas is usually among the first books purchased by new residents. Unlike most other textbook purchases, the atlas is expected to last and to be consulted over an entire surgical career. It is used to orient residents to unfamiliar procedures. At a later period in the career of a surgeon, it is a "refresher" course the night before an operation done only occasionally. It frequently has readers' notes in the margin, reflecting yet a further refinement or maneuver revealed to the surgeon who has performed the operation with the atlas as a blueprint.

This *Atlas* will predictably accompany many surgeons through decades of practice to the usefulness of our profession and the benefit of many patients.

GEORGE F. SHELDON, M.D., F.A.C.S.
Zack D. Owens Professor and Chairman
Department of Surgery
University of North Carolina
Chapel Hill, North Carolina

PREFACE

"The operating room is the surgeon's laboratory."
WILLIAM S. HALSTED

The concept underlying this *Atlas of General Surgery* is to make available to the surgical profession a complete and thorough presentation of contemporary procedures used in general surgery. Much emphasis has been placed on stepwise illustrations of these procedures, accompanied by depiction and narration in considerable detail. With such an approach, it is possible for surgical residents as well as practicing surgeons to follow in a detailed manner the exact technique employed for specific operations.

The *Atlas* is divided into 16 major sections with 125 chapters and more than a thousand illustrations. In the first portion, *Abdominal Incisions, Vascular Procedures, Hernias,* and the *Breast* are considered, followed by a lengthy section on *Abdominal Operations.* The *Liver, Pancreas,* and *Spleen* are individually presented with extensive drawings. *Endocrine Surgery, Head and Neck Procedures, Gynecology,* and *Transplantation of Organs* are discussed with a host of additional detailed illustrations. *Amputations* are reviewed, as well as a number of miscellaneous procedures including insertion of a variety of intravenous catheters for prolonged use.

During the past several years, *laparoscopic* surgical techniques have become extensively employed, and this approach is carefully described in the *Atlas* with specific illustrative procedures for *hernia, cholecystectomy, appendectomy, jejunostomy, fundoplication for esophageal hiatal hernia, truncal vagotomy, ileocolectomy,* and *colostomy.* The 72 individual drawings of laparoscopic procedure, with careful descriptions of each, thoroughly familiarize the surgeon with these very important contemporary techniques.

The illustrations have been meticulously drawn by a brilliant and skillful medical artist, Mr. Robert G. Gordon, M.F.A. It is exceedingly fortunate that over the past two years, he has drawn *every* illustration in the text. It is easy to predict that much praise will be heard in the future of Gordon's remarkable work. Thoroughly committed to his profession, he is an unusually conscientious and skilled medical artist with an original art form that is quite engaging and is uniformly characterized by its clarity. The editor is deeply grateful for his unique contributions to this *Atlas.*

Praise is also due the members of the faculty in the Department of Surgery at the Duke University Medical Center for their contributions. Their uniform commitment to the principles of the *Atlas* are gratefully acknowledged. Several other former members of the faculty who now hold academic positions at other centers have also contributed to this *Atlas* and are gratefully acknowledged.

The procedures described in this *Atlas* are those performed, endorsed, and in many instances devised by the members of the surgical staff of the Duke University Medical Center. The success of these techniques has been demonstrated in numerous patients, and they can be recommended as both safe and effective.

DAVID C. SABISTON, JR., M.D.

ACKNOWLEDGMENTS

The editor is deeply indebted to each of the contributors to this *Atlas* and especially for their enthusiasm and attention to every detail. Special recognition is due Robert G. Gordon, M.F.A., for his splendid artwork throughout the text and for his loyal and undivided commitment to this project during the past two years.

Appreciation is due also to Ms. Lisette Bralow, Vice President and Editor-in-Chief of Medical Books at W.B. Saunders Company, for her ever-present assistance, beginning with the conceptual plans and through each step of the development of this work until its final completion. Her interest and enthusiasm throughout are gratefully acknowledged. As in the past, the staff at the W.B. Saunders Company has been unflagging in their support throughout the production of this *Atlas*. Thanks are due Ms. Carolyn Naylor, Production Manager, for her thoughtful advice and continuous assistance in all aspects of the text. Her experience and judgment have meant much in this undertaking.

Special thanks and appreciation are due Ms. Tzipora Sofare, my editorial assistant, for her outstanding abilities and talent in editorial preparation and her impressive attention to detail. She has been an essential part of the preparation of this text, and her loyal commitment to all aspects of this *Atlas* are deeply appreciated. Thanks also go to Mrs. Patricia W. Jordan, who has prepared much of the correspondence and computer-driven production of the manuscripts.

Each of these colleagues is deserving of my enduring thanks. With their help and enthusiasm, this *Atlas* has become a reality.

CONTENTS

SECTION III
Hernias

SECTION IV
The Breast

SECTION V
Abdominal Operations

SECTION VI
Colon

S E C T I O N   X V I
Miscellaneous Procedures

Abdominal Incisions

1

Midline Incision Opening and Closing

ONYE E. AKWARI, M.D.

The advantages of a midline incision are

1. It is almost bloodless.
2. No muscle fibers are divided.
3. No nerves are injured.
4. It provides good access to abdominal viscera.
5. It can be made quickly.

The disadvantage is that access to the stomach, duodenum, gallbladder, and spleen may be unsatisfactory in patients who are massively obese, who have a wide costal margin, or in whom the distance from the xiphoid to the pubis is unusually short.

FIGURE 1–1. The incision is placed exactly in the midline, above and below the umbilicus, from the tip of the xiphoid process to the pubis. It is deflected around the umbilicus to the right or left at the discretion of the surgeon, depending on the side involved by the disease process. In addition, consideration is given to the placement of ostomies: the incision is generally made to deflect around the umbilicus opposite the site of the ostomy. This helps minimize spillover from the ostomy into the wound during the early postoperative period, when ostomy diarrhea and care are most problematic for the patient.

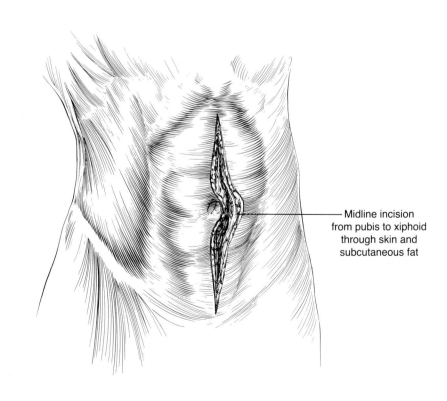

Midline incision from pubis to xiphoid through skin and subcutaneous fat

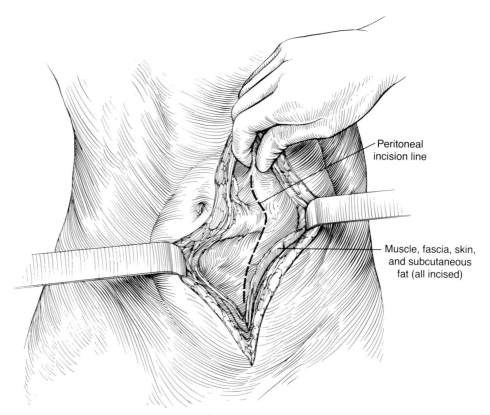

Peritoneal
incision line

Muscle, fascia, skin,
and subcutaneous
fat (all incised)

FIGURE 1–2

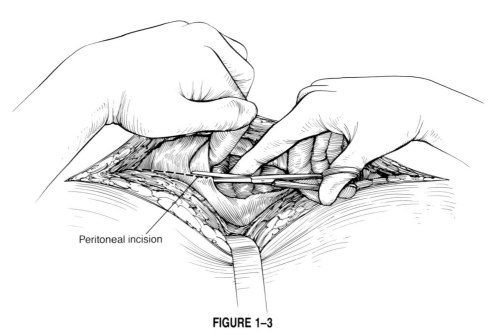

Peritoneal incision

FIGURE 1–3

FIGURES 1–2 and 1–3. The incision divides skin, subcutaneous tissues, extraperitoneal fat, and peritoneum. The extraperitoneal fat is abundant and vascular in the upper third of the incision. The suspensory ligament of the liver is avoided and is usually divided between two clamps and completely excised.

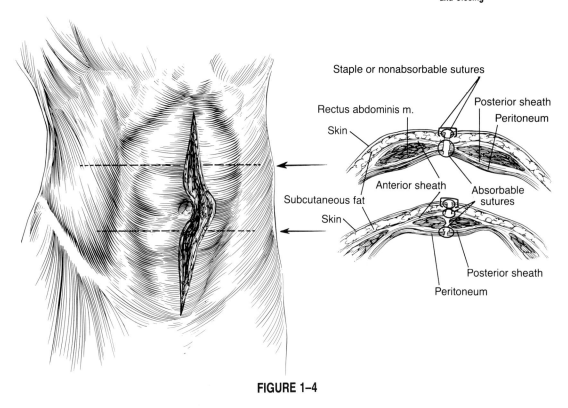

FIGURE 1–4

FIGURES 1–4 and 1–5. Wound closure is accomplished using interrupted or running 1 nonabsorbable suture in the midline fascia above the umbilicus. Below the umbilicus, the posterior fascia and then the anterior fascia of the rectus abdominis muscle are closed as separate layers. The subcutaneous fatty layer is approximated with skin sutures of interrupted No. 30 nonabsorbable suture. Interrupted stainless steel staples may be used on the skin before sterile dressings are applied.

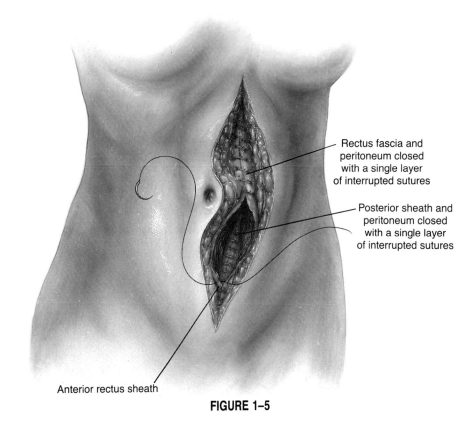

FIGURE 1–5

Vascular Procedures

2

Excision of Iliac Arterial Aneurysm

RICHARD L. McCANN, M.D.

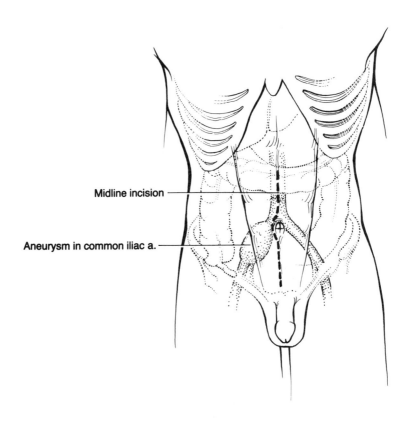

Midline incision

Aneurysm in common iliac a.

FIGURE 2–1. A midline incision is preferred for the excellent exposure and flexibility that it affords. The small bowel is retracted to the right, and the sigmoid colon to the left; these are protected with moist laparotomy pads. The aortic bifurcation and proximal iliac vessels are exposed.

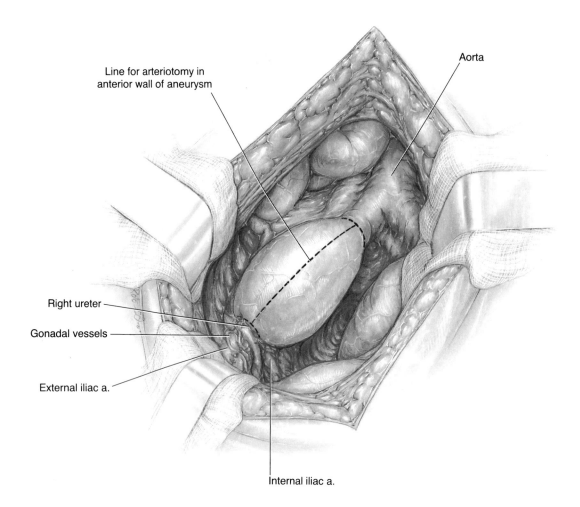

Line for arteriotomy in
anterior wall of aneurysm

Aorta

Right ureter

Gonadal vessels

External iliac a.

Internal iliac a.

FIGURE 2–2. The posterior parietal peritoneum is incised with care to identify the ureters and to mobilize them laterally. Most aneurysms end at the bifurcation of the common iliac artery. The neck of the aneurysm at the level of the terminal aorta is prepared for clamping, and the external and internal iliac vessels are individually controlled as well. The patient is heparinized and clamps are applied. The aneurysm is opened, and any thrombus or atherosclerotic material is removed. An appropriately sized Dacron graft, either woven or knitted, according to the surgeon's preference, is used.

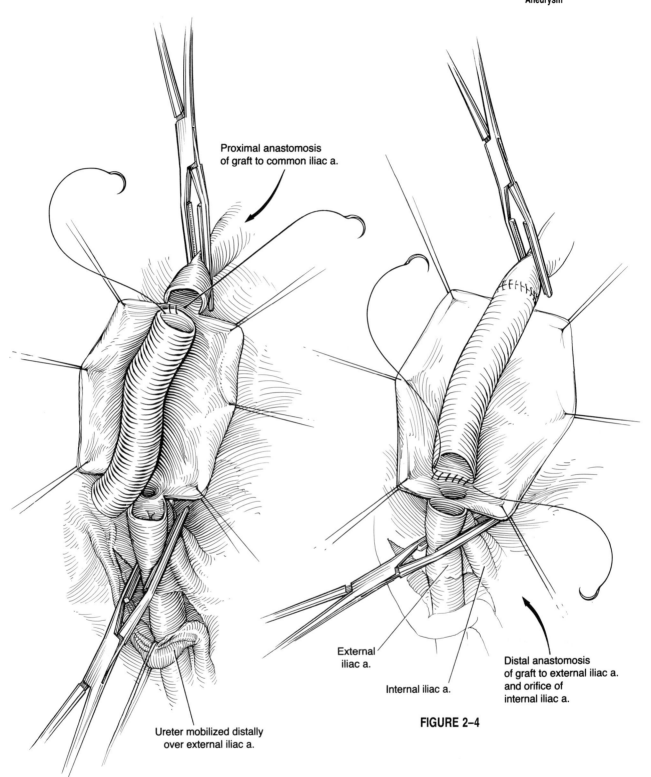

Proximal anastomosis
of graft to common iliac a.

Ureter mobilized distally
over external iliac a.

External
iliac a.

Internal iliac a.

Distal anastomosis
of graft to external iliac a.
and orifice of
internal iliac a.

FIGURE 2–4

FIGURE 2–3

FIGURE 2–3. The proximal anastomosis is done first using a continuous nonabsorbable vascular suture. After completion of the proximal anastomosis, the clamp is temporarily released to distend the graft under arterial pressure, and the appropriate length can be determined.

FIGURE 2–4. After sizing the graft, a single distal anastomosis is made between the two orifices of the internal and external iliac vessels. Every effort is made to preserve flow to the pelvic organs through the hypogastric artery.

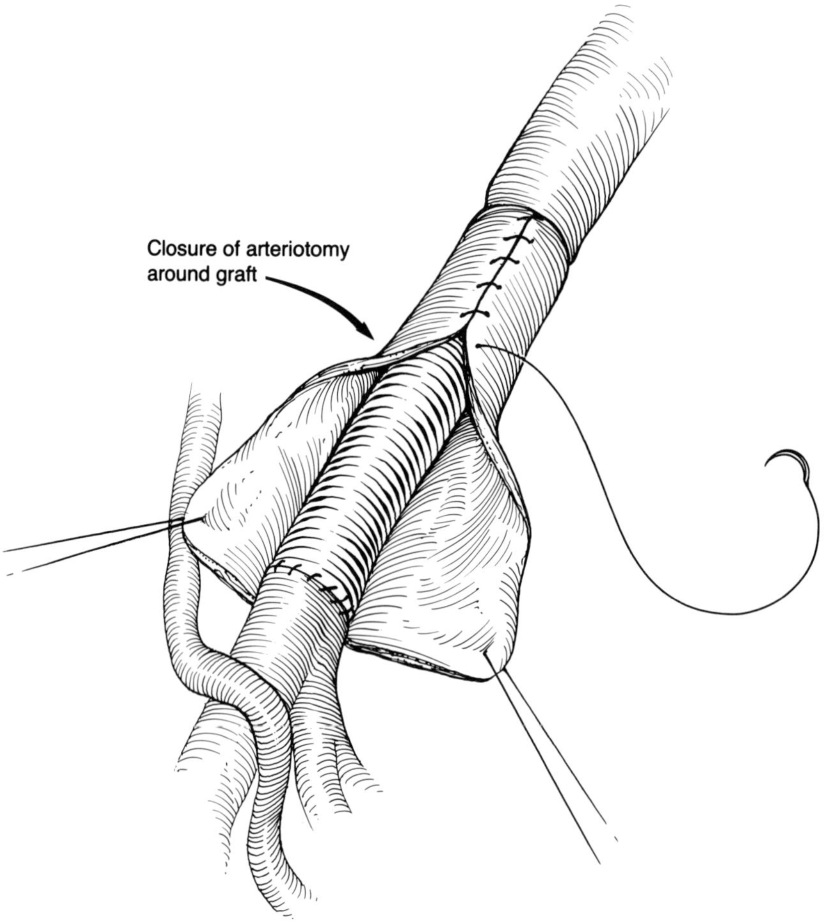

Closure of arteriotomy around graft

FIGURE 2–5. After release of the clamps, the pulse is palpated in the groin. If it is found to be satisfactory, the walls of the aneurysm are closed over the graft to isolate the prosthesis from the abdominal viscera. The peritoneum is repaired with an absorbable suture. After irrigation, the abdominal midline wound is closed by approximating the linea alba with interrupted nonabsorbable sutures and the skin is approximated with staples.

3

Excision of Femoral Arterial Aneurysm

DAVID C. SABISTON, JR., M.D.

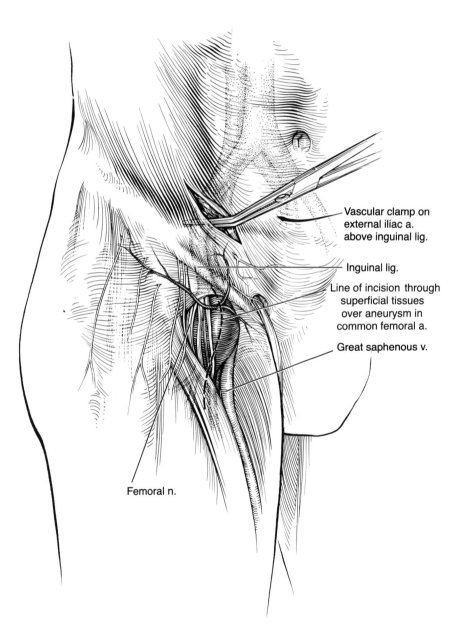

Vascular clamp on
external iliac a.
above inguinal lig.

Inguinal lig.

Line of incision through
superficial tissues
over aneurysm in
common femoral a.

Great saphenous v.

Femoral n.

FIGURE 3–1. A vertical incision is made in the groin to expose the aneurysm. A second incision is made just above the inguinal ligament to expose the femoral artery proximally.

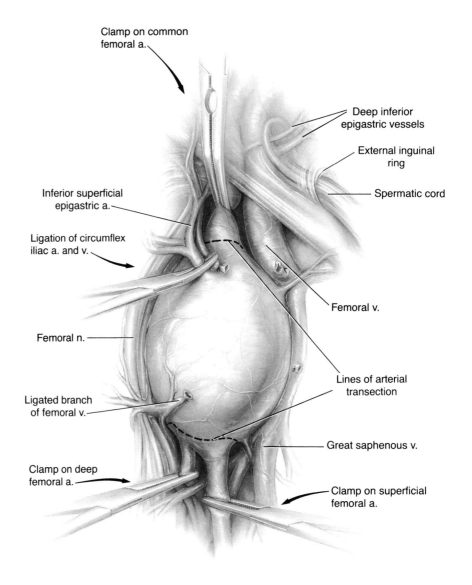

Clamp on common
femoral a.

Deep inferior
epigastric vessels

External inguinal
ring

Spermatic cord

Inferior superficial
epigastric a.

Ligation of circumflex
iliac a. and v.

Femoral v.

Femoral n.

Lines of arterial
transection

Ligated branch
of femoral v.

Great saphenous v.

Clamp on deep
femoral a.

Clamp on superficial
femoral a.

FIGURE 3–2. A woven Dacron graft of appropriate size is selected and preclotted with the patient's blood. A saphenous vein autograft can also be used if one of appropriate size is available. Heparin (5000 μ) is administered intravenously. The femoral artery is occluded proximally and distally, and the aneurysm is excised.

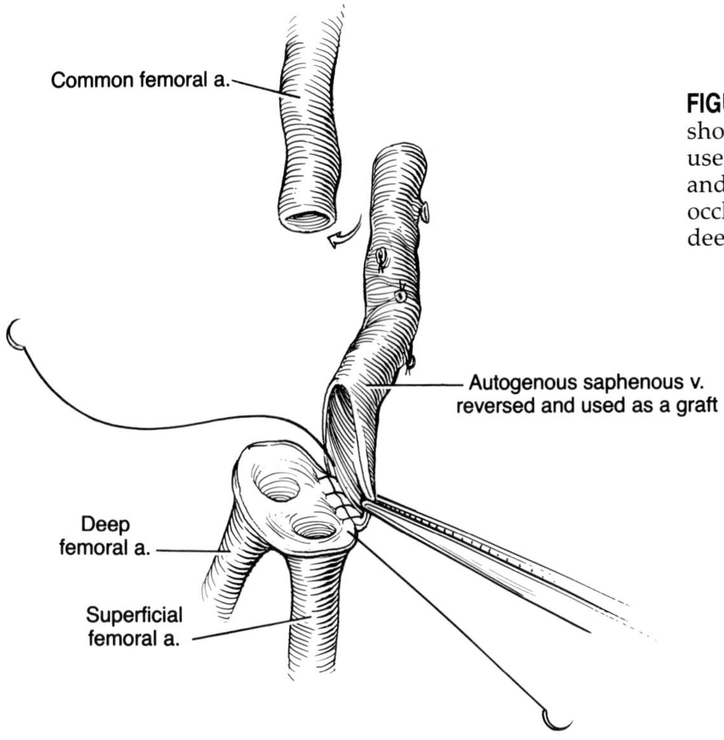

PREFERRED METHOD

Common femoral a.

Autogenous saphenous v.
reversed and used as a graft

Deep
femoral a.

Superficial
femoral a.

FIGURE 3–3. The proximal anastomosis is made as shown with 4–0 Prolene. The vein graft can also be used and is shown being inserted end-to-end proximally and distally through a button of the femoral artery, occluding the orifices of both the superficial and the deep femoral arteries.

FIGURE 3–3

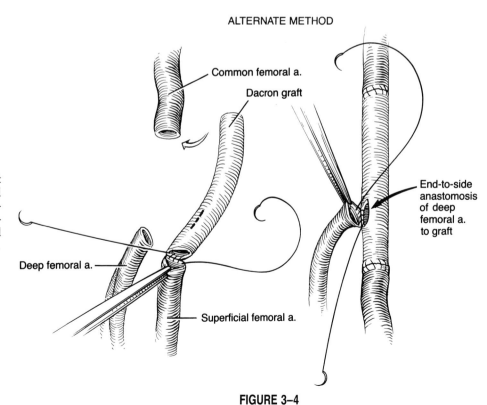

ALTERNATE METHOD

Common femoral a.

Dacron graft

End-to-side
anastomosis
of deep
femoral a.
to graft

Deep femoral a.

Superficial femoral a.

FIGURE 3–4. A Dacron graft also can be used and inserted end-to-end. It may be necessary to anastomose separately the distal deep femoral artery to the side of the graft.

FIGURE 3–4

4

Resection of Abdominal Aortic Aneurysm

DAVID C. SABISTON, JR., M.D.

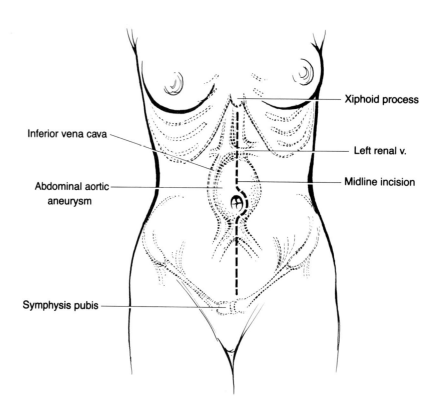

FIGURE 4–1. Aneurysms of the infrarenal abdominal aorta and of the iliac arteries are approachable *either* through a midline incision or through a left lateral approach. Most aneurysms of the abdominal aorta are managed through a midline incision extending from the xiphoid process to the symphysis pubis.

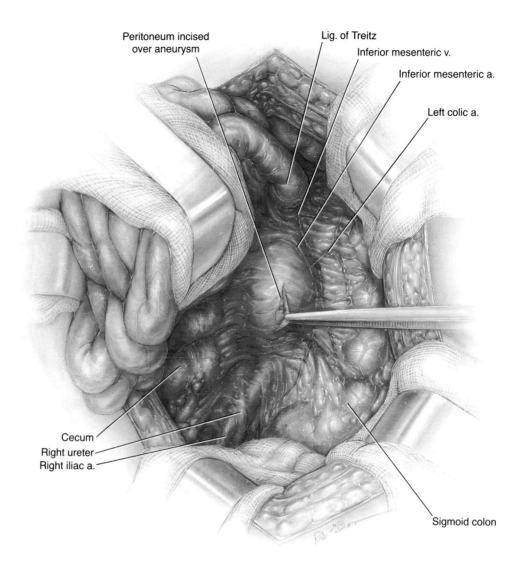

Peritoneum incised
over aneurysm

Lig. of Treitz

Inferior mesenteric v.

Inferior mesenteric a.

Left colic a.

Cecum

Right ureter

Right iliac a.

Sigmoid colon

FIGURE 4–2. The linea alba is incised, exposing the peritoneum, which is then opened, and a self-retaining retractor is placed. The abdominal cavity and its contents are carefully explored for any coexisting lesions. The small bowel is retracted toward the right and carefully protected by moist abdominal pads to prevent injury. The small bowel contents can be placed in a Lahey plastic bag and removed from the peritoneal cavity to provide more adequate exposure if needed. The transverse colon is retracted superiorly, and the posterior peritoneum is then exposed, identifying the ligament of Treitz and the fourth portion of the duodenum.

An incision is made in the retroperitoneum directly over the abdominal aneurysm and extended inferiorly beyond the bifurcation of the aorta and superiorly along the abdominal aorta to a point between the duodenum and the inferior mesenteric vein. This provides access to the abdominal aorta below the renal arteries and exposure of the left renal vein. The latter courses anterior to the aorta in approximately 95 per cent of patients, but, in the remaining 5 per cent, it is posterior and should be identified to be certain that it is not injured during subsequent dissection. At this point, it is appropriate to view the field carefully for proper exposure with the use of indwelling retractors, including the ring-shaped type, which allows retraction in all parts of the field, perhaps supplemented by appropriately placed Deaver retractors.

The infrarenal abdominal aorta is then dissected laterally on each side, as well as the two common iliac arteries, if necessary. Heparin is administered intravenously (100 I.U./kg.). A vascular clamp is applied proximally to the infrarenal aorta and across the aorta distally (or across both iliac arteries, as determined by the extent of the aneurysm).

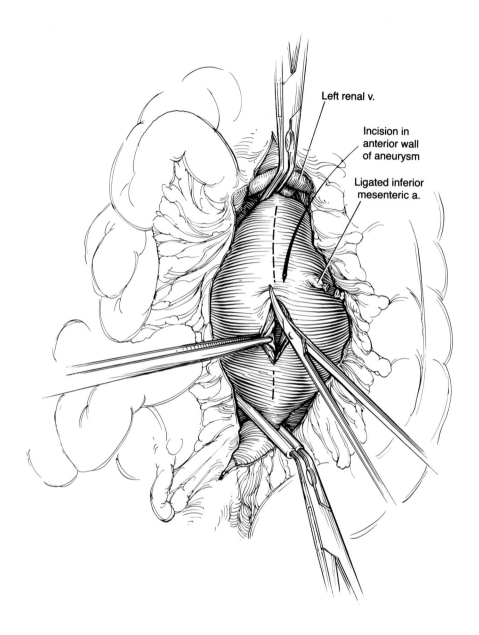

Left renal v.

Incision in anterior wall of aneurysm

Ligated inferior mesenteric a.

FIGURE 4–3. An incision is made in the midportion of the aortic abdominal aneurysm, and the lumen of the aneurysm is then opened and aspirated. Usually, considerable thrombus is present in the aneurysm, and this is removed.

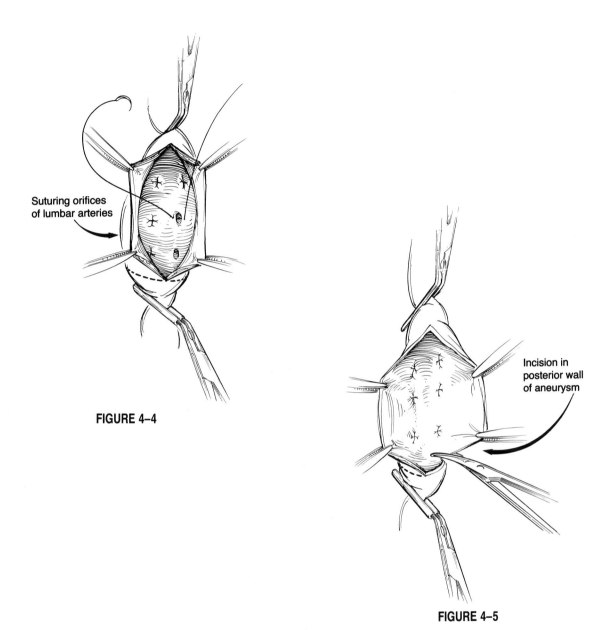

**Suturing orifices
of lumbar arteries**

FIGURE 4–4

**Incision in
posterior wall
of aneurysm**

FIGURE 4–5

FIGURES 4–4 and 4–5. At this point, *retrograde* bleeding is generally encountered from the lumbar arteries, and they are transfixed for control. The use of a cell saver may be advantageous to minimize the need for transfusion of blood. The inferior mesenteric artery can be safely ligated in the vast majority of cases because it is usually quite stenotic or totally occluded at its origin from the aneurysm. If the inferior mesenteric artery is large, it may be patent with only a small amount of backbleeding, and consideration can be given its reimplantation into the wall of the aortic graft. It is important to inspect the sigmoid colon carefully at the end of the procedure to be certain that it has adequate blood supply before closing the abdomen. If not, the inferior mesenteric artery should definitely be anastomosed to the aortic graft.

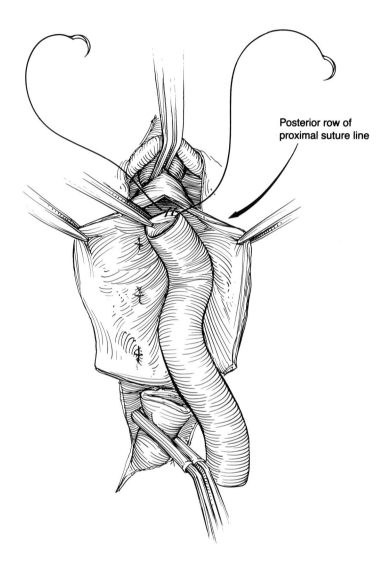

Posterior row of
proximal suture line

FIGURE 4–6. Suturing of the graft generally begins proximally at six o'clock posteriorly, extending on each side to twelve o'clock, with sutures of 2–0 polypropylene on large needles.

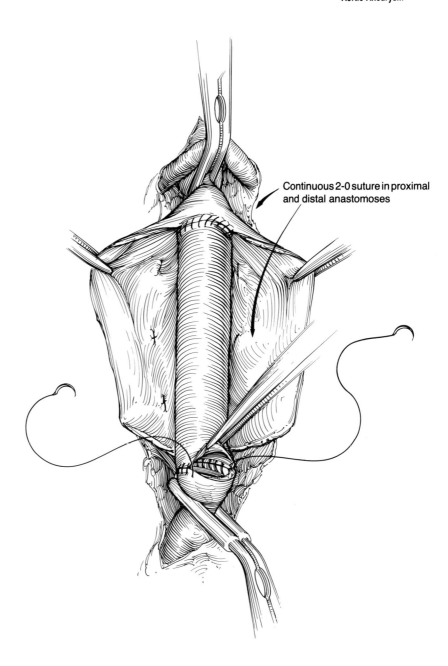

Continuous 2-0 suture in proximal
and distal anastomoses

FIGURE 4–7. After the proximal anastomosis is completed, a similar anastomosis is made to the distal aorta or to the iliac arteries, depending on the extent of the aneurysm.

Before the last suture is tied, the distal clamps on the iliac vessels should be individually released to be certain of backflow and also to flush out any thrombi or debris that may be present. Similarly, the proximal clamp is slowly released to flush the graft through the distal suture line.

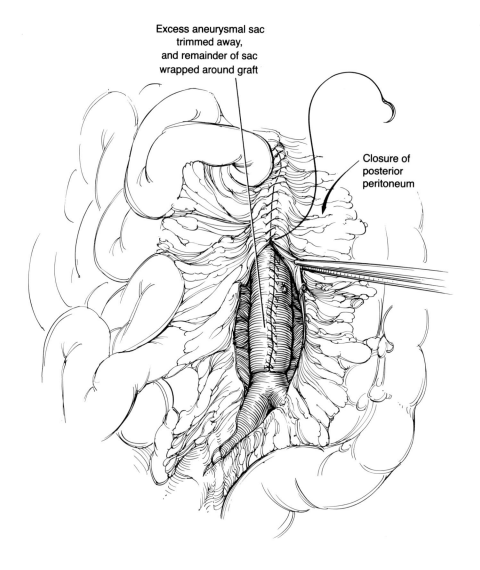

Excess aneurysmal sac
trimmed away,
and remainder of sac
wrapped around graft

Closure of
posterior
peritoneum

FIGURE 4–8. The excess aneurysmal sac is then trimmed away, and the remaining sac is closed over the graft to protect it from contact with the duodenum and jejunum. The posterior peritoneum is closed.

Careful exploration should be made for any bleeding points and for viability of the sigmoid colon. The incision is closed with interrupted sutures. The heparin is then reversed with protamine.

5

Aortofemoral Bypass Graft for Occlusive Disease (LERICHE'S SYNDROME)

DAVID C. SABISTON, JR., M.D.

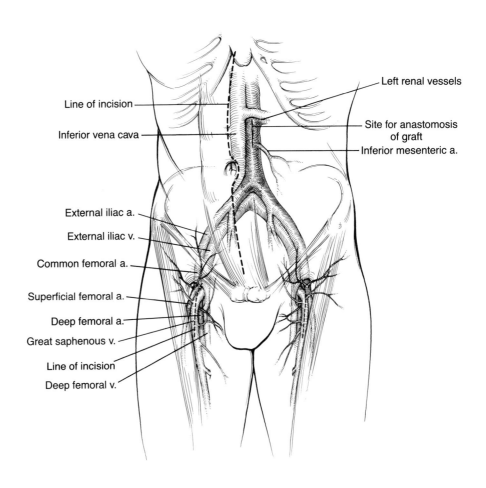

FIGURE 5–1. A midline incision is made from the xiphoid process to the symphysis pubis, and the peritoneal cavity is entered through the linea alba.

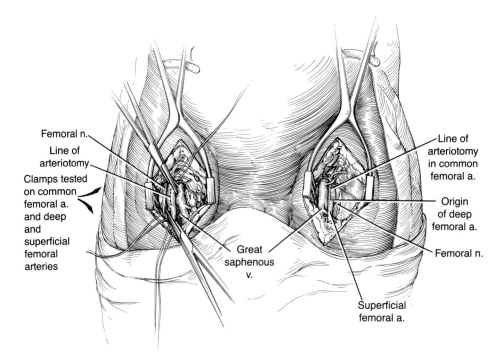

Femoral n.

Line of
arteriotomy

Clamps tested
on common
femoral a.
and deep
and
superficial
femoral
arteries

Great
saphenous
v.

Line of
arteriotomy
in common
femoral a.

Origin
of deep
femoral a.

Femoral n.

Superficial
femoral a.

FIGURE 5–2. Vertical incisions are made in both groins, crossing the inguinal crease to expose the femoral arteries.

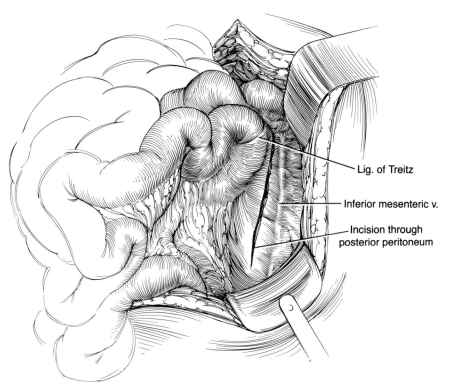

Lig. of Treitz

Inferior mesenteric v.

Incision through
posterior peritoneum

FIGURE 5–3. The small intestine is retracted laterally (or placed in a Lahey plastic bag and withdrawn through the incision for maximal exposure). An incision is made in the retroperitoneum overlying the abdominal aorta.

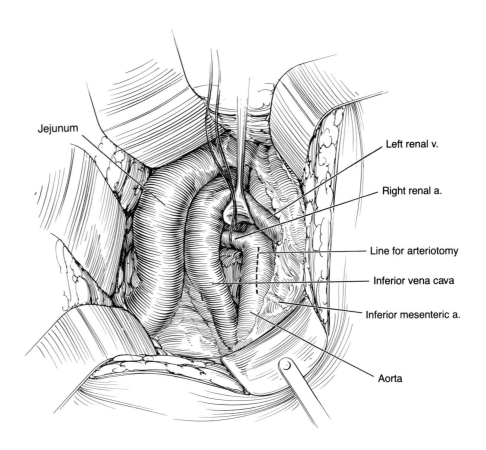

Jejunum

Left renal v.

Right renal a.

Line for arteriotomy

Inferior vena cava

Inferior mesenteric a.

Aorta

FIGURE 5–4. Appropriate exposure is obtained by the use of a Balfour-type or ring retractor and appropriate placement of Deaver retractors. If the thrombotic occlusion of the aorta is proximally located, the left renal vein is dissected and retracted superiorly. A partial occlusion arterial clamp is placed longitudinally, and an incision is then made in the aortic wall preparatory to anastomosis of the graft.

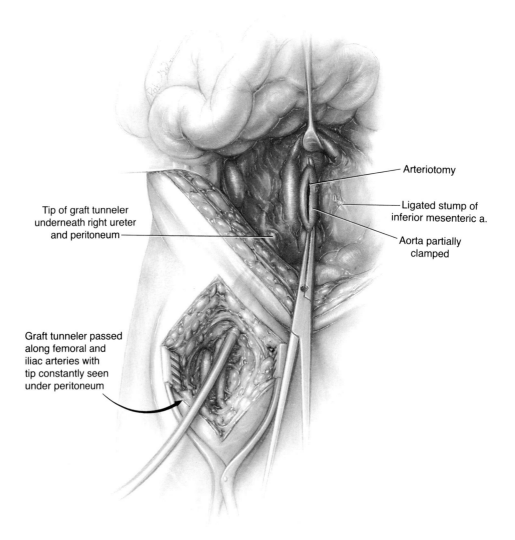

Arteriotomy

Ligated stump of
inferior mesenteric a.

Aorta partially
clamped

Tip of graft tunneler
underneath right ureter
and peritoneum

Graft tunneler passed
along femoral and
iliac arteries with
tip constantly seen
under peritoneum

FIGURE 5–5. Retaining retractors are then placed in the inguinal incisions. A tunneler is passed anterior to the femoral artery to the retroperitoneum, with constant vision from within the peritoneal cavity of the tunneler as it progresses toward the abdominal aorta to prevent injury.

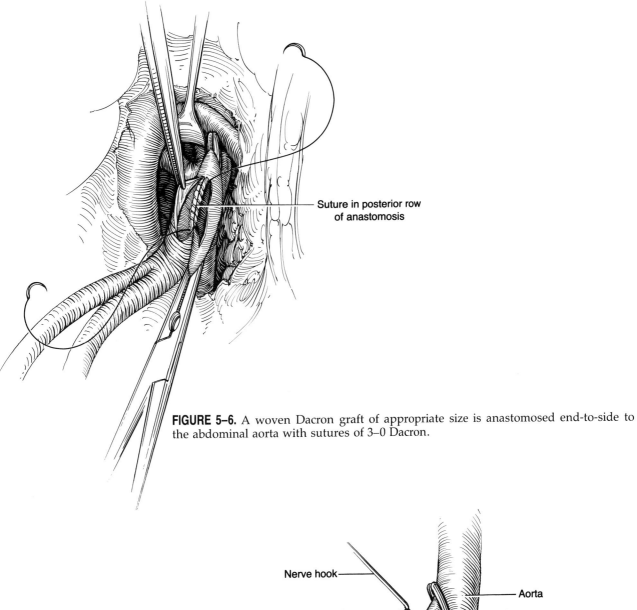

FIGURE 5–6. A woven Dacron graft of appropriate size is anastomosed end-to-side to the abdominal aorta with sutures of 3–0 Dacron.

Suture in posterior row
of anastomosis

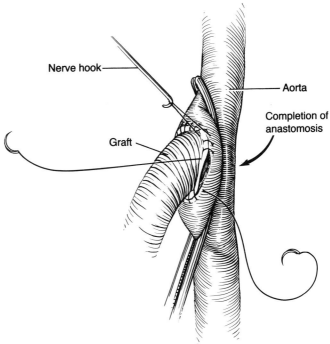

Nerve hook

Aorta

Completion of
anastomosis

Graft

FIGURE 5–7. A nerve hook is used to tighten the suture line as shown.

ALTERNATE METHOD OF ANASTOMOSIS WITH
COMPLETE TRANSECTION OF AORTA

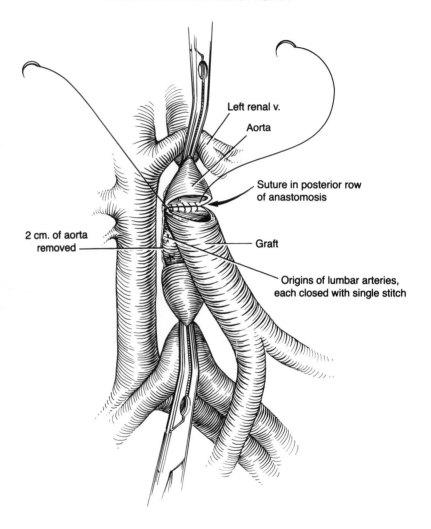

Left renal v.

Aorta

Suture in posterior row
of anastomosis

2 cm. of aorta
removed

Graft

Origins of lumbar arteries,
each closed with single stitch

FIGURE 5–8. An alternative technique for the proximal anastomosis is division of the
abdominal aorta with an end-to-end anastomosis to the graft.

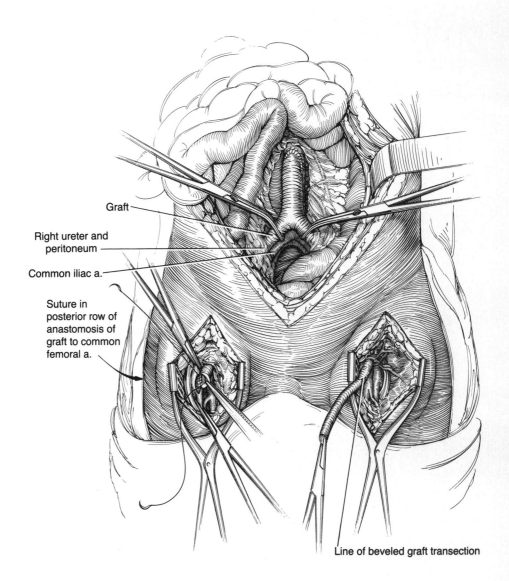

Graft

Right ureter and
peritoneum

Common iliac a.

Suture in
posterior row of
anastomosis of
graft to common
femoral a.

Line of beveled graft transection

FIGURE 5–9. The iliac limbs of the graft are drawn through the retroperitoneal tunnel into the inguinal region. Anastomoses are then made to the femoral arteries end-to-side with sutures of 4–0 Dacron. The retroperitoneum is reconstituted, and the incisions are closed in layers.

6

Excision of Thoracoabdominal Aneurysms

RICHARD L. McCANN, M.D.

Excision of thoracoabdominal and pararenal aortic aneurysms involves occluding the aorta proximal to the origin of the visceral vessels. The surgical technique is directed toward minimizing the visceral ischemic time and ensuring adequate visceral perfusion postoperatively.

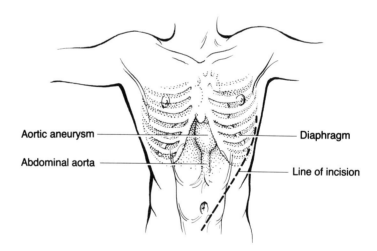

Aortic aneurysm

Abdominal aorta

Diaphragm

Line of incision

FIGURE 6–1. The upper abdominal aorta and origins of the visceral vessels are best approached through a thoracoabdominal or thoracoretroperitoneal incision. The patient is positioned with the left flank elevated, and the lower left thorax is included in the field. The incision extends from the region of the umbilicus through the eighth, ninth, or tenth intercostal space. The incision is made lower for iliac involvement and higher if the lower thoracic aorta is involved. The oblique muscles and the anterior rectus sheath are divided, and the intercostal space is entered. The rib may be resected if additional exposure is required; however, if the aneurysm extends only to the level of the diaphragm, division of one rib posteriorly usually provides satisfactory exposure.

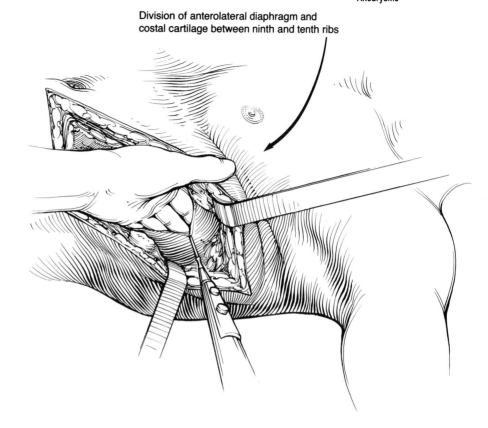

Division of anterolateral diaphragm and
costal cartilage between ninth and tenth ribs

FIGURE 6–2. The diaphragm is incised radially several centimeters away from its insertion. This provides entry into the retroperitoneal space.

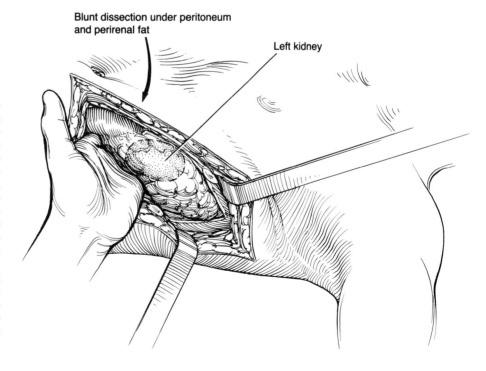

Blunt dissection under peritoneum
and perirenal fat

Left kidney

FIGURE 6–3. The plane anterior to the lumbar muscles is developed, and the peritoneum and posterior Gerota's fascia are dissected from the posterior muscles. The peritoneum is carefully dissected from the diaphragm. The advantage of keeping the peritoneal membrane intact is that the intestines are more easily retracted medially; however, this is not essential, and entry into the peritoneal cavity may be necessary if the peritoneum is not easily dissected away. Care is taken to identify the left ureter as the kidney is elevated.

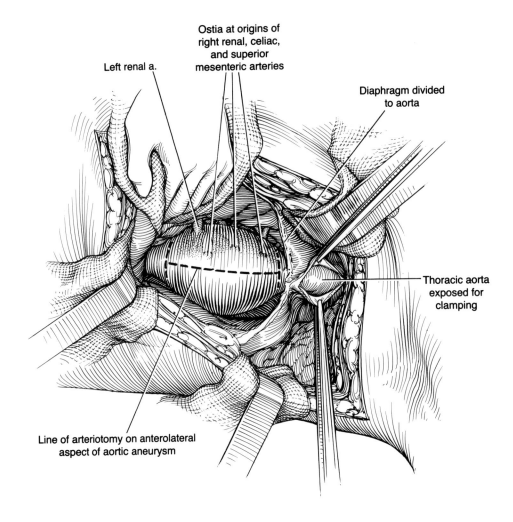

FIGURE 6–4. The lateral and posterior portion of the aneurysm is identified and the posterolateral aspect is prepared for incision. The normal aorta superiorly is exposed in preparation for clamping, care being taken to avoid injury to the overlying esophagus and phrenic nerve. The dissection is extended as far distally as required, depending on the extent of the aneurysm. If the iliac arteries are not involved, only the distal aorta needs to be identified. If the proximal iliac vessels are involved, they require exposure by continuing the dissection distally.

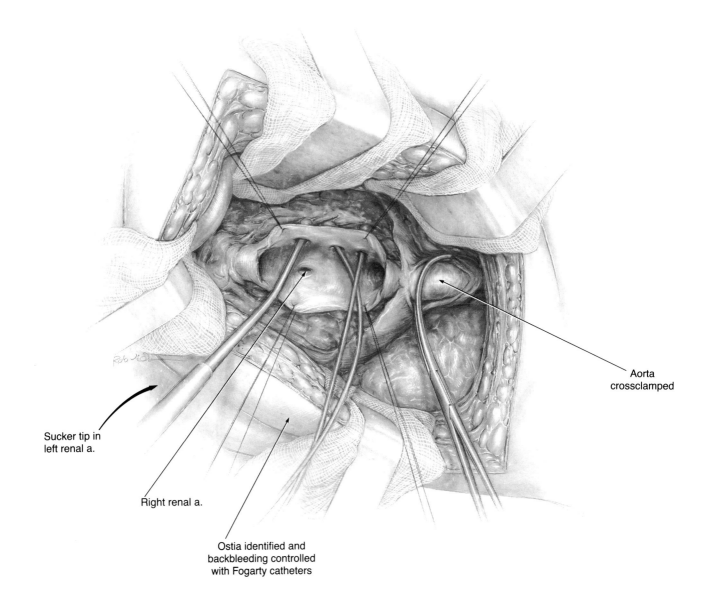

Sucker tip in
left renal a.

Right renal a.

Ostia identified and
backbleeding controlled
with Fogarty catheters

Aorta
crossclamped

FIGURE 6–5. Radial division of the diaphragm is continued to the aortic hiatus, and the distal thoracic aorta is exposed in preparation for placement of the aortic crossclamp. In elective cases, the patient is heparinized and the proximal crossclamp is slowly applied while the arterial pressure is monitored. Vasodilators are usually required, and it is helpful to monitor cardiac performance with transesophageal echocardiography during this phase of the procedure. The origins of the visceral vessels are anterior to the dissection and are usually not visualized until the aorta has been opened. After placement of the proximal crossclamp, the aorta is incised and the blood from backbleeding of the visceral vessels and the lower extremities is collected with a blood-scavenging apparatus and reinfused. Backbleeding from the celiac, superior mesenteric, and two renal vessels is controlled by insertion of balloon catheters. If necessary, ostial endarterectomy can be performed on these vessels. A distal clamp is usually not required, as backbleeding from the iliac vessels is minimal. Intraluminal Fogarty catheters can be used in the iliac arteries if desired.

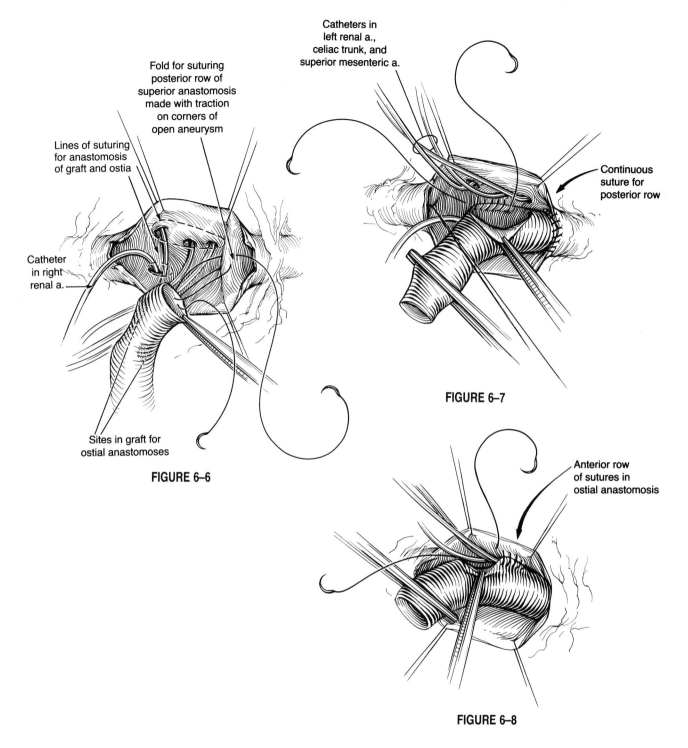

Lines of suturing
for anastomosis
of graft and ostia

Fold for suturing
posterior row of
superior anastomosis
made with traction
on corners of
open aneurysm

Catheters in
left renal a.,
celiac trunk, and
superior mesenteric a.

Catheter
in right
renal a.

Continuous
suture for
posterior row

Sites in graft for
ostial anastomoses

FIGURE 6–6

FIGURE 6–7

Anterior row
of sutures in
ostial anastomosis

FIGURE 6–8

FIGURE 6–6. After the mural thrombus has been removed and the neck of the aneurysm identified, the proximal anastomosis is begun with a woven Dacron graft, and the proximal anastomosis is made using a running vascular suture.

FIGURES 6–7 and 6–8. At the completion of the proximal anastomosis, reimplantation of the visceral vessels is begun. Usually, several vessels can be incorporated into a single island; however, if one vessel is separated from the others by a significant distance, it may be necessary to reimplant it separately. Openings in the graft are sewn to the aortic wall around the orifices of the visceral vessels sequentially. As soon as feasible, flow is restored to the visceral vessels, and ischemic time can usually be kept to less than 60 minutes.

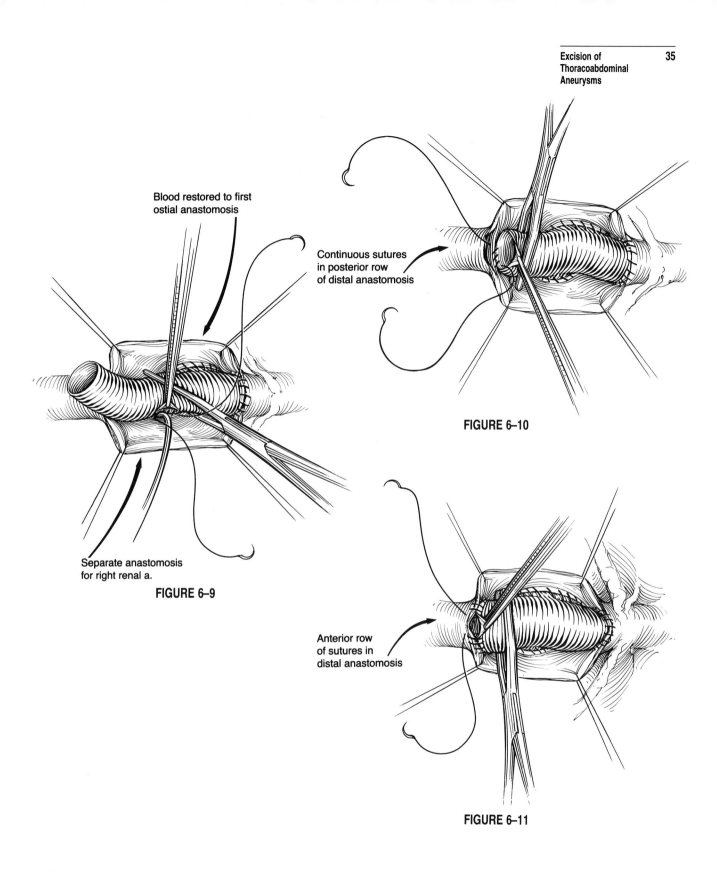

Blood restored to first
ostial anastomosis

Continuous sutures
in posterior row
of distal anastomosis

FIGURE 6–10

Separate anastomosis
for right renal a.

FIGURE 6–9

Anterior row
of sutures in
distal anastomosis

FIGURE 6–11

FIGURES 6–9 to 6–11. After complete visceral revascularization, the distal anastomosis is made either to the iliac or to the aortic bifurcation, as required. After release of the final crossclamp, perfusion is restored to the lower extremities.

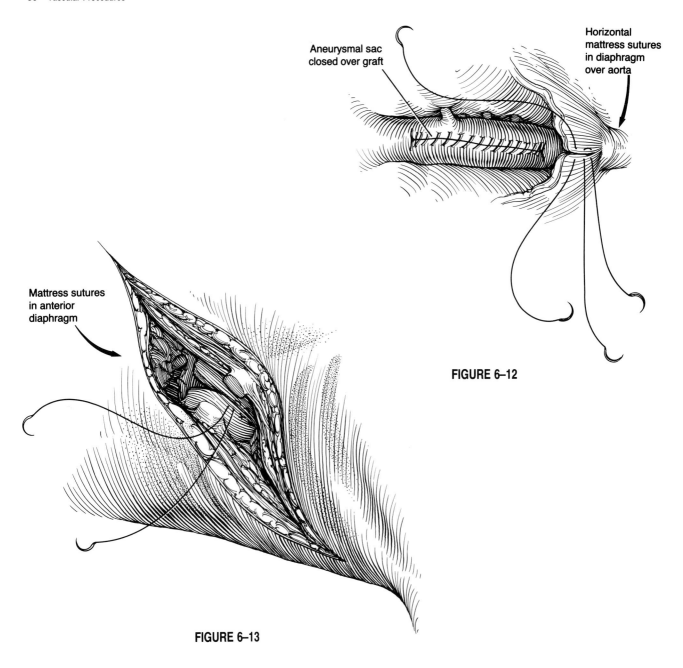

Aneurysmal sac
closed over graft

Horizontal
mattress sutures
in diaphragm
over aorta

FIGURE 6–12

Mattress sutures
in anterior
diaphragm

FIGURE 6–13

FIGURE 6–12. The remaining wall of the aneurysm is closed over the graft with a continuous suture. The abdominal viscera are allowed to return to their anatomic position. The chest is drained with an anterior and posterior tube for air and fluid, respectively. The abdomen is closed by approximating the muscle layers anatomically.

FIGURE 6–13. The diaphragm is closed with a continuous suture, which may be reinforced with interrupted horizontal mattress sutures.

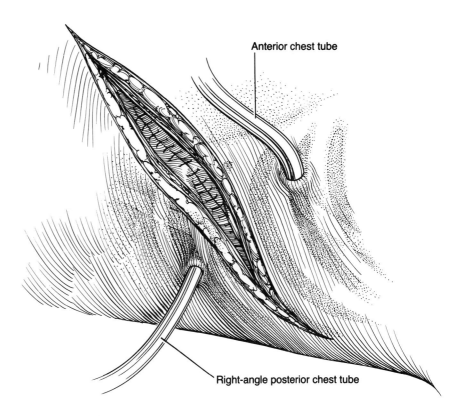

Anterior chest tube

Right-angle posterior chest tube

FIGURE 6–14. Chest tubes are placed in the anterior axillary line and may be exited above or below the incision. The chest tubes are removed when no longer draining, usually by the second or third postoperative day. Mechanical ventilation is usually continued through the first night and, if pulmonary function is satisfactory, can often be discontinued by the first postoperative day.

7

Carotid Endarterectomy (WITH INTERNAL SHUNT)

RICHARD L. McCANN, M.D.

Carotid endarterectomy is a technically demanding procedure. Although local or regional anesthesia can be used successfully, general anesthesia is preferred because it provides the best control of hemodynamic parameters. Positioning of the patient is critical. It is imperative that the neck be extended and turned as much as possible to the contralateral side.

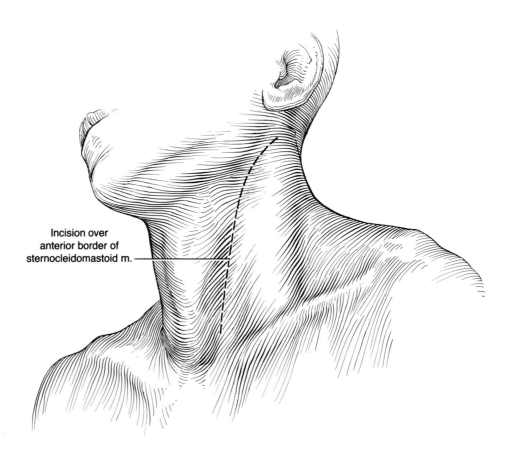

Incision over
anterior border of
sternocleidomastoid m.

FIGURE 7–1. The skin incision is made obliquely along the anterior border of the sternocleidomastoid muscle. It is important to stay at least 1 cm. distant from the angle of the mandible to avoid injury to the marginal mandibular branch of the seventh cranial nerve. If necessary, the incision can be curved posteriorly, particularly if a prominent skin crease is present.

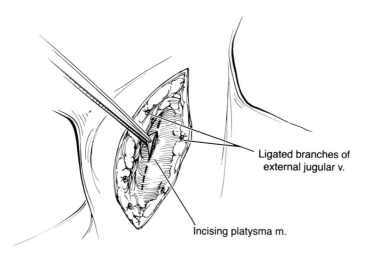

Ligated branches of
external jugular v.

Incising platysma m.

FIGURE 7–2. The platysma is divided, and the sternocleidomastoid muscle is mobilized laterally.

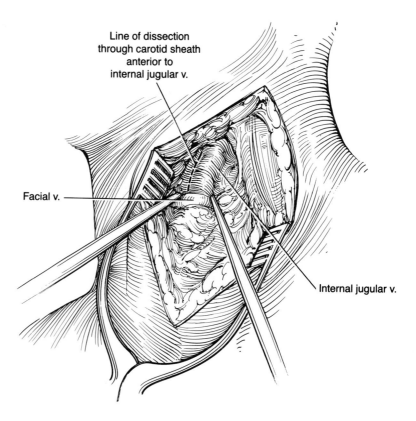

Line of dissection
through carotid sheath
anterior to
internal jugular v.

Facial v.

Internal jugular v.

FIGURE 7–3. The carotid sheath is exposed, and a self-retraining retractor is inserted. The facial branch of the internal jugular vein often crosses the carotid artery near the level of the bifurcation.

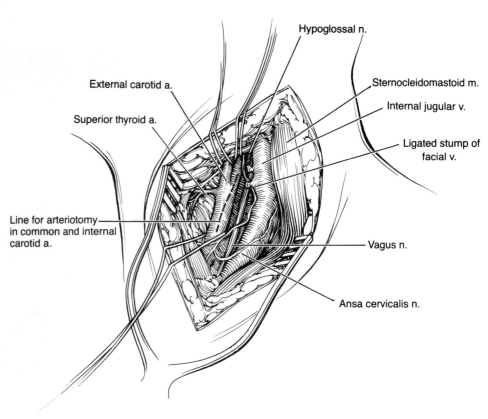

FIGURE 7–4. Dissection above the bifurcation is done carefully to prevent injury to the twelfth cranial nerve. This usually crosses anterior to the carotid and may be as low as the bifurcation. If the lesion is particularly high and the dissection extends superior to the digastric muscle, the ninth cranial nerve also must be identified and preserved. The ansa cervicalis nerve is often encountered and can be traced superiorly as a guide to the hypoglossal nerve. The distal common carotid, the bifurcation, and the proximal internal and external carotid vessels are then dissected free of surrounding structures.

Hypoglossal n.

External carotid a.

Sternocleidomastoid m.

Superior thyroid a.

Internal jugular v.

Ligated stump of facial v.

Line for arteriotomy in common and internal carotid a.

Vagus n.

Ansa cervicalis n.

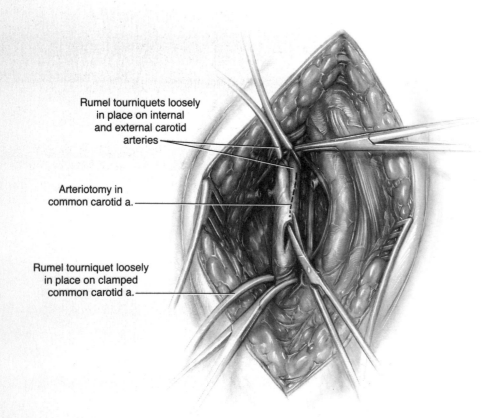

Rumel tourniquets loosely in place on internal and external carotid arteries

Arteriotomy in common carotid a.

Rumel tourniquet loosely in place on clamped common carotid a.

FIGURE 7–5. It is imperative to dissect the internal carotid superiorly until essentially normal vessel is encountered. Rumel tourniquets are placed around each of the vessels in preparation for clamping. If the superior thyroid artery is patent, it may be saved by using a Potts ligature for occlusion. The patient is given heparin intravenously, and the internal carotid is clamped first. This is followed by the external carotid and, finally, the common carotid. An opening is made on the anterior surface of the vessel and extended superiorly into the proximal internal carotid until normal vessel is encountered. It is important that the arteriotomy not encroach upon the orifice of the external carotid.

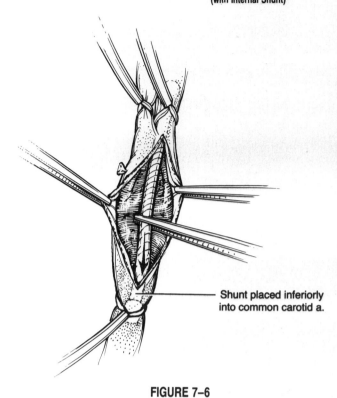

— Shunt placed inferiorly
into common carotid a.

FIGURE 7–6

Insertion of shunt into
internal carotid a.

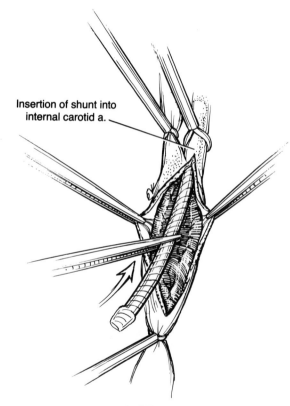

FIGURE 7–7

FIGURES 7–6 and 7–7. Usually, a heparin-bonded Silastic shunt (Sundt) is inserted first into the internal carotid and then into the common carotid, restoring cerebral perfusion, with a clamp time of usually less than 1 minute for the insertion.

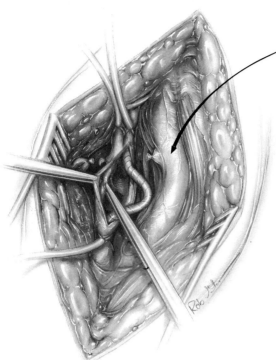

Removal of plaque with shunt in place

FIGURE 7–8. An endarterectomy plane is established at an appropriate location, and the distal common carotid, the bulb, the orifice of the external carotid, and the proximal internal carotid are cleared of plaque material. The vessel is liberally irrigated with heparin solution to loosen and remove debris.

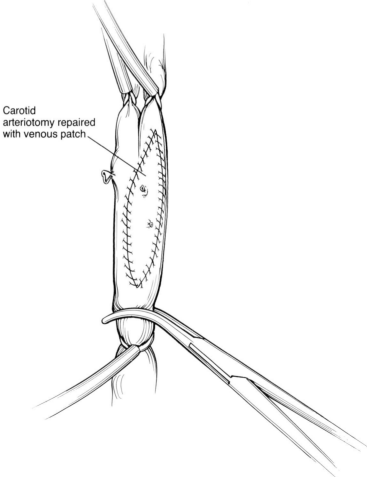

Carotid arteriotomy repaired with venous patch

FIGURE 7–9. The arteriotomy is closed either primarily or with a vein patch. A patch is preferred in women, in patients with small vessels, and in procedures done for recurrent stenosis.

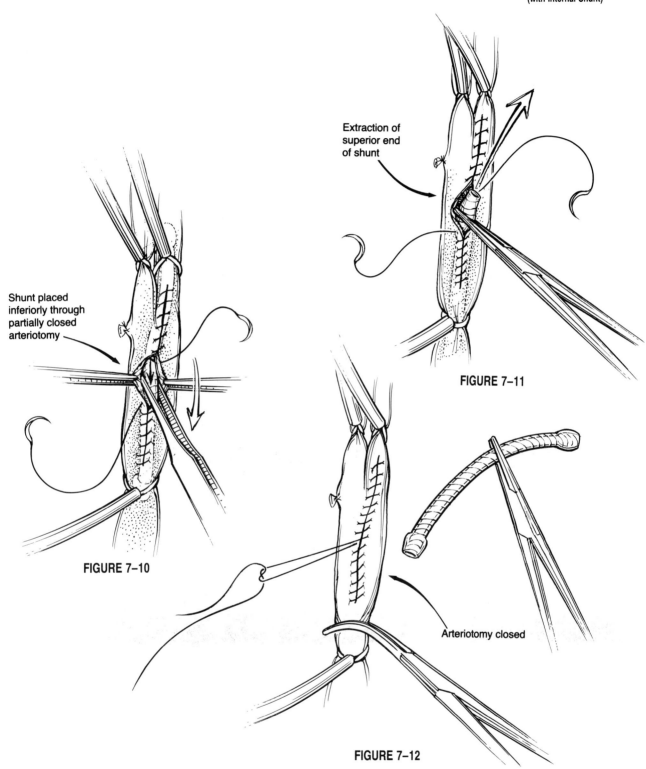

Extraction of
superior end
of shunt

FIGURE 7–11

Shunt placed
inferiorly through
partially closed
arteriotomy

FIGURE 7–10

Arteriotomy closed

FIGURE 7–12

FIGURES 7–10 to 7–12. Just prior to completing the suture line, the vessels are reclamped and the shunt is removed. If much thrombus or plaque is present proximal to the arteriotomy, the proximal end of the shunt may be removed first instead of the distal end first as shown. Backbleeding is allowed from the internal carotid to ensure that no debris is washed into the cerebral circulation. The suture line is rapidly completed, and flow is established to the external carotid and subsequently to the internal carotid. An operative arteriogram is preferred in all cases to ensure the absence of a distal flap and a satisfactory endarterectomy.

8

Excision of Carotid Body Tumor

W. GLENN YOUNG, JR., M.D.

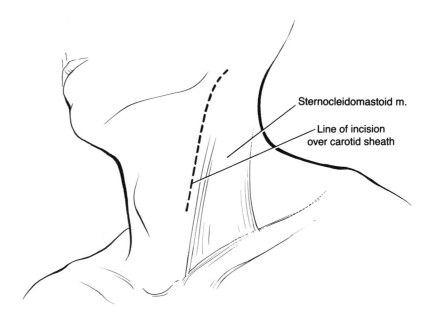

Sternocleidomastoid m.

Line of incision
over carotid sheath

FIGURE 8–1. An oblique incision, similar to that used for carotid endarterectomy, that parallels the anterior border of the sternocleidomastoid muscle is made. The tumor usually arises within the bifurcation of the common carotid artery, where it splays apart the internal and external carotid arteries. This very vascular tumor receives its blood supply through the periadventitia of the carotid vessels; as it enlarges, it may actually surround the external and internal carotid vessels. Occasionally, the external carotid artery may be divided to aid in the removal of the tumor. Rarely is it necessary to divide the internal carotid artery, but an intraluminal shunt and vein graft may be needed in appropriate cases.

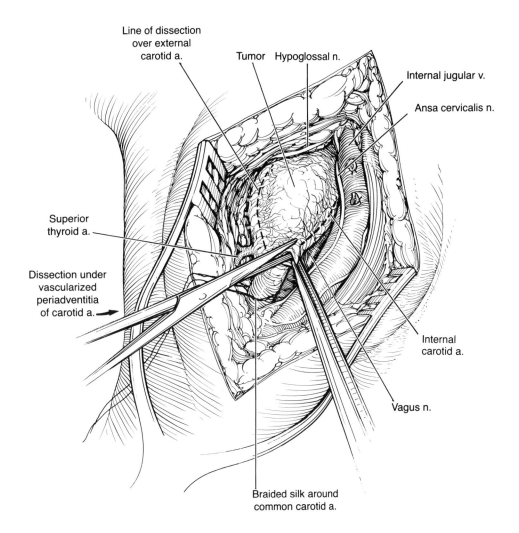

Line of dissection
over external
carotid a.

Tumor   Hypoglossal n.

Internal jugular v.

Ansa cervicalis n.

Superior
thyroid a.

Dissection under
vascularized
periadventitia
of carotid a. ➤

Internal
carotid a.

Vagus n.

Braided silk around
common carotid a.

FIGURE 8–2. The common carotid artery is exposed and encircled with a tape. The dissection is extended superiorly, exposing the tumor, with identification and protection of the hypoglossal nerve above the lesion. To dissect the artery from its intimate relationship with the carotid vessels, it is necessary to extend the dissection beneath the periadventitia of the vessels, as illustrated.

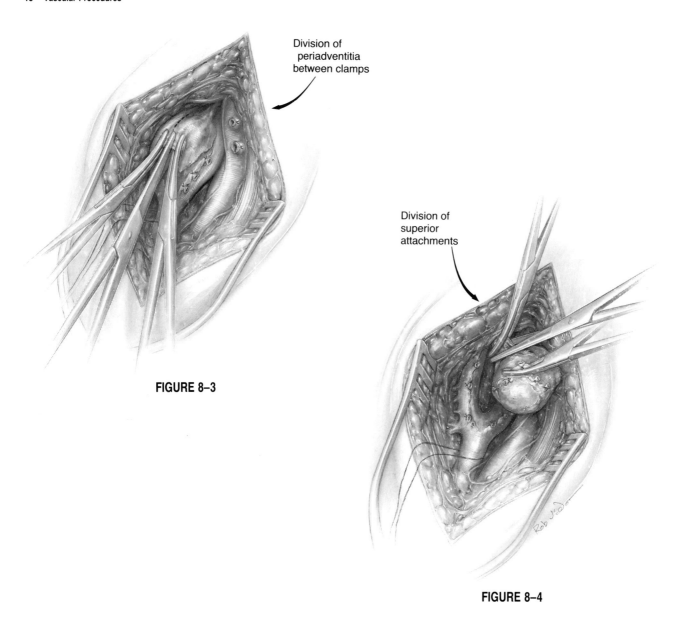

Division of
periadventitia
between clamps

FIGURE 8–3

Division of
superior
attachments

FIGURE 8–4

FIGURES 8–3 and 8–4. With careful and tedious dissection, using small Halsted clamps and judicious use of the cautery, the tumor is first separated from the external carotid branch and the internal carotid artery. As these attachments are divided and ligated, the tumor becomes less vascular and, finally, the small nerves and fibrous bands arising from the tumor and coursing up into the cranium are divided.

Recently, preoperative embolization of the vascular supply from the external carotid artery has been advocated as a means to decrease the vascularity of the tumor. Whether this will prove to be useful and cost-effective has not been determined.

9

Femoropopliteal Bypass

RICHARD L. McCANN, M.D.

Femoropopliteal bypass is one of the most frequently performed vascular procedures and requires meticulous technique to be consistently successful. It has been conclusively demonstrated that the autogenous vein graft is the best conduit and that prosthetic material should be used only in *unusual* circumstances. When necessary, two or more segments of vein may be joined together to obtain sufficient length for the bypass. Whereas some surgeons prefer the saphenous vein graft by the *in situ* technique, others favor the traditional reversed vein graft. Each technique has advantages and disadvantages, and both are illustrated (see also Chapter 10).

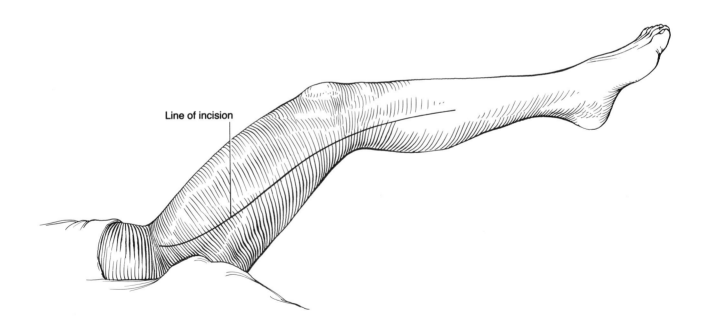

Line of incision

FIGURE 9–1. For a standard reversed saphenous vein graft, it is important to expose and evaluate the saphenous vein first. It may be necessary to tailor the operation to the quantity of available vein. In harvesting the vein, it is critical that the incision be made directly over the vein because a large subcutaneous flap in the thigh may slough, and such wound complications may jeopardize the success of the procedure. It is also critical to dissect the vein gently, and it should never be stretched or pulled.

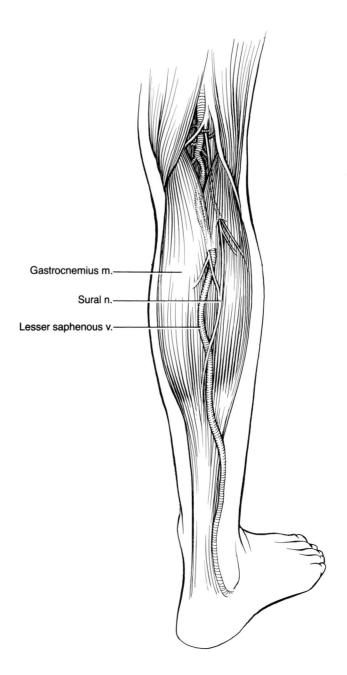

Gastrocnemius m.———

Sural n.———

Lesser saphenous v.———

FIGURE 9–2. The lesser saphenous vein is the conduit of second choice if adequate greater saphenous vein is not available. It is exposed posteriorly, and long segments may be harvested by turning the patient to the prone position. Care should be taken not to injure the adjacent sural nerve.

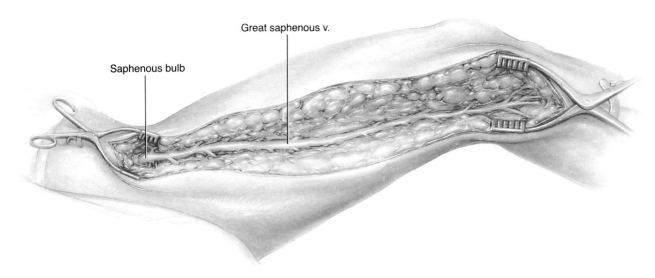

Saphenous bulb

Great saphenous v.

FIGURE 9–3. After the vein is exposed for its entire length, the side branches are ligated flush with the main channel. The temptation to use clips should be resisted (particularly on the larger branches) if the graft is going to be passed through a blind tunnel because the clips may become detached, causing a hematoma. The side branches are ligated, with attention paid to avoiding constriction from ligating them too close to the saphenous vein. One or more side branches are left long to be used as sites for contrast injection following completion of the anastomosis.

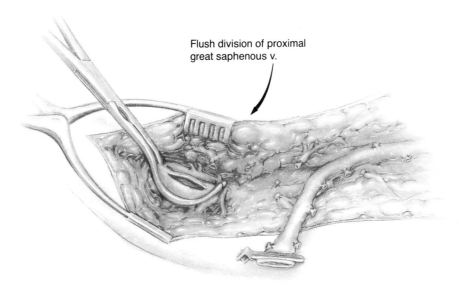

Flush division of proximal great saphenous v.

FIGURE 9–4. Maximum length is achieved by taking the saphenous bulb flush with the femoral vein and closing the opening in the femoral vein with a vascular suture.

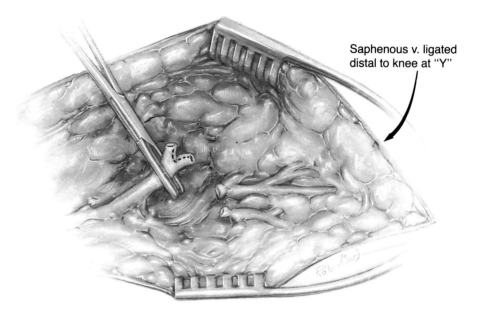

Saphenous v. ligated
distal to knee at "Y"

FIGURE 9–5

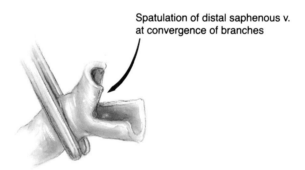

Spatulation of distal saphenous v.
at convergence of branches

FIGURE 9–6

FIGURES 9–5 and 9–6. When convenient, it is helpful to use a side branch distally to spatulate the proximal anastomosis.

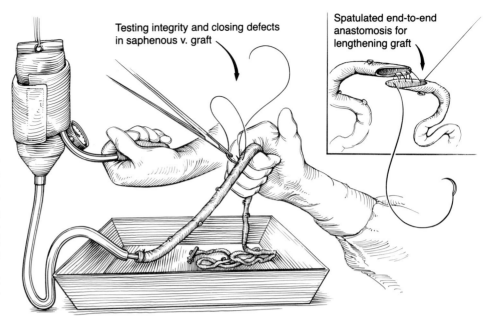

FIGURE 9–7. After an adequate length of vein is procured, it is gently dilated by hydrostatic pressure, and any leaks are repaired with fine vascular sutures. Some surgeons prefer heparinized blood, and others advocate a balanced electrolyte solution. The important aspect of graft dilation is avoidance of excessive intraluminal pressure.

Testing integrity and closing defects in saphenous v. graft

Spatulated end-to-end anastomosis for lengthening graft

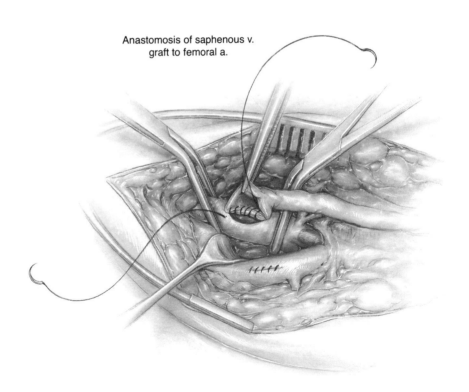

Anastomosis of saphenous v. graft to femoral a.

FIGURE 9–8. The proximal anastomosis is done first. A widely spatulated anastomosis is created by incising through a side branch, creating a large opening for the anastomosis. When maximal length is critical, the bulb can be cut flush with the femoral vein and that opening closed with a vascular suture. The most distal site with normal flow on the angiogram and with an acceptable arterial wall is chosen for the proximal anastomosis. This is performed with a continuous 5–0 or 6–0 vascular suture.

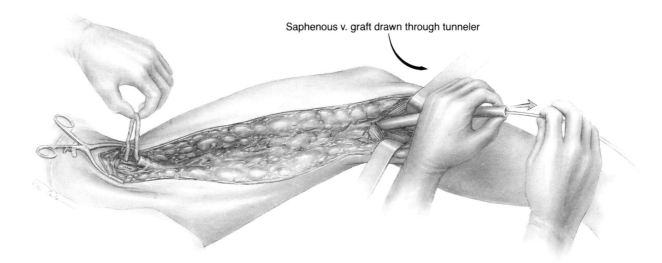

Saphenous v. graft drawn through tunneler

FIGURE 9–9. The graft is then passed in a subsartorial or subcutaneous tunnel using a tunneling apparatus consisting of a plastic sheath and metal obturator. With the obturator in place, the instrument is passed bluntly in the plane desired. After passage, the obturator is removed, and a long passer is used to pull the vein gently through the plastic sheath, which is then withdrawn leaving the graft in place. This location of the graft protects it in the event of wound healing complications of the medial thigh incision.

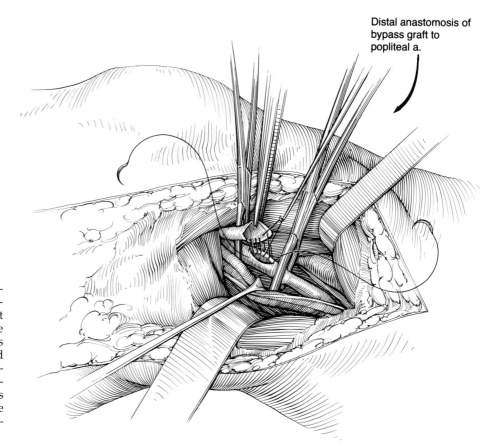

Distal anastomosis of bypass graft to popliteal a.

FIGURE 9–10. The distal anastomosis is performed end-to-side using 6–0 monofilament vascular suture. After release of the clamps, blood flow is measured in the graft, and operative angiography is performed to document a satisfactory distal anastomosis and appropriate status of the runoff for follow-up purposes.

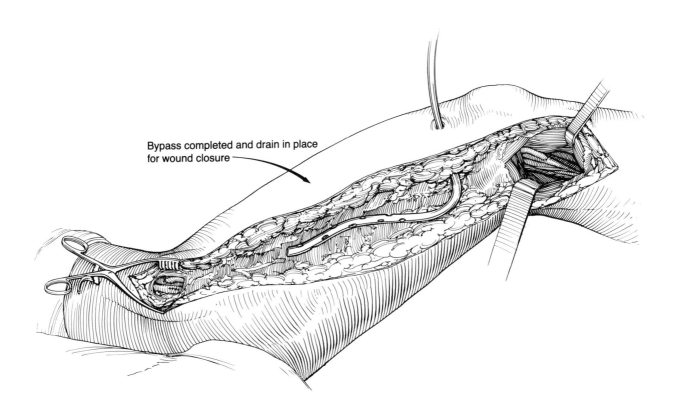

Bypass completed and drain in place
for wound closure

FIGURE 9–11. Because the patient has been heparinized, a drain may be placed in the bed of the harvested vein prior to closure and removed in 24 hours. The graft remains protected by its deep position. Patients remain in bed until the first operative day and are allowed up after the drain is removed.

10

Femoropopliteal Bypass *(IN SITU)*

RICHARD L. McCANN, M.D.

Preparation of the saphenous vein by the *in situ* technique has several advantages. The large end of the vein is sutured to the larger artery while the smaller, more delicate end of the vein is sutured to the smaller vessel distally. Because the vein remains intact in its bed, kinking, length discrepancy, and twisting are avoided. The disadvantages of the technique are that it requires lysis of the valves and closure of major tributaries to avoid persistent arteriovenous fistulas.

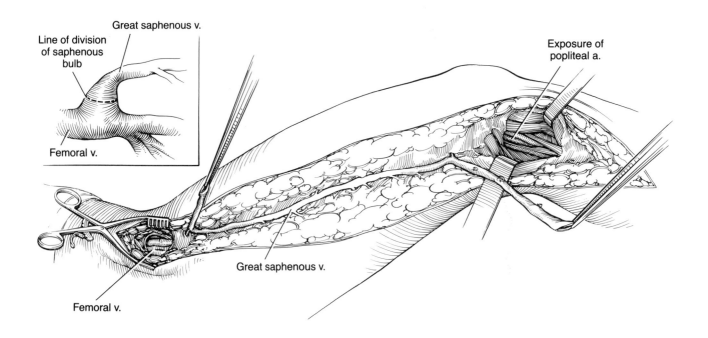

FIGURE 10–1. Most surgeons expose the vein at least on its anterior surface through a continuous medial thigh incision. If the proximal anastomosis must be done to the common femoral or proximal superficial femoral artery, the bulb must be completely mobilized and the vein divided flush with the femoral vein.

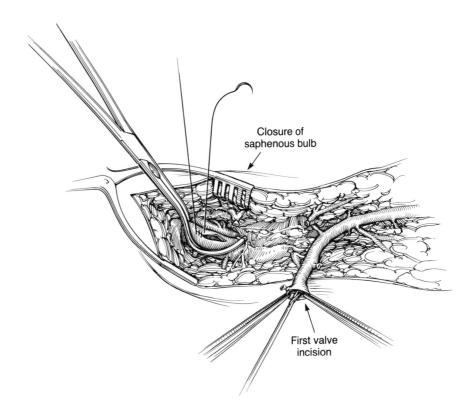

Closure of
saphenous bulb

First valve
incision

FIGURE 10–2. The opening in the femoral vein is closed with a continuous vascular suture. The first valve is excised under direct vision, and the valve scissors may be inserted into the vein lumen and advanced with the jaws open until the second valve is engaged in the jaws of the scissors, which are then closed, incising the valve leaflets and rendering the valve incompetent. Because the valve leaflets are parallel to the skin surface, the scissors and valvulotomes need to be oriented perpendicular to this plane to engage and incise the leaflets.

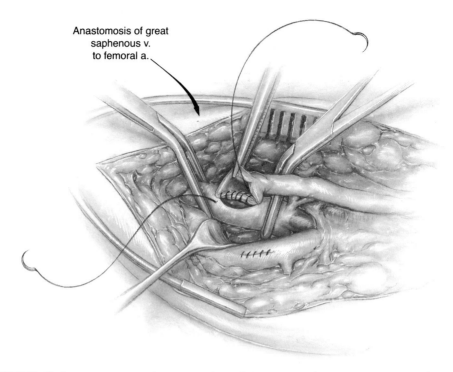

Anastomosis of great
saphenous v.
to femoral a.

FIGURE 10–3. The patient is heparinized, and the proximal anastomosis is made to a convenient site.

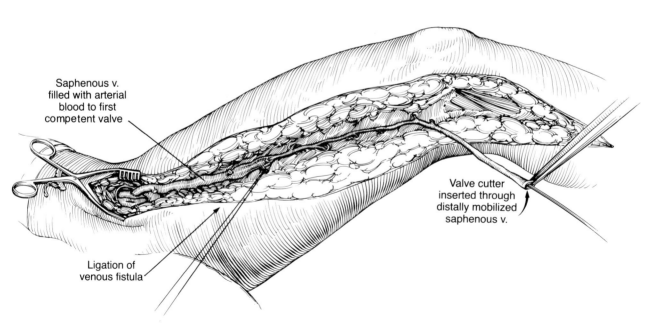

Saphenous v.
filled with arterial
blood to first
competent valve

Valve cutter
inserted through
distally mobilized
saphenous v.

Ligation of
venous fistula

FIGURE 10–4. Arterial blood is allowed to enter the vein; it flows distally until flow is interrupted by the first remaining competent valve. The distal end of the vein is then cannulated with one of several commercially available valvulotomes. The valvulotome is advanced into the dilated pressurized proximal portion of the graft.

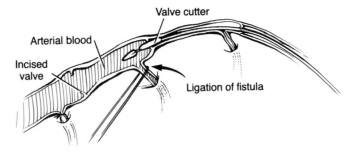

FIGURE 10–5

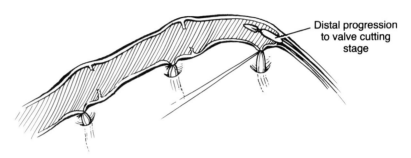

FIGURE 10–6

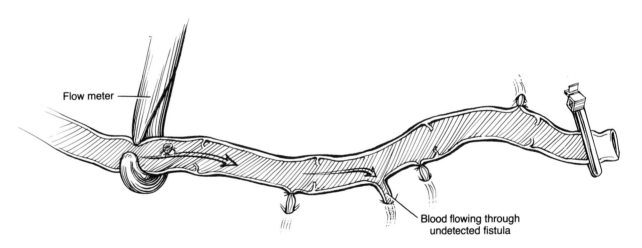

FIGURE 10–7

FIGURE 10–5. The valvulotome is retrieved. Upon retrieval, the blades engage any competent valves remaining in the graft. This process is performed *slowly*, allowing the arterial pressure to dilate each vein segment as the valve is cut. Good pulsatile arterial flow must be achieved at the distal end for the graft to be successful.

FIGURE 10–6. The distal mobilized end of the vein graft is secured with a vascular clamp while any arteriovenous fistulas are ligated. The side branches are usually ligated in continuity, as it is not necessary to divide them.

FIGURE 10–7. A flowmeter or Doppler flowmeter is used and is placed on the proximal vein segment. The graft is then occluded with the forefinger, and the occlusion is moved distally while the flow is monitored. As soon as the occlusion passes a patent branch, flow will increase from zero to a recordable volume. This locates the site of a patent side branch, which is a potential arteriovenous fistula, and the branch is ligated. This process is repeated down the length of the vein so that each potential fistula is secured.

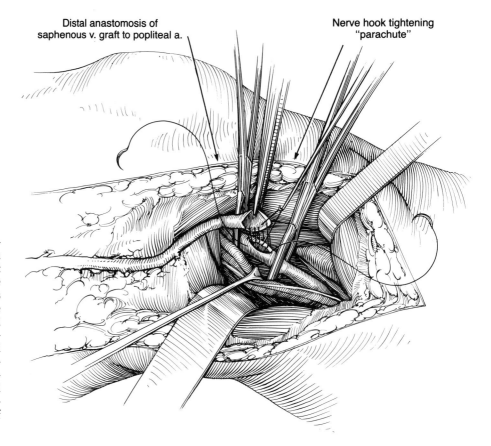

Distal anastomosis of
saphenous v. graft to popliteal a.

Nerve hook tightening
"parachute"

FIGURE 10–8. At the conclusion of this procedure, with the distal end of the graft clamped, the flow should be nil. The distal anastomosis is then made end-to-side to the appropriate vessel, and all clamps are released. A postbypass arteriogram is useful to confirm the absence of patent branches and to demonstrate patency of the distal anastomosis as well as to record the status of the runoff for follow-up purposes.

11

Femorotibial and Peroneal Bypass

RICHARD L. McCANN, M.D.

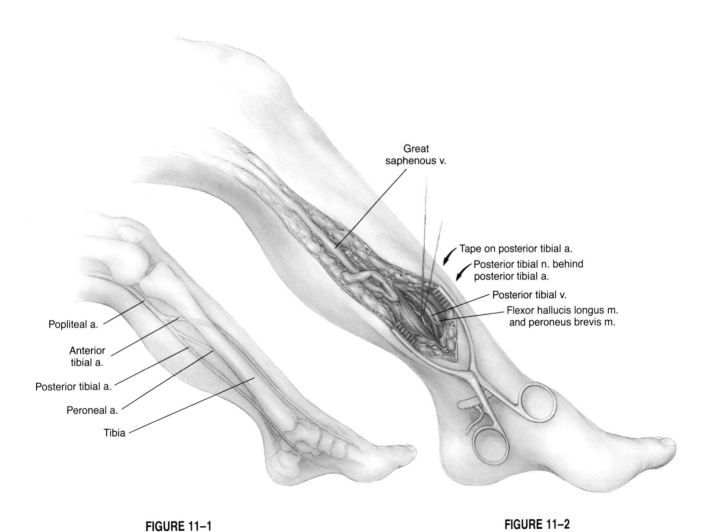

Great
saphenous v.

Tape on posterior tibial a.

Posterior tibial n. behind
posterior tibial a.

Posterior tibial v.

Flexor hallucis longus m.
and peroneus brevis m.

Popliteal a.

Anterior
tibial a.

Posterior tibial a.

Peroneal a.

Tibia

FIGURE 11–1

FIGURE 11–2

FIGURES 11–1 and 11–2. The posterior tibial vessel is exposed through a direct medial incision and is close to the surface at the medial malleolus.

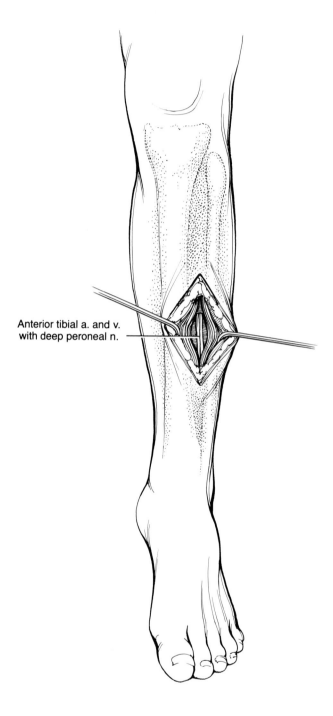

Anterior tibial a. and v.
with deep peroneal n.

FIGURE 11–3. The anterior tibial vessel is found on the surface of the interosseous membrane after splitting the muscles of the anterior compartment. Exposure is facilitated by flexion of the knee.

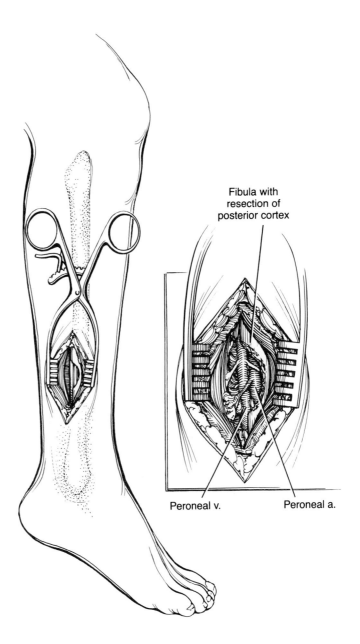

Fibula with
resection of
posterior cortex

Peroneal v.   Peroneal a.

FIGURE 11–4. The peroneal artery is the most difficult vessel to expose. In the thin calf, it is approached from the medial aspect; however, in the large leg, and if the distal portion is required, a lateral approach may be preferred. When this is required, removal of the posterior cortex of the fibula may improve exposure.

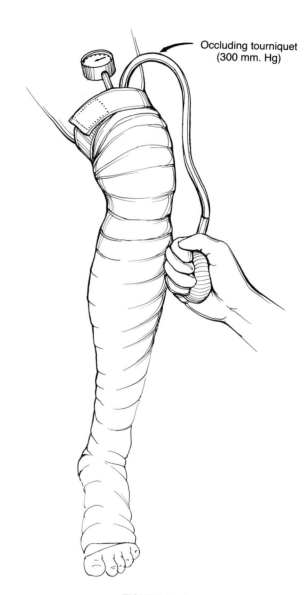

Occluding tourniquet
(300 mm. Hg)

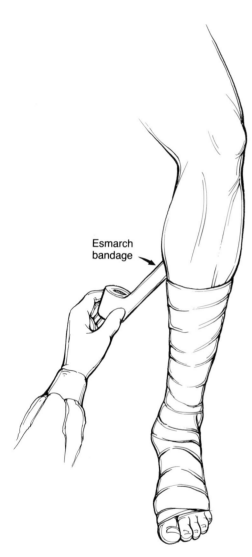

Esmarch
bandage

FIGURE 11–5

FIGURE 11–6

FIGURES 11–5 and 11–6. Because of the small size of the tibial and peroneal vessels, the distal anastomosis is performed using a different technique to avoid placing clamps on these fragile vessels. After exposure of the target vessel, an occluding tourniquet is placed on the thigh or upper calf, as appropriate. The distal limb is freed of blood by elevation and application of an elastic Esmarch bandage. The tourniquet is inflated to 300 mm. Hg pressure, which is tolerated for periods of up to an hour or more. The distal anastomosis can then be performed in an asanguinous field without clamps, and only the anterior surface of the target vessel need be exposed. This anastomosis requires coaxial lighting using a headlight and optical magnification with loops or, occasionally, an operating microscope. The anastomosis is made with a continuous 7–0 or 8–0 monofilament suture. After release of the tourniquet, an operative arteriogram is helpful to document the status of the anastomosis and the runoff.

12

Hepatorenal Bypass

RICHARD L. McCANN, M.D.

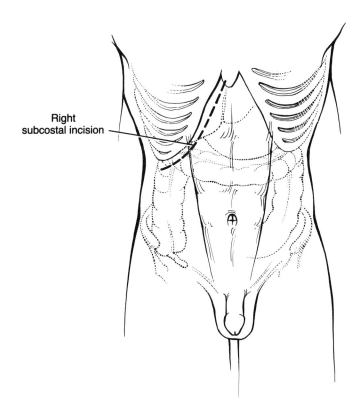

FIGURE 12–1. For hepatorenal reconstruction, a standard right subcostal incision is made and extended into the flank for adequate renal exposure. The peritoneal cavity is entered, and, after general exploration, the foramen of Winslow is identified and the portal triad exposed. The hepatic artery at the level of the gastroduodenal branch is dissected; it is usually large and should be quite soft at this location in order for it to be a satisfactory origin for a bypass graft.

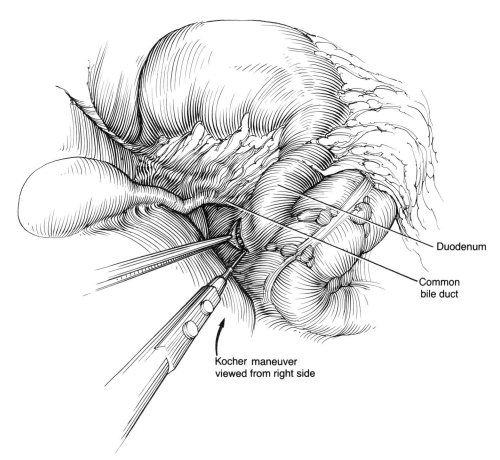

FIGURE 12–2. After exposure of the hepatic artery, a generous Kocher maneuver is performed to expose the inferior vena cava and the right renal vein.

FIGURE 12–3. The right renal arteries are identified deep to the renal vein, and an appropriate segment is prepared for the anastomosis. The main renal artery is usually posterior to the inferior vena cava, and considerable mobilization of the cava may be required for its complete exposure.

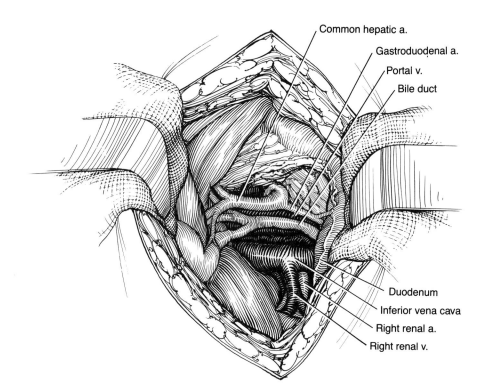

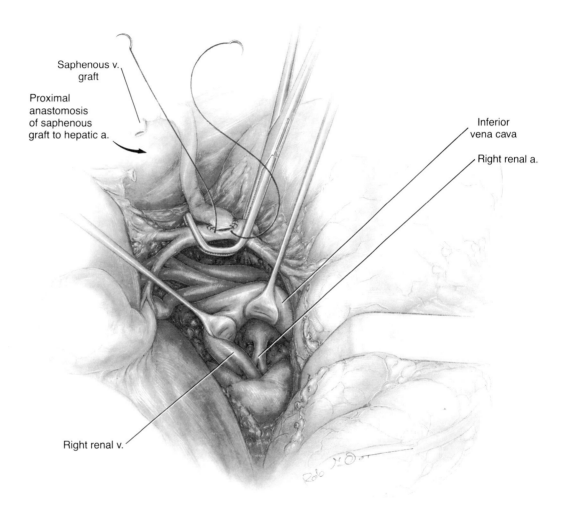

Saphenous v.
graft

Proximal
anastomosis
of saphenous
graft to hepatic a.

Inferior
vena cava

Right renal a.

Right renal v.

FIGURE 12–4. A saphenous vein graft is harvested from the thigh. An attempt is made to use a side branch of the vein for spatulation of the proximal anastomosis. After heparinization, the hepatic artery is clamped and the proximal anastomosis is made end-to-side. Depending on the size and location of the gastroduodenal artery, the proximal anastomosis can be placed in the gastroduodenal artery or in the hepatic artery just proximal or distal to the gastroduodenal takeoff. After completion of the anastomosis, the graft is sized under arterial pressure.

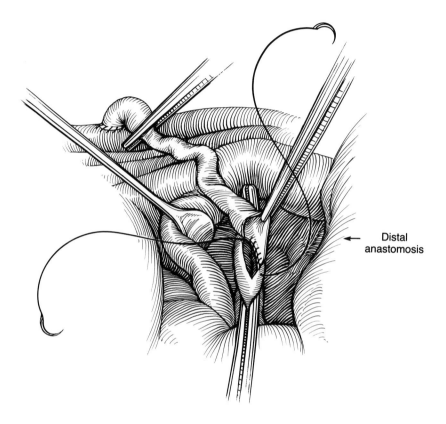

Distal
anastomosis

FIGURE 12–5. The distal anastomosis should not be made too far under the vena cava, as kinking is a potential problem. The distal anastomosis can be made in end-to-end or end-to-side fashion, depending on preference. Renal ischemia time should be no more than 15 minutes. If a longer period of renal ischemia is anticipated, preservation of renal function may be enhanced by injection of cold electrolyte solution into the renal artery to cool the kidney during performance of the anastomosis.

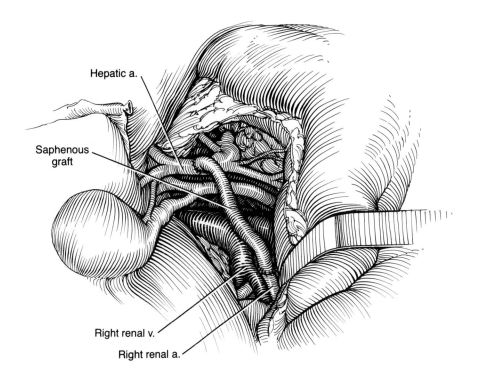

Hepatic a.

Saphenous
graft

Right renal v.

Right renal a.

FIGURE 12–6. After release of the clamp, the kidney is inspected for color and turgor to assure that adequate revascularization has been achieved. A healthy pink color and firm consistency suggest a successful revascularization. The course of the graft should be almost directly posterior, and its length is critical to avoid kinking. The viscera are allowed to return into place, and the subcostal incision is closed in layers. The patient is monitored in the intensive care unit postoperatively until the blood pressure is stable.

13

Aortorenal Revascularization

RICHARD L. McCANN, M.D.

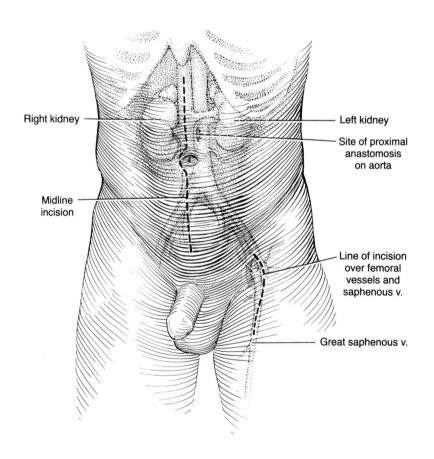

FIGURE 13–1. For aortorenal revascularization, a midline incision is usually used, although a transverse abdominal incision is also satisfactory. The thighs are prepared into the field to allow harvesting of the saphenous vein graft or grafts.

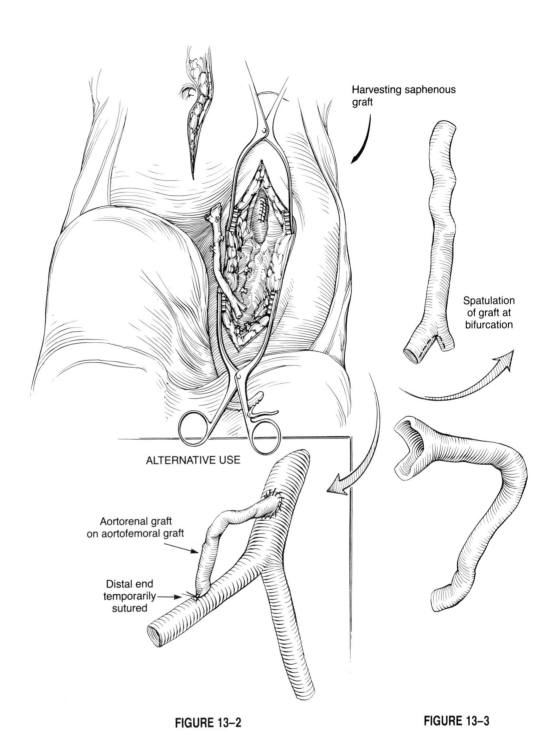

Harvesting saphenous
graft

Spatulation
of graft at
bifurcation

ALTERNATIVE USE

Aortorenal graft
on aortofemoral graft

Distal end
temporarily
sutured

FIGURE 13–2   **FIGURE 13–3**

FIGURES 13–2 and 13–3. The saphenous veins are often harvested using a side branch
to spatulate the proximal anastomosis. If simultaneous aortofemoral reconstruction is
being performed, the saphenous vein is attached to the Dacron graft as a preliminary
maneuver.

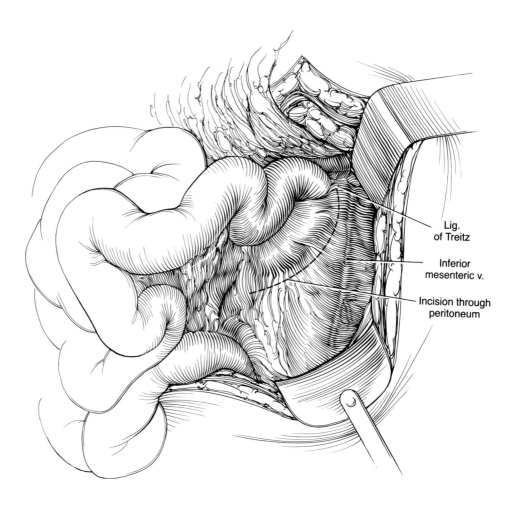

Lig.
of Treitz

Inferior
mesenteric v.

Incision through
peritoneum

FIGURE 13–4. After abdominal exploration, the viscera are displaced to the right and the posterior parietal peritoneum is incised, mobilizing the ligament of Treitz.

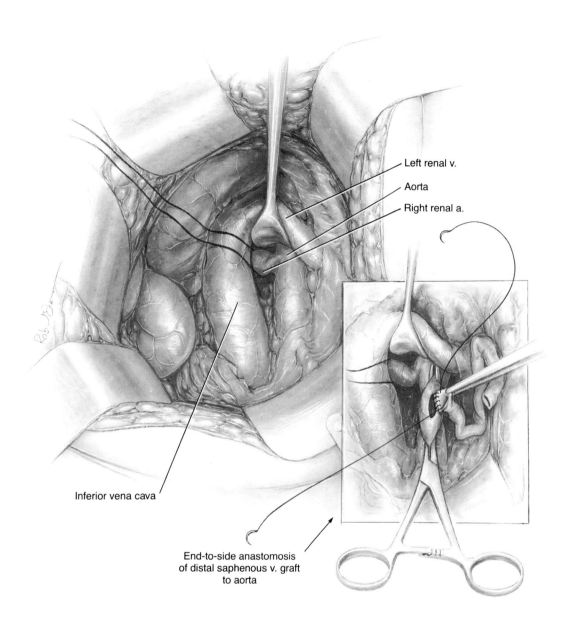

Left renal v.

Aorta

Right renal a.

Inferior vena cava

End-to-side anastomosis of distal saphenous v. graft to aorta

FIGURE 13–5. The aorta just inferior to the crossing of the left renal vein is the preferred site for the proximal anastomosis if free of significant atherosclerotic disease. Alternative sites include the supraceliac aorta and the common iliac artery if the aorta is not suitable.

FIGURE 13–6. After heparinization, the aorta is clamped, and, if it is large and minimally diseased, a partially occluding clamp can be used to isolate a sufficient area to perform the proximal anastomosis. An effort is made to use a spatulated segment of the vein to ensure an adequate orifice. Care is taken in sizing the graft and trimming it to an appropriate length to avoid kinking. The sizing should be done with the graft under arterial pressure.

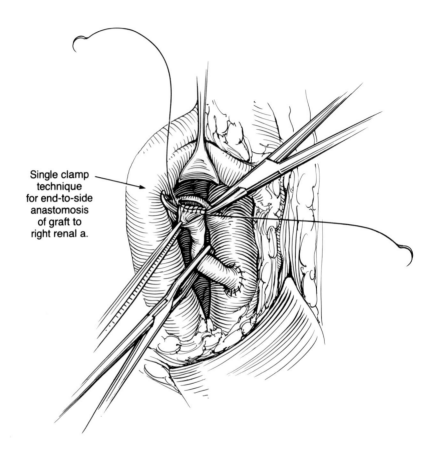

Single clamp
technique
for end-to-side
anastomosis
of graft to
right renal a.

FIGURE 13–7. The distal anastomosis can then be done end-to-end or end-to-side, according to preference. The anastomosis is done with a running vascular suture, and renal ischemic time should be limited to 15 to 20 minutes. Following release of the clamps, the color and turgor of the kidney are examined to ensure that satisfactory revascularization has been achieved. The retroperitoneum is reconstructed with a running absorbable suture, and the midline incision is closed in the standard manner. The patient is observed in the intensive care unit postoperatively until the blood pressure has stabilized. A postoperative angiogram prior to discharge is recommended to document satisfactory revascularization and to serve as a baseline for future examinations.

14

Splenorenal Anastomosis

RICHARD L. McCANN, M.D.

The splenic artery can be used to revascularize the left kidney, particularly in instances in which the aorta is severely diseased or has been the site of a previous operation. Even though the splenic artery is divided, the spleen can be left in place, as it will be sufficiently nourished by the short gastric vessels. Another advantage of this technique is that it can be performed entirely in the retroperitoneal plane, minimizing the problem of postoperative ileus and convalescence.

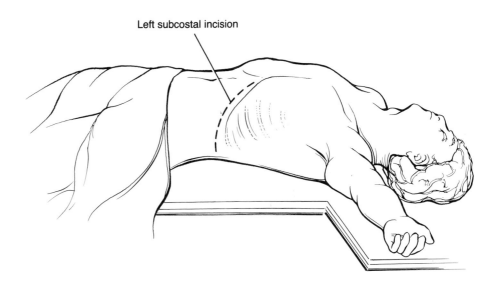

Left subcostal incision

FIGURE 14–1. The patient is positioned with the left flank elevated. The incision is extended through the anterior rectus sheath and the oblique muscles, but an effort is made to keep the peritoneal membrane intact. Usually, the lateral half of the rectus muscle is also divided as the peritoneum is swept away from the undersurface of the anterior abdominal wall, the diaphragm, and the flank. The peritoneal membrane may be thin anteriorly, and scissor dissection may be required to keep it intact. It is important to clear the peritoneum from a considerable portion of the diaphragm and the anterior abdominal wall to provide sufficient exposure. Posteriorly, the plane between Gerota's fascia and the peritoneum is identified and developed. The dissection is extended anterior to the kidney, sweeping the peritoneum from the anterior aspect of the left kidney. The intestines remain within the peritoneal envelope, facilitating their retraction.

FIGURE 14–2. The left renal vein is identified, and the dissection is extended medially as far as the aortic pulse. Self-retaining retractors are inserted while the renal hilum is dissected. The artery is usually located deep and cephalad to the vein. Careful correlation with the preoperative arteriogram is required at this point to avoid revascularizing the wrong vessel. If there is early branching, it is easy to expose a segmental artery rather than the main vessel. This is less important if an end-to-side anastomosis is planned. Superiorly, the lower edge of the pancreas is identified and is rotated anteriorly to expose the under-surface. The splenic vein and then the artery are encountered beneath the pancreas.

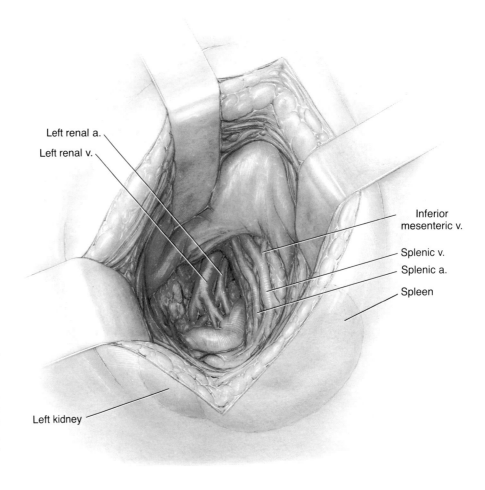

Left renal a.

Left renal v.

Inferior mesenteric v.

Splenic v.

Splenic a.

Spleen

Left kidney

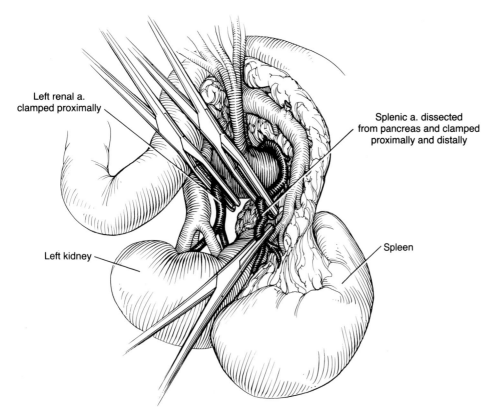

Left renal a. clamped proximally

Splenic a. dissected from pancreas and clamped proximally and distally

Left kidney

Spleen

FIGURE 14–3. The splenic artery is dissected distally as far as its first major branch and proximally as far as practicable. Small branches often penetrate the pancreas and require ligation and division. After heparinization, the splenic artery is clamped proximally and divided distally.

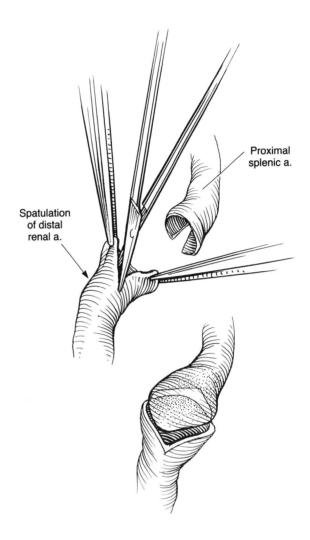

Proximal
splenic a.

Spatulation
of distal
renal a.

FIGURE 14–4. It is often feasible to use the first major branching of the splenic artery as a spatulation to widen the anastomosis. The artery is rotated inferiorly to meet the renal vessel.

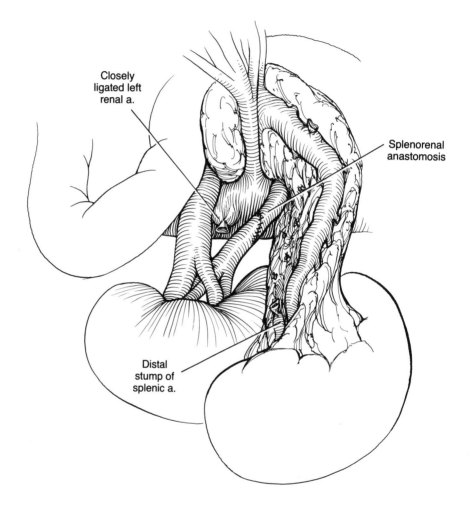

Closely
ligated left
renal a.

Splenorenal
anastomosis

Distal
stump of
splenic a.

FIGURE 14–5. Either end-to-end or end-to-side anastomosis can be performed as dictated by local anatomy. If exposure is adequate, renal ischemic time should be an acceptable 15 to 20 minutes. If a longer ischemic time is anticipated, it may be wise to cool the kidney by injection of a cold electrolyte solution and clamping of the vein. After restoration of blood flow, the color and turgor of the kidney are observed to evaluate the success of the revascularization.

Occasionally, in elderly hypertensive patients, the splenic artery is quite tortuous and the wall is excessively stiff and may be calcified. This type of vessel does not easily rotate inferiorly, and there is a high likelihood of kinking. In this instance, one can occasionally resort to the use of a short saphenous vein interposition graft, which allows the splenic artery to remain in its normal location.

After being satisfied that a successful revascularization has been achieved, the abdominal viscera are allowed to return to their normal position. The muscle layers of the abdominal wall are closed anatomically. A nasogastric tube is seldom required, and bowel function is expected to return promptly.

15

Portocaval Shunt

RICHARD L. McCANN, M.D.

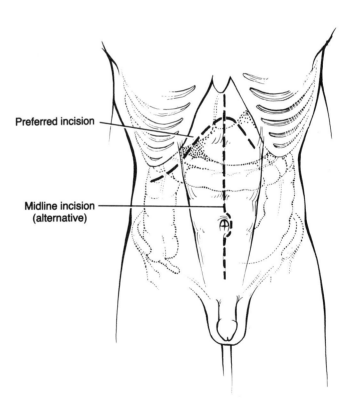

FIGURE 15–1. For a portocaval shunt, an asymmetric bilateral subcostal incision with a longer limb on the right side is preferred. This allows easy access to the portal vein. For a splenorenal anastomosis, a midline incision is made, allowing access to both the splenic vein and the coronary vein, which often must be ligated within the lesser sac.

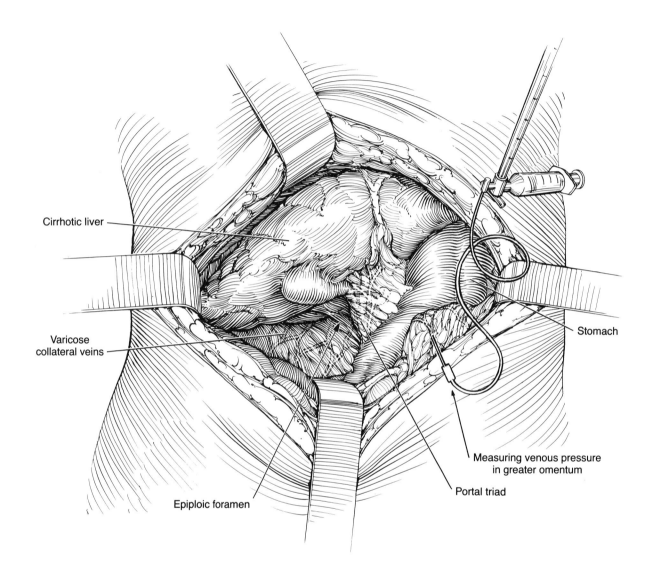

Cirrhotic liver

Varicose
collateral veins

Epiploic foramen

Stomach

Measuring venous pressure
in greater omentum

Portal triad

FIGURE 15–2. After opening the abdomen, a general exploration with drainage of ascites is performed. Biopsy of the liver can be done if required for documentation. It is also important to measure the portal pressure to confirm the presence of portal hypertension and to judge the efficacy of the shunt in portal decompression. Portal vein pressure can conveniently be measured by cannulating an omental vein and using a simple water manometer. The level of the right atrium is estimated and is used as the reference point. This vein is then ligated and another vein cannulated after completing the shunt to assess the pre- and postshunt difference.

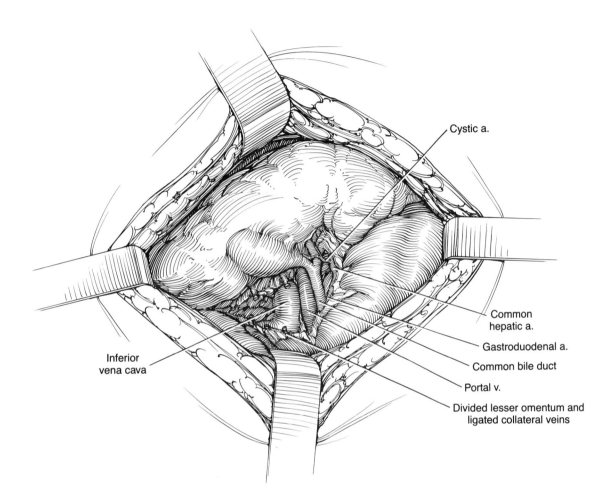

Cystic a.

Common
hepatic a.

Gastroduodenal a.

Common bile duct

Portal v.

Divided lesser omentum and
ligated collateral veins

Inferior
vena cava

FIGURE 15–3. After determining the portal pressure, the portal triad is exposed. All tissues must be individually doubly clamped and ligated to minimize bleeding when the portal pressure is high and the tissues are traversed by engorged venous collaterals. Use of the electrocautery should be minimized. As much of the portal vein as is feasible is exposed in the hilum of the liver.

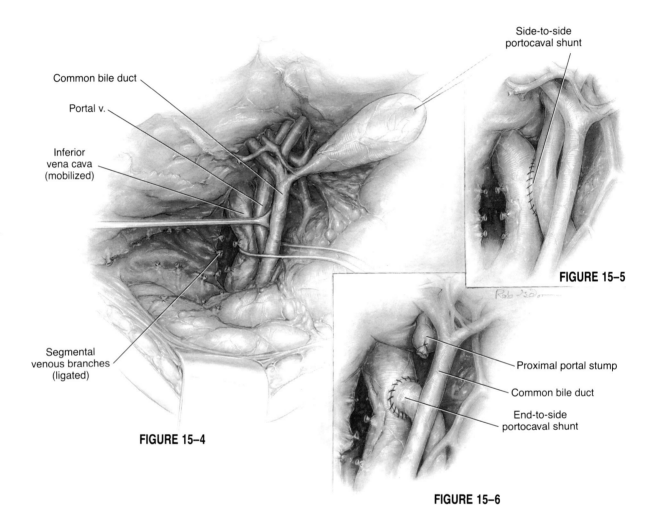

Common bile duct

Portal v.

Inferior
vena cava
(mobilized)

Segmental
venous branches
(ligated)

FIGURE 15–4

Side-to-side
portocaval shunt

FIGURE 15–5

Proximal portal stump

Common bile duct

End-to-side
portocaval shunt

FIGURE 15–6

FIGURE 15–4. An important technical feature is full mobilization of the vena cava to permit elevation to meet the portal vein, as well as extension of the portal vein inferiorly.

FIGURES 15–5 and 15–6. Side-to-side or end-to-side anastomosis can be performed as indicated. A running 4–0 vascular suture is used for the anastomosis. The pressure is measured in the portal system *following* release of the clamps, and substantial fall in portal pressure is expected. The abdomen is closed without drainage with use of running sutures to minimize the risk of ascitic leak postoperatively. It is important to be vigilant for hepatic encephalopathy and to treat it aggressively if it occurs postoperatively.

16

Distal Splenorenal Shunt (DISTAL AND PROXIMAL)

DAVID C. SABISTON, JR., M.D.

The splenorenal shunt is primarily designed to treat patients with portal hypertension and esophageal varices. If other means of therapy for bleeding varices are unsuccessful, splenorenal shunt becomes a logical choice, especially the *distal* splenorenal shunt described by Warren. In this procedure, portal perfusion pressure remains essentially unchanged postoperatively, whereas the pressure in the venous system supplying the esophageal varices *is* decompressed through flow into the left renal vein, thus reducing the likelihood of bleeding from esophageal varices.

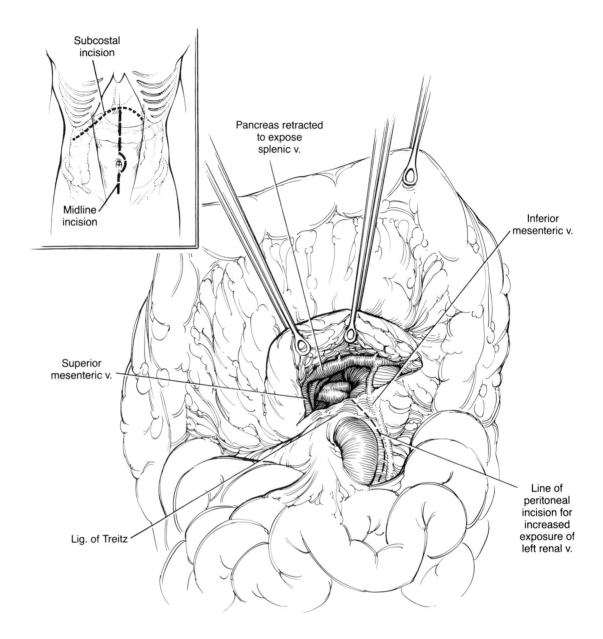

FIGURE 16–1. In the performance of a splenorenal shunt, it is essential to have *excellent* exposure. Either a midline or a bilateral subcostal approach may be used, depending somewhat on the patient's body habitus. In general, a longitudinal incision is preferable, extending from the xiphoid process, around the umbilicus, to approximately halfway from the umbilicus to the symphysis pubis. Upon entry into the peritoneal cavity, a careful examination is made of the abdominal contents, with particular attention given to the liver and to the presence of dilated venous collaterals within the abdomen. The venous pressure in the portal system is measured by cannulating an omental vein with the use of a water manometer. The small intestine is retracted to the right side and protected by moist abdominal pads or is placed in a Lahey plastic bag and temporarily removed from the abdominal cavity. The region of the ligament of Treitz is exposed, and an incision is made in the retroperitoneum to the left of the ligament beneath the left renal vein. The pancreas is retracted to expose the splenic vein, and its junction with the inferior mesenteric vein is identified.

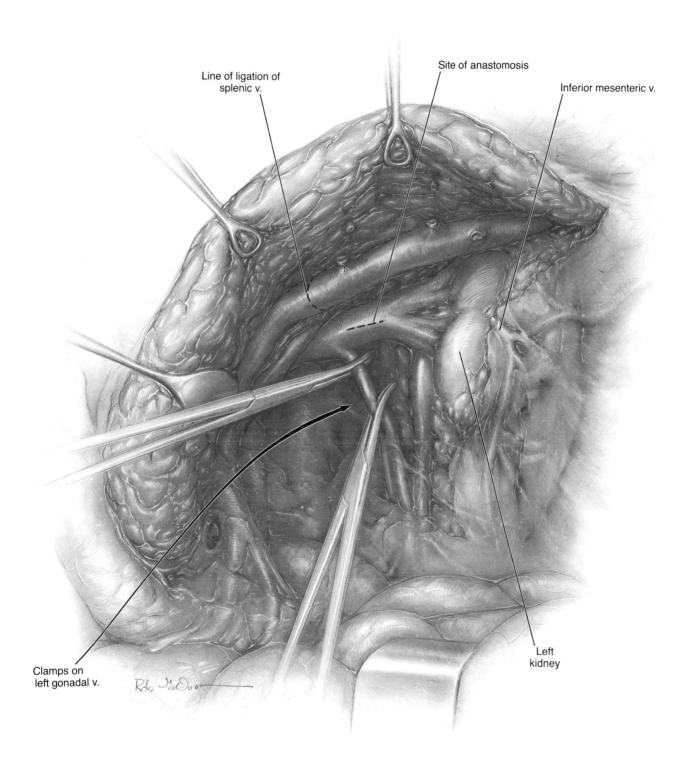

Line of ligation of
splenic v.

Site of anastomosis

Inferior mesenteric v.

Clamps on
left gonadal v.

Left
kidney

FIGURE 16–2. The left renal vein is exposed and is freed preparatory to the splenorenal
anastomosis.

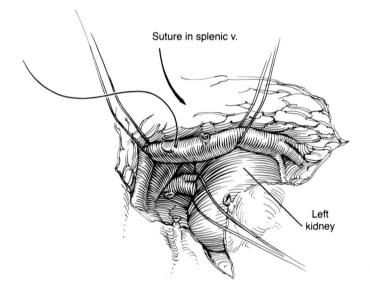

FIGURE 16–3. The splenic vein is mobilized, and the small branches are ligated and divided. A tape is passed beneath this vein proximally and distally.

TRANSFIXION
LIGATURE OF SPLENIC V.

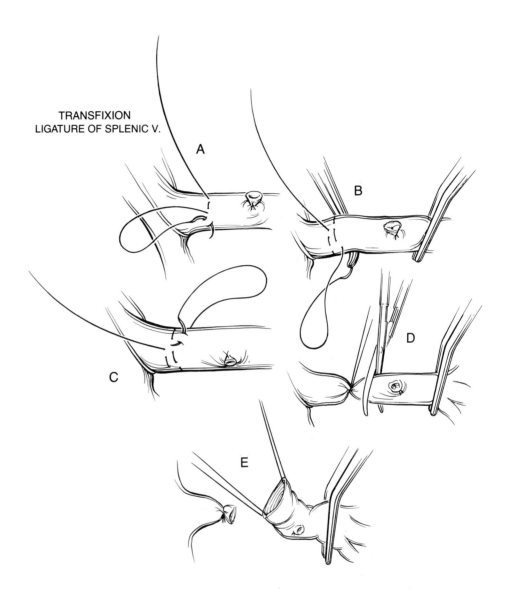

FIGURE 16–4. *A,* A transfixion ligature of 3–0 Prolene is placed at the proximal end of the splenic vein as it joins the portal system. *B,* A vascular occluding clamp is placed on the distal splenic vein, leaving sufficient length for reflecting of the vein to the left renal vein for anastomosis. *C,* The transfixion suture is completed and tied. *D,* The splenic vein is divided preparatory to anastomosis. *E,* The distal splenic vein is carefully examined, and the orifice of the divided end may be enlarged by spatulation if necessary.

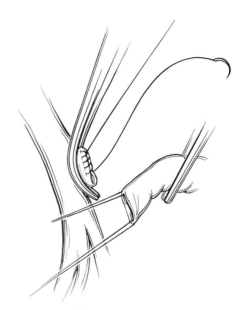

ALTERNATIVE TECHNIQUE FOR
LIGATION OF SPLENIC V.

FIGURE 16–5. Alternatively, the proximal end of the splenic vein at the site of division may be oversewn with a suture of 5–0 Prolene.

Continuous suture in posterior row of
end-to-side anastomosis of splenic v.
to left renal v.

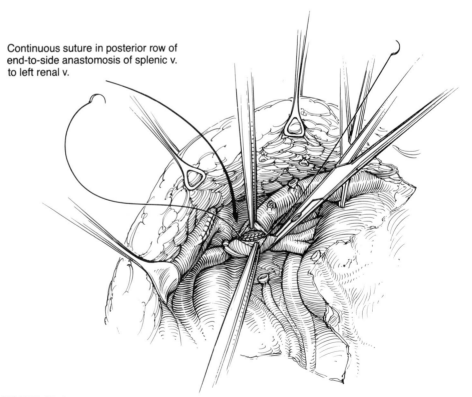

FIGURE 16–6. An end-to-side anastomosis is made between the end of the distal splenic vein and the side of the left renal vein using a continuous suture of 5–0 Prolene.

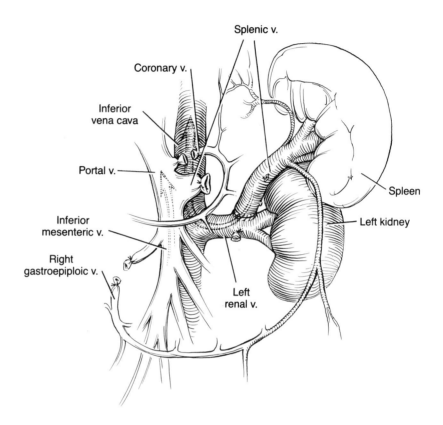

FIGURE 16–7. After the anastomosis is completed, additional venous collaterals, including the right gastroepiploic vein, the coronary vein, and others in the region, are ligated and divided. This point is strongly emphasized by Warren in describing the technical aspects of this operation.

The portal pressure is again obtained postoperatively through an omental vein. There is usually little change, and portal perfusion pressures are maintained at a high level through the liver to provide it with adequate blood flow and reduce the likelihood of hepatic encephalopathy. The incision is then closed in layers.

17

Ligation and Stripping of Varicose Veins

RICHARD L. McCANN, M.D.

Preoperatively, the leg is marked with an indelible pencil while the patient is standing. The tributaries are difficult to see when they are collapsed but are easily marked when the patient is upright. The course of each of the major tributaries is outlined on the skin for both the greater and the lesser saphenous systems. After the induction of anesthesia, the leg is prepared, taking care not to erase the marks.

FIGURE 17–1. The saphenous vein is exposed in the groin and at the ankle. The saphenous bulb is located one fingerbreadth medial to the pulse and one fingerbreadth below the inguinal ligament. The entire bulb is exposed, ligating all branches except the main trunk of the vein. The saphenous vein is ligated flush with the femoral vein.

FIGURES 17–2 and 17–3. A disposable plastic stripper is passed from the ankle to the groin. The vein is tied about the stripper. The smallest olive tip feasible is placed on the stripper, and the patient is placed in a head-down position. The vein is then bluntly stripped from the thigh distally. Hemostasis is achieved by gentle pressure, and incisions are then made directly over the tributaries that have previously been marked. These branches are carefully but bluntly dissected from the subcutaneous tissues.

The wounds are closed in layers, usually with subcuticular sutures such that suture removal is not required. The leg is wrapped in elastic bandage, and bedrest is maintained for 2 or 3 days postoperatively except for bathroom privileges. Gradual ambulation with elastic support is encouraged after removal of the dressings on the third day.

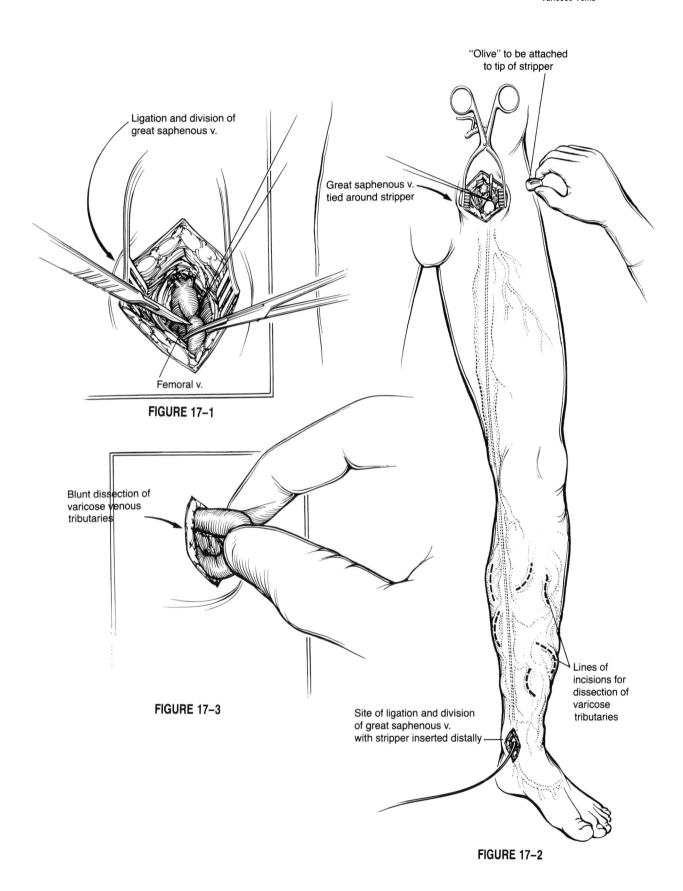

"Olive" to be attached
to tip of stripper

Ligation and division of
great saphenous v.

Great saphenous v.
tied around stripper

Femoral v.

FIGURE 17–1

Blunt dissection of
varicose venous
tributaries

FIGURE 17–3

Lines of
incisions for
dissection of
varicose
tributaries

Site of ligation and division
of great saphenous v.
with stripper inserted distally

FIGURE 17–2

18

Renal Dialysis Access Procedures

DELFORD L. STICKEL, M.D.

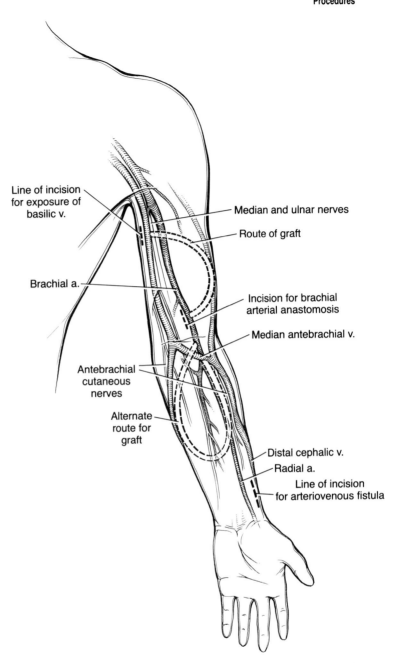

Line of incision
for exposure of
basilic v.

Median and ulnar nerves

Route of graft

Brachial a.

Incision for brachial
arterial anastomosis

Median antebrachial v.

Antebrachial
cutaneous
nerves

Alternate
route for
graft

Distal cephalic v.

Radial a.

Line of incision
for arteriovenous fistula

FIGURE 18–1. If the vessels are adequate, a primary radiocephalic arteriovenous fistula is the procedure of choice. Physical examination will have demonstrated a normal cephalic vein throughout the forearm and normal brachial, radial,* and ulnar pulses. The incision is made midway between the radial artery and the cephalic vein and is centered approximately 5 cm. proximal to the wrist joint. The nondominant forearm is used unless the other arm has noticeably better vessels.

If the vessels are inadequate for a radiocephalic fistula, an arteriovenous polytetra-fluoroethylene (PTFE) graft is necessary. The author prefers to use the upper arm because of the large, single-vein outflow; however, others prefer to use a forearm loop. Regardless of site, skin incisions are planned to obviate their lying directly over any part of the graft.

*The congenital anomaly of an absent or hypoplastic radial artery in the forearm can be associated with a palpable "radial" pulse at the wrist joint, the pulse being transmitted via the ulnar artery and the palmar arches. In order to avoid a surprise encounter with this anomaly intraoperatively, one demonstrates preoperatively that the radial pulsation at the selected site is fully normal and not diminished by point pressure occluding the ulnar artery or distal radial artery.

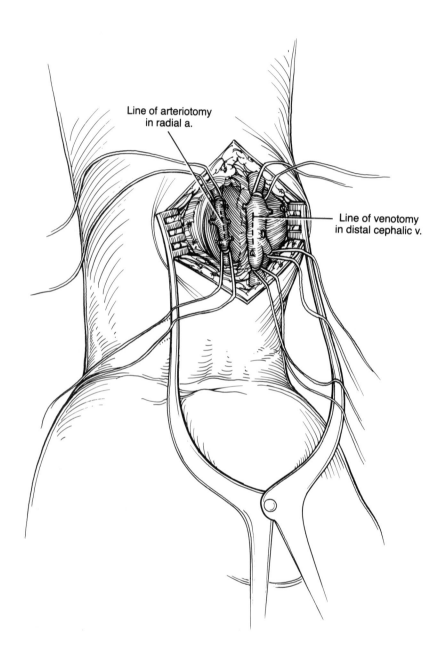

Line of arteriotomy
in radial a.

Line of venotomy
in distal cephalic v.

FIGURE 18–2. Under local anesthesia, the radial artery and the cephalic vein are mobilized sufficiently to bring them together without angulation or tension. Small cutaneous nerves, variable in exact location, are protected from cautery and other injury. Each vessel branch or tributary is ligated at least a millimeter away from the main vessel in order to prevent adventitial entrapment, which can manifest as main channel stenosis after the vessel dilates. With Potts ties of smooth rubber tapes in place and with the lumen containing blood, the vein is gently distended with 1 per cent plain lidocaine and incised longitudinally with a pointed blade. The incision is then extended to 7 to 9 mm. with tenotomy scissors. Adequacy of outflow is tested by a forcible injection of heparinized saline into the proximal vein. An arteriotomy is then made similarly. The patient is not anticoagulated.

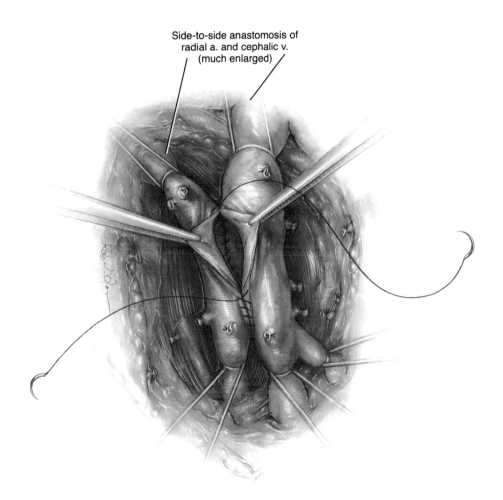

Side-to-side anastomosis of
radial a. and cephalic v.
(much enlarged)

FIGURE 18–3. One continuous 7–0 suture is used to create a side-to-side anastomosis. The back wall is sutured first from within the vessels. Upon completion of the anastomosis, the knot will lie near the midpoint anteriorly. Just prior to completion of the suture line, adequacy of inflow is tested by momentary release of the proximal arterial tape. The immediate signs of a well-functioning fistula are (1) a palpable thrill and (2) a *soft* pulse that noticeably hardens during momentary occlusion of the proximal outflow vein. The wound is closed with subcuticular sutures.

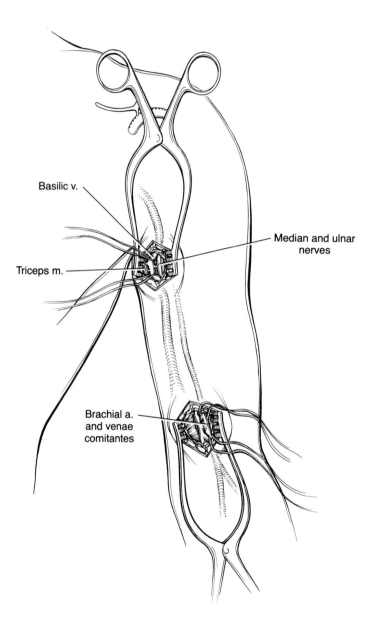

Basilic v.

Median and ulnar
nerves

Triceps m.

Brachial a.
and venae
comitantes

FIGURE 18–4. Under local anesthesia, 4 to 5 cm. of the basilic vein and brachial artery is dissected free. The largest and most superficial vein in the proximal upper arm is usually the basilic. It lies near the edge of the triceps muscle. If it is less than 5 mm. in diameter, a search for a larger brachial vein is worthwhile. In either event, the major nerves are protected from the pressure of retractors and from other injury.

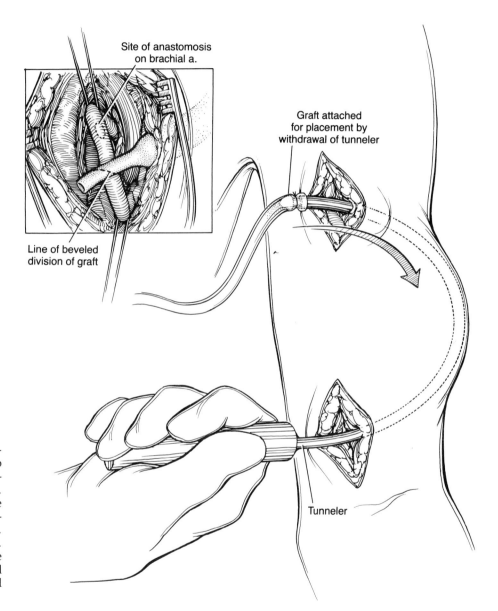

Site of anastomosis
on brachial a.

Line of beveled
division of graft

Graft attached
for placement by
withdrawal of tunneler

Tunneler

FIGURE 18–5. A rigid semicircular tunneler is used to make a subdermal tunnel between the two skin incisions. Care is taken to make the tunnel superficial to all subcutaneous fat. Either a 6-mm. graft or a tapered 4- to 7-mm. graft is drawn through the tunnel. The beveled arterial end of the graft is directed somewhat cephalad.

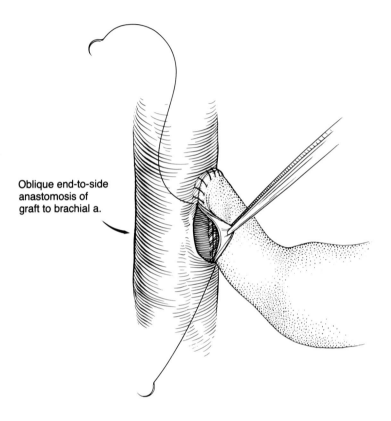

Oblique end-to-side anastomosis of graft to brachial a.

FIGURE 18–6. The anastomosis to the brachial artery is made with a running 6–0 monofilament suture.

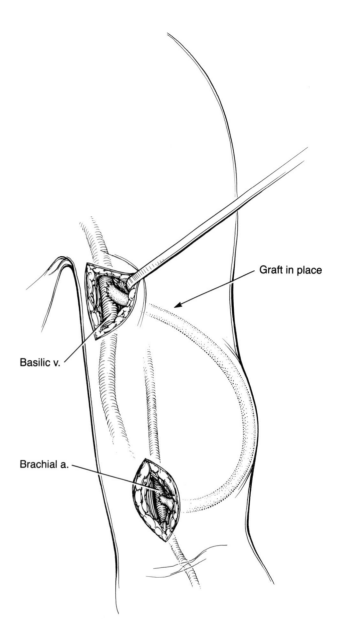

Graft in place

Basilic v.

Brachial a.

FIGURE 18–7. Both ends of the graft are obliquely directed cephalad. The reason for this configuration is the need for future thrombectomy catheters to pass cephalad. Wound closure is with subcuticular sutures.

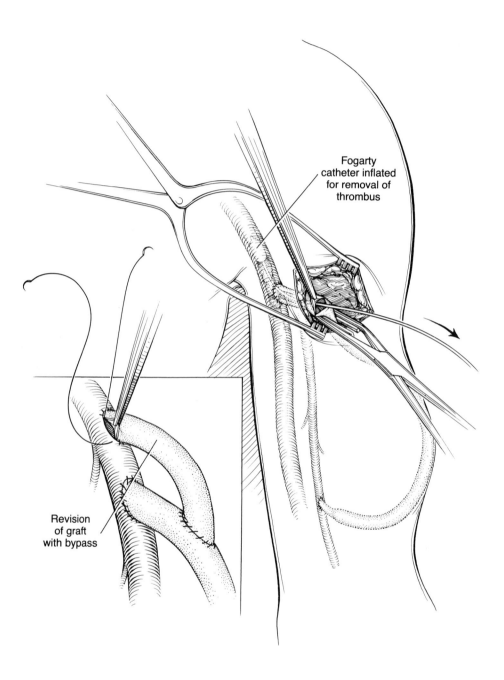

Fogarty
catheter inflated
for removal of
thrombus

Revision
of graft
with bypass

FIGURE 18–8. Graft thrombosis is treated by Fogarty catheter thrombectomy through an incision beside the venous end of the graft, under local anesthesia. Notice again that no part of the incision directly overlies the graft. The incision is placed at the venous end because stenosis of the venous anastomosis and stenosis of the outflow vein are the most common underlying causes of thrombosis. Through this incision, vascular dilators (not shown) can be used to assess the extent of stenosis. The graft is closed with running or interrupted 5–0 monofilament sutures.

If the outflow lumen is less than 3.0 to 3.5 mm. in diameter, revision is advisable. Bypass of the stenosis with a new segment of PTFE graft is usually simpler than revision with an onlay patch. The anastomoses may be either side-to-side as shown or end-to-end.

19

Insertion of Tenckhoff Catheter

DELFORD L. STICKEL, M.D.

An open approach to catheter insertion, such as this approach, is particularly indicated when adhesions from previous abdominal surgery increase the risk of bowel perforation during blind insertion through a trocar or introducer sheath.

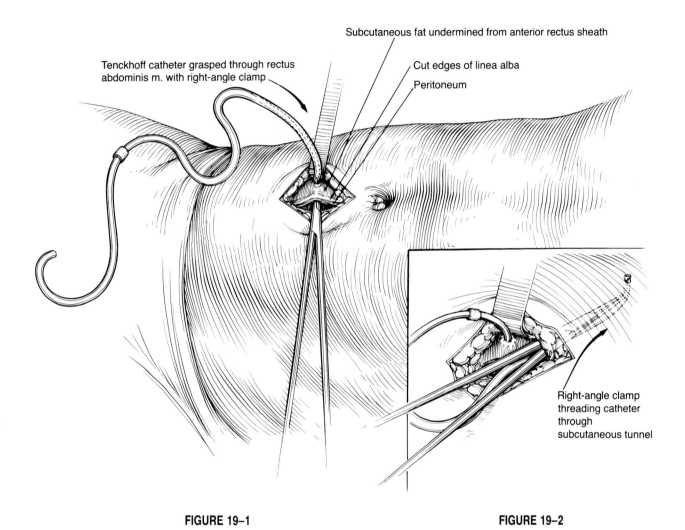

Tenckhoff catheter grasped through rectus abdominis m. with right-angle clamp

Subcutaneous fat undermined from anterior rectus sheath

Cut edges of linea alba

Peritoneum

Right-angle clamp threading catheter through subcutaneous tunnel

FIGURE 19–1

FIGURE 19–2

FIGURE 19–1. Under local anesthesia, the abdomen is entered through a short infraumbilical incision, and subcutaneous fat is dissected off the anterior rectus fascia. A separate puncture is made through the peritoneum, rectus muscle, and rectus fascia with a fine right-angle clamp used to grasp the internal tip of a single-cuff Tenckhoff catheter. A long Kelly clamp (not shown) is then used to direct the tip of the catheter to the bottom of the true pelvis. A pursestring suture in the anterior rectus fascia is snugly tied around the catheter. The peritoneum and linea alba are tightly closed. A liter of heparinized electrolyte solution is instilled into the peritoneal cavity, and its free return through the catheter is confirmed before the end of the procedure.

FIGURE 19–2. With a fine-tipped right-angle clamp, the external end of the catheter is threaded beneath subcutaneous fat and through a separate skin incision that is no larger than the catheter. *No* suture is placed at the skin exit site.

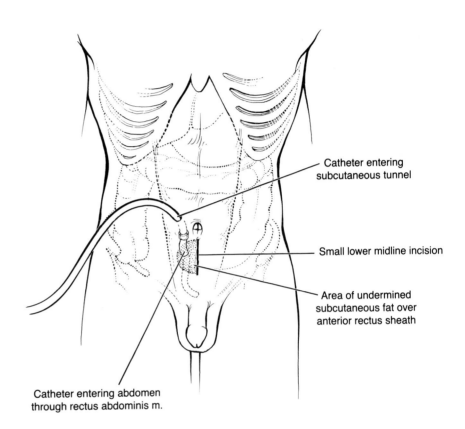

Catheter entering
subcutaneous tunnel

Small lower midline incision

Area of undermined
subcutaneous fat over
anterior rectus sheath

Catheter entering abdomen
through rectus abdominis m.

FIGURE 19–3. At the conclusion of the procedure, the midline incision is tightly closed, and the catheter passes through an entirely separate track to the right (or left) of the midline. A subcuticular skin closure is used so that there are no exposed sutures at either the midline incision or the skin exit site.

20

Insertion of Peritoneal Shunts

ROBERT C. HARLAND, M.D.

The patient with ascites refractory to medical therapy and free of bacterial peritonitis is an appropriate candidate for placement of a peritoneovenous shunt. The presence of malignant ascites is a relative contraindication, although in certain circumstances is acceptable despite the risk of hematogenous seeding of tumor cells.

The patient is placed supine on the operating table. A roll placed under the selected side aids exposure of the lateral costal margin. Local or general anesthesia is used. The placement of a Foley urinary catheter aids in volume management in the postoperative period.

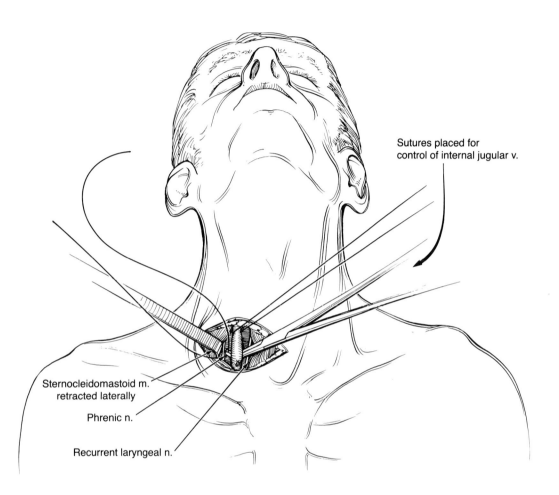

Sutures placed for
control of internal jugular v.

Sternocleidomastoid m.
retracted laterally

Phrenic n.

Recurrent laryngeal n.

FIGURE 20–1. The internal jugular vein is exposed through a transverse cervical incision 1 cm. superior to the clavicle. The clavicular head of the sternocleidomastoid muscle is retracted laterally. Care is taken to avoid the nerves in the area. A pursestring suture of 5-0 polypropylene is placed on the anterior aspect of the vein.

A transverse incision is placed 2 to 5 cm. inferior to the costal margin, avoiding the prominent angle of the anterolateral aspect of the ribs. The Denver shunt requires creation of a pocket placed over the ribs to provide a stable platform for active pumping of the shunt valve. The LeVeen valve is placed under the oblique muscles.

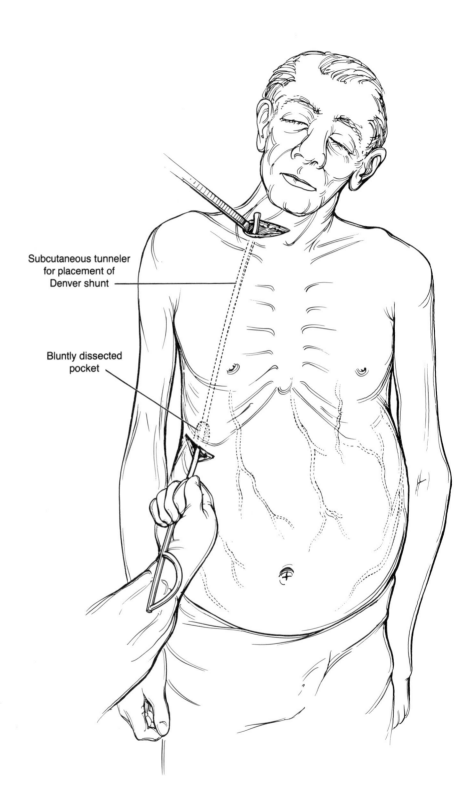

Subcutaneous tunneler
for placement of
Denver shunt

Bluntly dissected
pocket

FIGURE 20–2. The shunt tubing is passed through the subcutaneous tissue to the neck incision. Patency is ensured and air embolism is avoided by filling the shunt with heparinized saline.

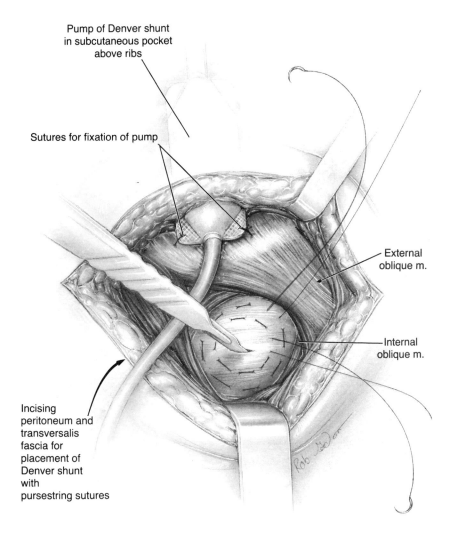

Pump of Denver shunt
in subcutaneous pocket
above ribs

Sutures for fixation of pump

External
oblique m.

Internal
oblique m.

Incising
peritoneum and
transversalis
fascia for
placement of
Denver shunt
with
pursestring sutures

FIGURE 20–3. After the shunt valve is secured to the fascia with monofilament sutures, the peritoneum is exposed by splitting the external and internal oblique muscles in the direction of their fibers. Two concentric pursestrings of 3-0 PDS are placed in the peritoneum and transversalis fascia, and an opening is made into the peritoneal cavity. Removal of 1 to 2 liters of ascites fluid from the abdomen prior to insertion of the catheter helps to limit rapid infusion of fluid into the circulation. The catheter is passed into the peritoneal cavity, directed toward the gutter, and secured with the pursestring sutures.

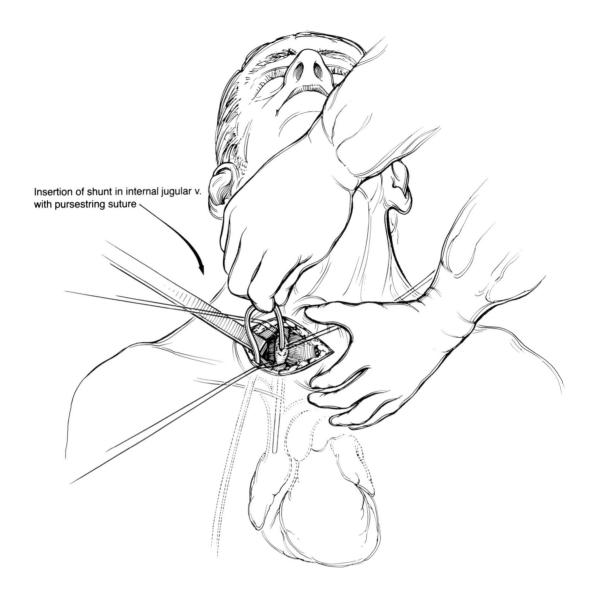

Insertion of shunt in internal jugular v.
with pursestring suture

FIGURE 20–4. After being cut to length, the venous end of the catheter is inserted through the pursestring in the jugular vein and directed into the superior vena cava. The tip should lie at the junction of the superior vena cava and the right atrium. Care is taken to avoid kinking the tubing.

Meticulous attention is given to hemostasis, especially in patients with coagulopathy. The wounds are irrigated with an antibiotic solution and closed in several layers with absorbable sutures. A subcuticular skin stitch is used.

Postoperative care: A chest film is obtained to document appropriate placement. A dose of intravenous diuretic is administered at the conclusion of the procedure. During the first 12 to 24 hours, frequent examinations are required to detect volume overload of the patient, which may be treated with diuretics and by elevating the head of the bed, thus limiting flow through the shunt.

Patients in whom a Denver shunt is placed should be instructed to pump the valve chamber 50 to 100 times at least 4 times per day in order to maintain patency. Pumping is not required with a LeVeen shunt.

Shunt dysfunction can be diagnosed by pumping the Denver shunt and assessing ease of filling and resistance to emptying. All shunts can be tested with a radionuclide test measuring clearance of radiolabeled tracer from the peritoneal cavity into the blood stream. The occluded portion of the shunt can be replaced, or a new shunt may be placed on the opposite side.

21

Insertion of Right Atrial Catheters for Chemotherapy, Antibiotics, and Hyperalimentation

JOHN P. GRANT, M.D.

A number of manufacturers produce external and totally implantable long-term vascular access catheters. The selection is a matter of personal choice, and placement is similar for all devices. The procedure is best performed in the operating room to ensure optimal sterility.

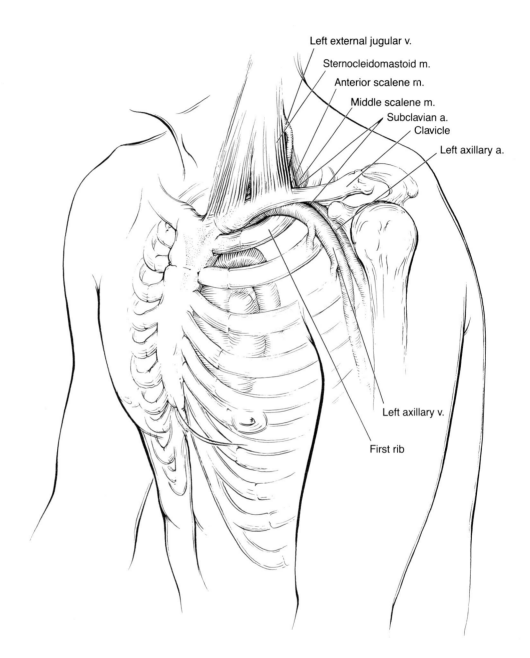

Left external jugular v.

Sternocleidomastoid m.

Anterior scalene m.

Middle scalene m.

Subclavian a.

Clavicle

Left axillary a.

Left axillary v.

First rib

FIGURE 21–1. The subclavian vein begins at the lateral border of the first rib. It arches behind the clavicle and over the first rib anterior to the insertion of the anterior scalene muscle. At the medial border of the anterior scalene muscle, the subclavian vein joins the internal jugular vein to form the brachiocephalic (innominate) vein. Anteriorly, the subclavian vein is covered in its entire course by the clavicle, the costoclavicular ligament, and the subclavius muscle. Inferiorly, the vein rests on the first rib laterally and on the cupola of the lung medially. Posteriorly, as the subclavian vein crosses the first rib, it is separated from the subclavian artery by the anterior scalene muscle, which is usually about 1 cm. thick. The thoracic duct enters the internal jugular vein near its junction with the left subclavian vein, passing anterior to the subclavian artery and its branches and posterior to the internal jugular vein.

The subclavian vein adheres to the adjacent ligaments, fasciae, and periosteum through an extension of the fascia colli media. Because of these attachments, it is not easily displaced and does not collapse, even in shock or death.

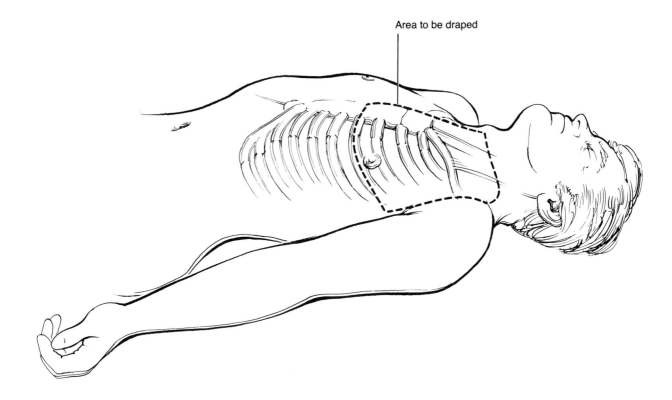

Area to be draped

FIGURE 21–2. The patient is positioned supine on the operating table with the arms drawn toward the feet and secured at the side. If the shoulders are in a shrugged position, the vein is at a variable distance below the lower edge of the clavicle and may take a tortuous course.

A rectangular area from the midneck to below the nipple line and from the anterior axillary line to just across the sternum is thoroughly cleansed with povidone-iodine soap, alcohol, and then povidone-iodine solution. Sterile drapes are placed.

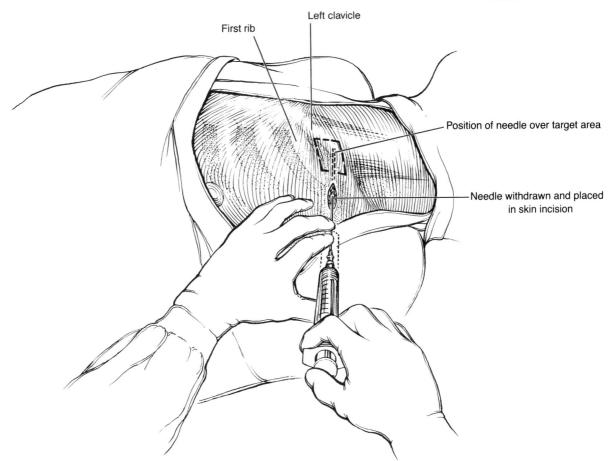

First rib

Left clavicle

Position of needle over target area

Needle withdrawn and placed
in skin incision

FIGURE 21–3. Either the right or the left subclavian vein may be used. If there has been a previous mastectomy, fractured clavicle, or infected or injured skin, use of the vein on the opposite side is preferable, as is use of the opposite side when a catheter is already in place in the internal jugular vein. If none of the above is of concern, the left subclavian vein is preferred because it has a straighter course. The lateral edge of the clavicular head of the sternocleidomastoid muscle as it inserts on the clavicle can usually be easily seen. The anterior scalene muscle lies just under the clavicular head of the sternocleidomastoid muscle, passes under the clavicle, and inserts on the tubercle of the first rib. By passing a finger behind the clavicle along the anterior scalene muscle, one can sometimes palpate the subclavian artery posteriorly. The target for subclavian vein catheterization is thus identified as a 2 × 2 cm. area bounded inferiorly by the first rib as marked by the lower edge of the clavicle, posteriorly by the anterior scalene muscle as it inserts on the tubercle of the first rib, anteriorly by the clavicle, and superiorly by the upper edge of the clavicle (see Fig. 21–1). The location of the subclavian vein in this area is very constant. If displaced, it is more cephalad only as the result of hyperinflation of the lung. A 2- to 2.5-inch 16-gauge needle is attached to a 10-ml. syringe and is tested to ensure that no air leaks are present by occluding the tip of the needle with a gloved finger while applying suction to the syringe. This procedure must be done so that no question arises during insertion of the needle as to whether the lung has been punctured if air is drawn into the syringe. The barrel of the syringe is placed in the deltopectoral groove, with the tip of the needle overlying the 2 × 2 cm. target zone. The needle and syringe are then drawn away laterally until the tip of the needle is approximately 2 cm. away from the inferior edge of the clavicle. Lidocaine (½ per cent) with epinephrine is injected at the chosen puncture site with a 25-gauge needle. The epinephrine additive is optional, but it reduces the incidence of exit site bleeding. No attempt should be made to anesthetize the subclavius muscle or periosteum of the clavicle. Complete anesthesia cannot be obtained, nor is it necessary, and the vein might be displaced by a large amount of fluid. A 1-cm. incision is placed, and the needle is inserted with its bevel directed anteriorly. The practice of "walking down the clavicle" is not necessary and should be avoided because it can be painful both immediately and for several days and because osteomyelitis of the clavicle following needle injury has been reported.

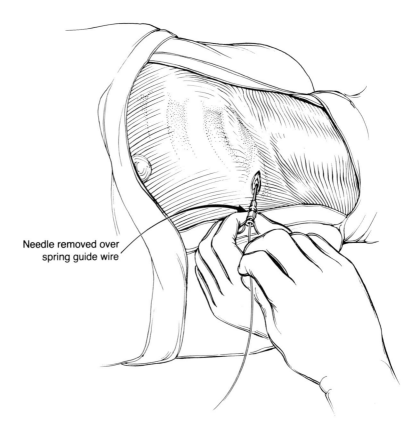

Needle removed over
spring guide wire

FIGURE 21–4. The needle should be slowly advanced toward the target area, with the syringe held against the patient's shoulder in a position horizontal to the floor. Frequent small aspirations, rather than constant suctioning, should be applied to the plunger of the syringe as the needle is advanced until a free flow of blood is obtained. Continuous aspiration may cause plugging of the needle with a core of soft tissue, masking entry into the vein. The vein is usually entered after 4 to 6 cm. of the needle has been inserted. If the vein is not entered, the needle should be removed slowly and completely with intermittent aspiration. If, as occasionally occurs, the vein has been punctured through-and-through without aspiration of blood, a return of blood into the syringe may be seen during withdrawal, and the catheter can often be inserted successfully. If no blood is aspirated during withdrawal of the needle, the needle should be completely removed and any plugs of tissue or blood flushed out with the plunger of the syringe. The target area should then be re-evaluated. A point slightly more cephalad on the anterior scalene muscle should be selected. The temptation to direct the needle more posteriorly should absolutely be avoided because the vein does not lie behind the anterior scalene muscle, but the subclavian artery and the cupola of the lung do. *At no time* should probing for the vein be done with short jabs of the needle in different directions. This markedly increases the risk of laceration of the subclavian vein or artery and increases the risk of pneumothorax. The needle should always be completely withdrawn and landmarks re-evaluated before making another pass.

Upon puncture of the subclavian vein and free return of blood into the syringe, the needle should be advanced approximately 0.5 cm. farther to ensure that the beveled tip lies entirely within the subclavian vein. A spring guide wire is advanced through the needle, and the needle is removed.

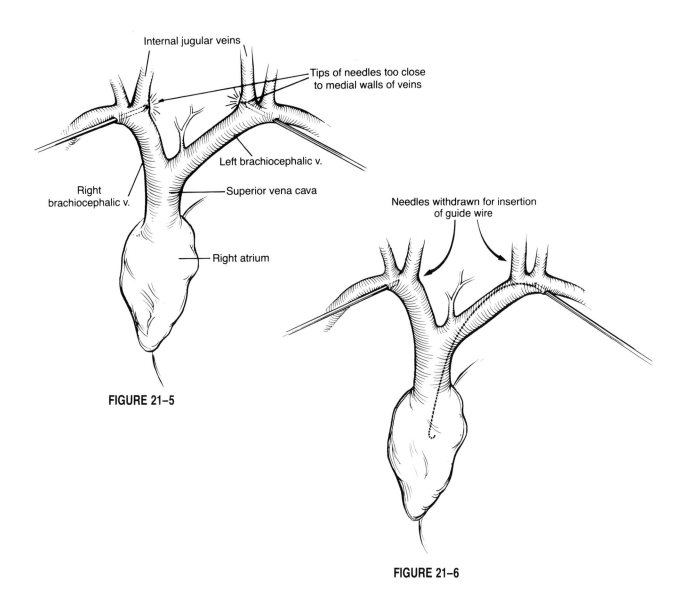

FIGURE 21–5

FIGURE 21–6

FIGURES 21–5 and 21–6. Failure of the guide wire to be advanced easily usually means that it is no longer within the vein or that it is against the vein's wall at the junction of the internal jugular and subclavian veins. In the latter case, withdrawal of the needle a short distance often allows free passage of the guide wire into the venous system. If the wire passes into the internal jugular vein, it cannot be fully advanced, and the patient often reports a noise or pain in the ear. Partial withdrawl of the guide wire and reinsertion should be done until the wire passes all the way in without resistance. The guide wire is advanced fully or until cardiac irritability is observed.

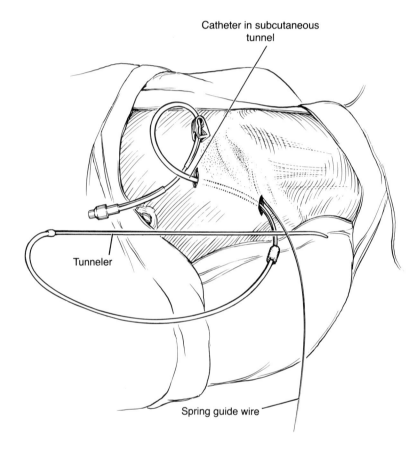

Catheter in subcutaneous
tunnel

Tunneler

Spring guide wire

FIGURE 21-7. The catheter is attached to a tunneler and passed through an incision placed just medial and above the breast, exiting out the incision at the clavicle. The tract is infiltrated with local anesthetic containing epinephrine just prior to passage of the tunneler to minimize pain and reduce bleeding. The catheter is cut to proper length.

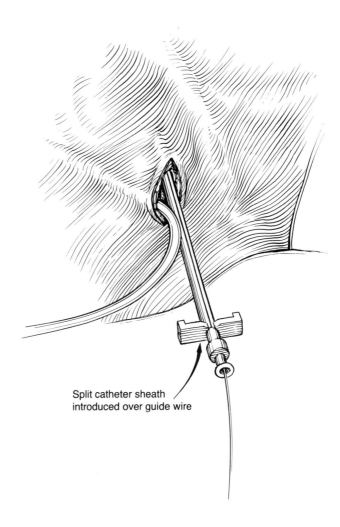

Split catheter sheath
introduced over guide wire

FIGURE 21–8. A split catheter sheath with introducer is passed over the guide wire and advanced into the innominate vein.

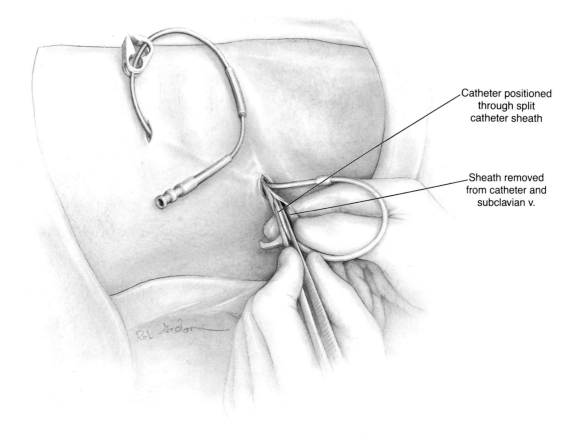

Catheter positioned
through split
catheter sheath

Sheath removed
from catheter and
subclavian v.

FIGURE 21–9. The trocar and guide wire are removed, and the catheter is passed through the split catheter sheath into the right atrium. The split catheter sheath is removed. The correct position of the catheter tip in the right atrium is confirmed by injection of contrast material under fluoroscopic observation.

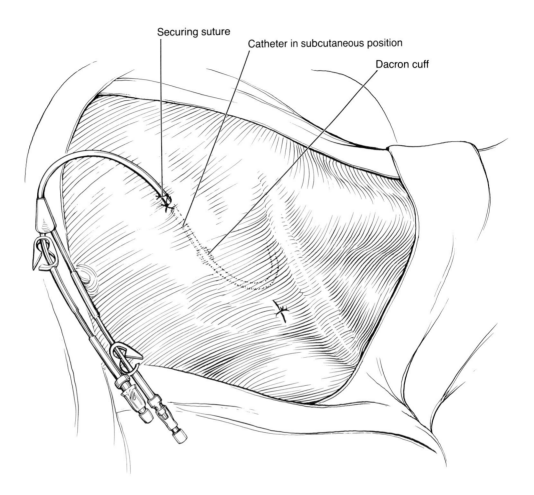

Securing suture

Catheter in subcutaneous position

Dacron cuff

FIGURE 21–10. The catheter is drawn out of the lower incision until all slack is removed, placing the Dacron cuff in the subcutaneous tract. The incisions are closed, and the catheter is retained by securing the ends of the lower suture about the catheter. Sterile dressings are applied.

A chest x-ray film should be obtained to confirm location of the catheter tip and to ensure no pneumothorax occurred with catheter placement.

Subcutaneous pocket bluntly dissected

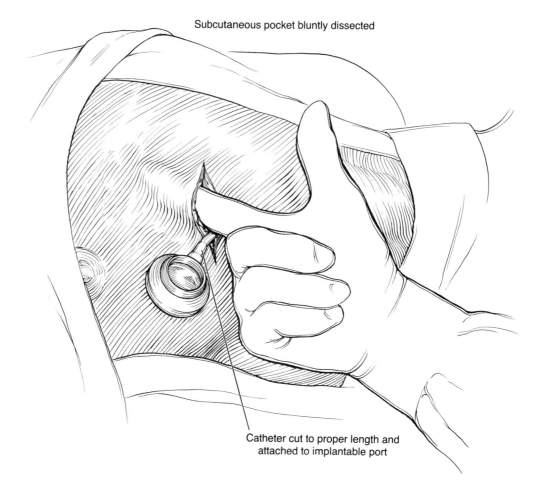

Catheter cut to proper length and
attached to implantable port

FIGURE 21–11. The catheter for a totally implantable device is placed as described for
the external type, cut to proper length, and attached to the chamber. A subcutaneous
pocket is created by blunt and sharp dissection just large enough to accept the chamber.
This pocket should be just above the breast in approximately the midclavicular line.

Port in subcutaneous pocket

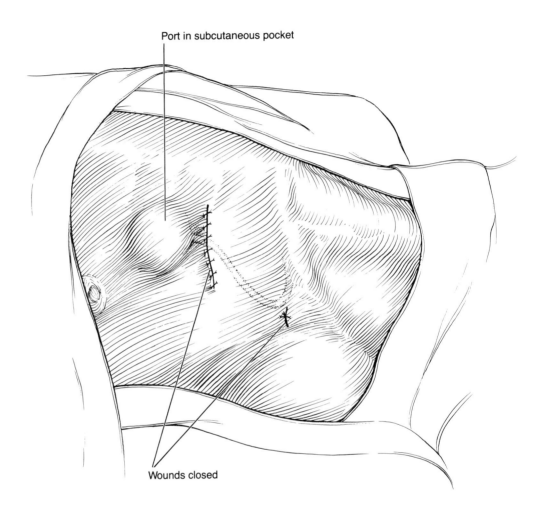

Wounds closed

FIGURE 21–12. The port is placed into the pocket, and the wounds are closed.

A chest film should be obtained to confirm location of the catheter tip and to ensure no pneumothorax occurred with catheter placement.

SECTION III
Hernias

22

Hernia Repair: General Principles

WILLIAM P. J. PEETE, M.D.

On the operating table, the patient is placed in a 15- to 20-degree Trendelenburg position. This maneuver flattens the operating field and simplifies the procedure by allowing easier reduction of a hernia, which can be maintained in a reduced condition. It also reduces the stasis of blood in the leg veins and serves as prophylaxis against thrombophlebitis and pulmonary embolism.

Local anesthesia can often be used. A curved in-the-skin-line incision is outlined from just above the pubic tubercle to beyond the internal opening laterally. If local anesthesia is used, a diamond-shaped field is outlined, and about 60 ml. of 0.5 per cent Xylocaine with epinephrine is administered, and a skin wheal is made laterally with a No. 27 needle. Eight to 10 ml. is then placed beneath the outlined incision with a No. 23 needle, and 8 to 10 ml. is used beneath each quadrant of the diamond. When anesthesia is ensured by testing, the skin incision is made and deepened through subcutaneous fascia and the external oblique aponeurosis.

Anesthesia is continued by injecting a small quantity in (or around) the ilioinguinal and iliohypogastric nerves laterally. A few milliliters are placed at the external and then the internal ring.

Often, 5 to 10 ml. of Xylocaine are inserted into the open sac. This permits a careful and painless dissection to delineate the anatomic features of the hernia, and the type of repair is determined on the basis of these findings.

When the repair is complete and before the external oblique aponeurosis is closed, 20 to 25 ml. of 0.25 per cent Marcaine may be placed in the field with reinjection of the nerves and subcutaneous tissue for prolonged analgesia. Interrupted *or* running sutures of 2–0 Prolene for Shouldice or Bassini repairs should be used. If a femoral hernia is present, the McVay repair is preferred by most surgeons.

Epinephrine tends to wear off, and small vessels may begin to bleed and thus create more ecchymosis with local anesthesia. Accordingly, the subcutaneous tissue is closed with a running 3–0 chromic catgut suture. The skin closure is usually accomplished with a subcuticular 4–0 catgut suture fortified with Steri-Strips and covered with either a collodion or an Op-Site dressing to make it reasonable for the patient to bathe soon after the operation.

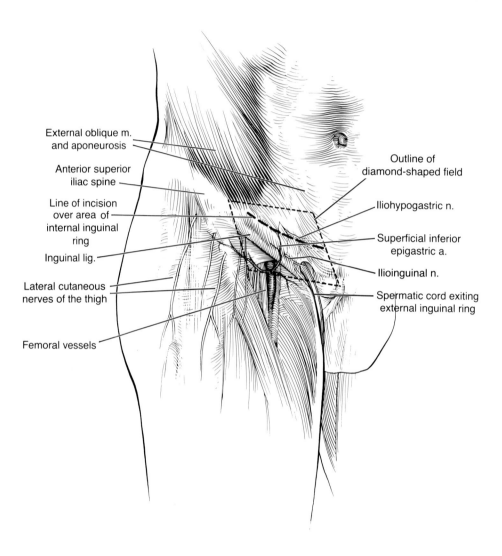

External oblique m.
and aponeurosis

Anterior superior
iliac spine

Line of incision
over area of
internal inguinal
ring

Inguinal lig.

Lateral cutaneous
nerves of the thigh

Femoral vessels

Outline of
diamond-shaped field

Iliohypogastric n.

Superficial inferior
epigastric a.

Ilioinguinal n.

Spermatic cord exiting
external inguinal ring

FIGURE 22–1

23

Inguinal Herniorrhaphy: Bassini (INGUINAL LIGAMENT)

JOSEPH A. MOYLAN, M.D.

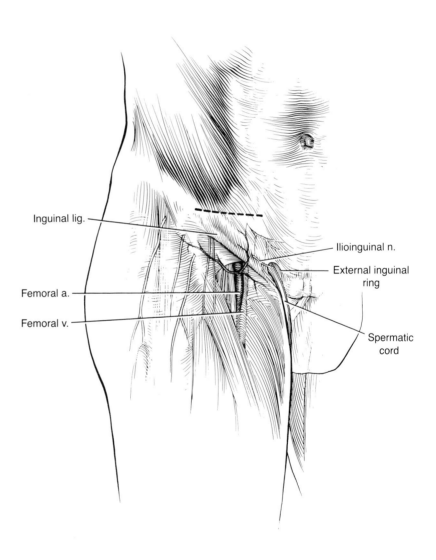

FIGURE 23–1. This illustration shows the topical anatomy of the inguinal area at the level of the abdominal wall. Important structures include the external inguinal ring, the ilioinguinal nerve, and the femoral vessels beneath the inguinal canal.

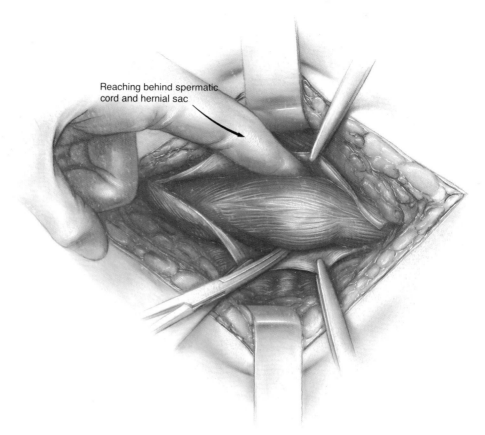

FIGURE 23–2. Through a transverse or slightly oblique incision, the external ring and external oblique fascia are opened and the cord is encircled.

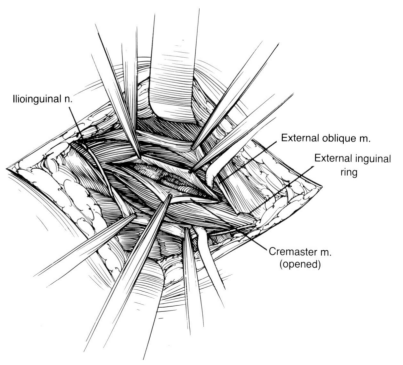

FIGURE 23–3. The cremaster muscle is carefully dissected off the medial aspect of the cord to identify the indirect sac.

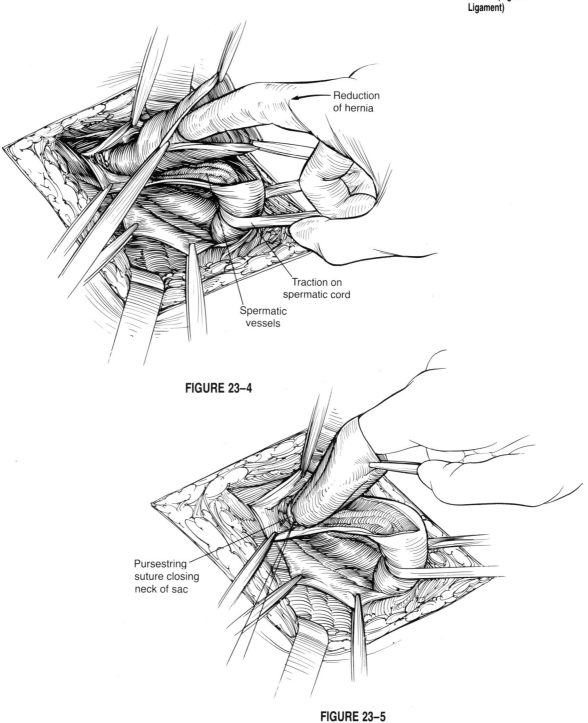

Reduction
of hernia

Traction on
spermatic cord

Spermatic
vessels

FIGURE 23–4

Pursestring
suture closing
neck of sac

FIGURE 23–5

FIGURE 23–4. After the sac has been dissected free to the level of the abdominal wall, it is opened and its contents are reduced.

FIGURE 23–5. The neck of the sac at the level of the abdominal wall is ligated, and the remaining distal sac is amputated.

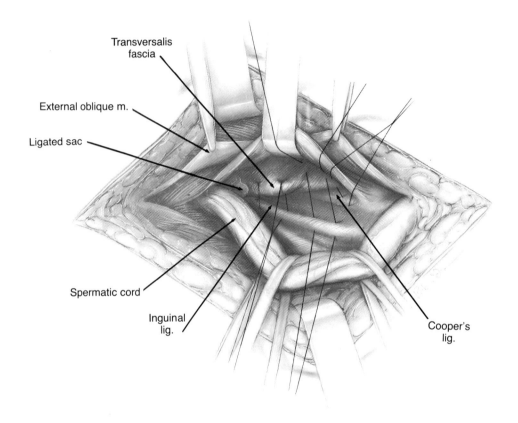

Transversalis
fascia

External oblique m.

Ligated sac

Spermatic cord

Inguinal
lig.

Cooper's
lig.

FIGURE 23–6. With serial sutures, the transversalis fascia is approximated to Cooper's ligament and then along the course of the iliopubic tract (the shelving portion of the inguinal ligament). Care is taken at the junction of the inguinal ligament and the symphysis pubis so that the transition suture between Cooper's ligament and the iliopubic tract ensures closure of this area.

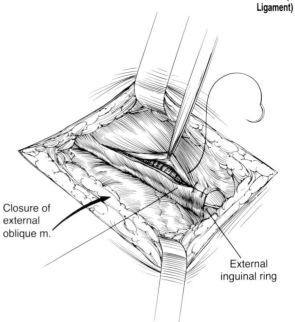

Closure of
external
oblique m.

External
inguinal ring

FIGURE 23–7. After completion of the approximation of the transversalis fascia to the iliopubic tract, the cord is returned to its anatomic position and the external oblique fascia is approximated over the cord down to the level of the previous external ring.

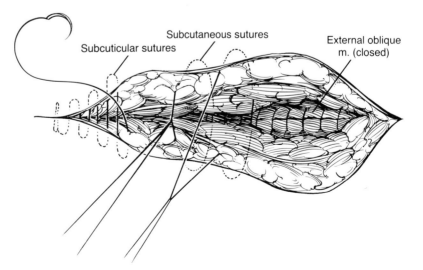

Subcutaneous sutures

Subcuticular sutures

External oblique
m. (closed)

FIGURE 23–8. The wound is irrigated and closed in layers using subcutaneous and subcuticular sutures.

24

Inguinal Herniorrhaphy: McVay (COOPER'S LIGAMENT)

WILLIAM P. J. PEETE, M.D.
(after ROBB H. RUTLEDGE, M.D.)

The decision to perform a Cooper's ligament (McVay) repair is made after careful dissection of the groin with identification of the anatomy. Generally, the technique described by Rutledge is followed, except that Prolene sutures are used instead of silk.* Rutledge employs a Cooper's ligament repair for all groin hernias, but it is usually performed for recurrent hernias, femoral hernias, and large mixed hernias.

---

*Rutledge, R. H.: Cooper's ligament repair. Surgical Rounds, pp. 17–30, January, 1989.

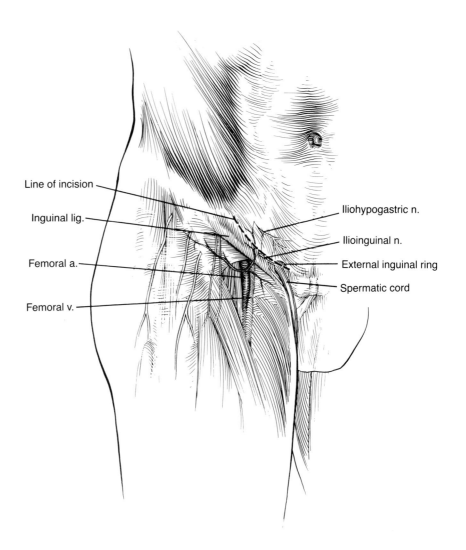

FIGURE 24–1. A curved incision is made in the skin crease from the pubic tubercle laterally beyond the internal ring.

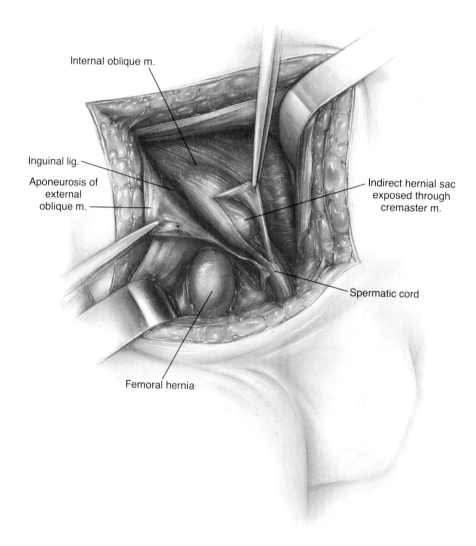

Internal oblique m.

Inguinal lig.

Aponeurosis of
external
oblique m.

Indirect hernial sac
exposed through
cremaster m.

Spermatic cord

Femoral hernia

FIGURE 24–2. The external oblique aponeurosis is opened through the external ring. The spermatic cord is mobilized, and both indirect and femoral hernias are demonstrated here.

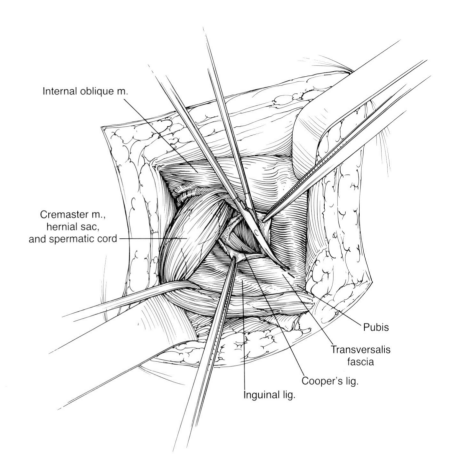

Internal oblique m.

Cremaster m.,
hernial sac,
and spermatic cord

Pubis

Transversalis
fascia

Cooper's lig.

Inguinal lig.

FIGURE 24–3. The posterior wall of the inguinal canal is incised, completely destroying
the internal ring. Cooper's ligament is dissected free.

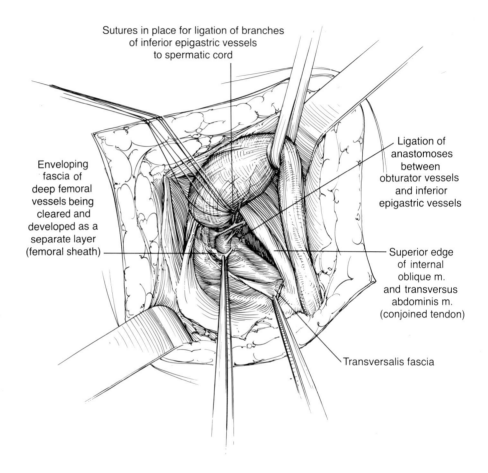

Sutures in place for ligation of branches
of inferior epigastric vessels
to spermatic cord

Enveloping
fascia of
deep femoral
vessels being
cleared and
developed as a
separate layer
(femoral sheath)

Ligation of
anastomoses
between
obturator vessels
and inferior
epigastric vessels

Superior edge
of internal
oblique m.
and transversus
abdominis m.
(conjoined tendon)

Transversalis fascia

FIGURE 24–4. The spermatic cord is retracted superiorly, and the deeper portion of Cooper's ligament is cleared. The anterior femoral fascia is developed, and the anterior surfaces of the femoral artery and vein are cleared. Working medially around the femoral vein, the surgeon clears the femoral canal; any anomalous connections to the obturator vessels are divided. The transversus abdominis arch is developed superiorly, and any weakened transversalis fascia and internal oblique muscle are excised. A 4-inch relaxing incision is made medially at the line of fusion of the external oblique aponeurosis and the rectus sheath beginning just above the pubic symphysis. This incision is lengthened if more relaxation is needed.

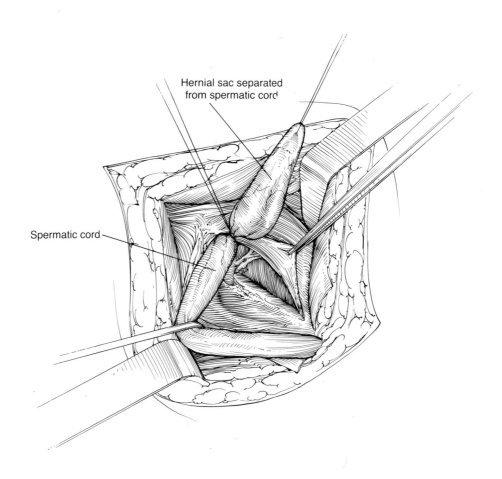

Hernial sac separated
from spermatic cord

Spermatic cord

FIGURE 24–5. The spermatic cord is opened, and the cremasteric fibers are divided at the internal ring. The external spermatic artery is divided to permit the cord to be moved laterally. Any indirect sac is dissected, opened, explored, and oversewn or suture-ligated flush with the peritoneum. Large indirect sacs are transected, and the distal portion of the sac is left in place to prevent damage to the spermatic cord. Combined indirect and direct sacs are joined by dividing the inferior epigastric vessels and closing the sacs as one peritoneal defect. The repair is begun by inverting all of the preperitoneal tissues with a continuous suture to reduce the tissues away from the main repair.

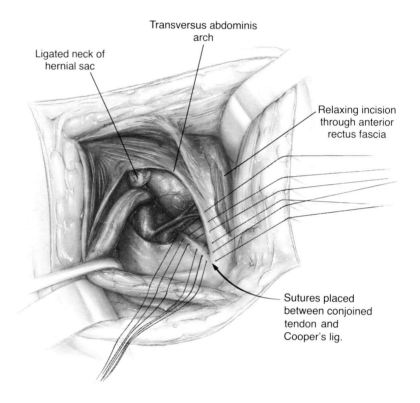

Ligated neck of
hernial sac

Transversus abdominis
arch

Relaxing incision
through anterior
rectus fascia

Sutures placed
between conjoined
tendon and
Cooper's lig.

FIGURE 24–6. Beginning at the pubic tubercle, a row of interrupted 1–0 Prolene sutures is placed and held between the transversus arch and Cooper's ligament. An Allis clamp may be used to grasp the transversus abdominis arch. Placement of the abdominis arch to Cooper's ligament sutures proceeds as far laterally as the medial edge of the femoral vein.

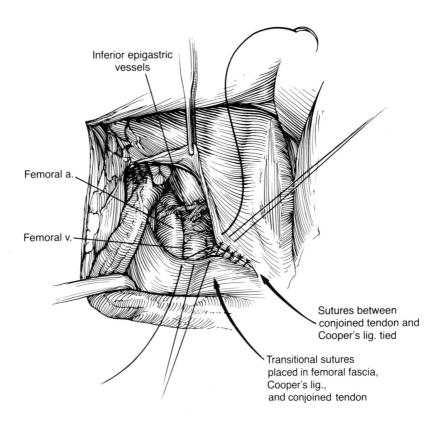

Inferior epigastric
vessels

Femoral a.

Femoral v.

Sutures between
conjoined tendon and
Cooper's lig. tied

Transitional sutures
placed in femoral fascia,
Cooper's lig.,
and conjoined tendon

FIGURE 24–7. The femoral canal is closed with three or four 2–0 Prolene sutures between Cooper's ligament and the anterior femoral fascia. Some of these sutures are placed between the lateralmost sutures in Cooper's ligament.

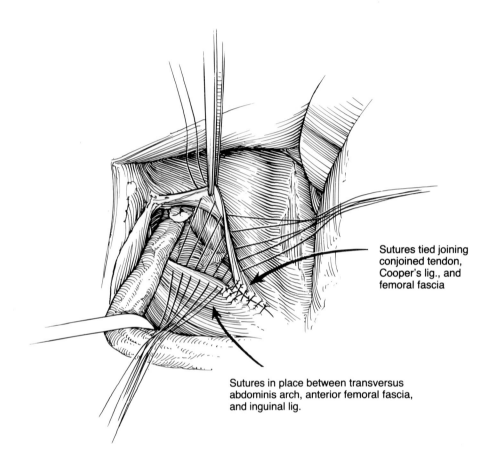

Sutures tied joining
conjoined tendon,
Cooper's lig., and
femoral fascia

Sutures in place between transversus
abdominis arch, anterior femoral fascia,
and inguinal lig.

FIGURE 24–8. The repair is continued by placing sutures between the transversus abdominis arch, the anterior femoral fascia, and the inguinal ligament, continuing laterally beyond any indirect sac so that the cord actually emerges obliquely laterally at the new internal ring. No sutures are placed lateral to the cord, thus allowing it to move laterally without constriction. This layer is accomplished with 1–0 Prolene or silk. The sutures are tied medial to lateral.

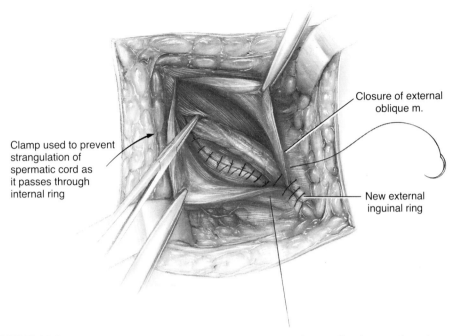

Closure of external
oblique m.

Clamp used to prevent
strangulation of
spermatic cord as
it passes through
internal ring

New external
inguinal ring

FIGURE 24–9. The new internal ring is snug and admits only a Kelly clamp. The relaxing incision may be secured in place with interrupted 2–0 Prolene sutures. If the area of the relaxing incision appears weak, it is patched with a piece of Marlex mesh sutured in place with 2–0 Prolene. Occasionally, a layer of Marlex mesh is sutured as a reinforcement above the basic layer. The external oblique aponeurosis is closed over the spermatic cord with a running 2–0 Prolene suture. The new external ring is *loose*.

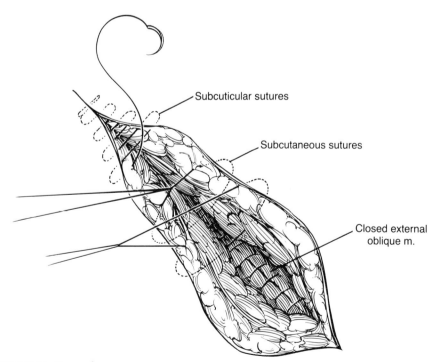

Subcuticular sutures

Subcutaneous sutures

Closed external
oblique m.

FIGURE 24–10. The soft tissue is closed with 3–0 chromic catgut, and the skin is closed with a subcuticular 4–0 chromic catgut. Steri-Strips are applied, and the area is dressed with collodion.

25

Inguinal Herniorrhaphy: Shouldice

WILLIAM P. J. PEETE, M.D.

For the repair of groin hernias, Shouldice emphasized a six-layer closure using fine running steel sutures, with the conviction that there is less tissue tear with running sutures. He further emphasized careful attention to the sac, imbrication of the transversalis fascia, suture of the transversus abdominis arch and/or conjoined tendon to the inguinal ligament, closure of the external oblique aponeurosis, and closure of the subcutaneous fascia and the skin.

Shouldice routinely advocated *local anesthesia* for its safety and because, with a *Valsalva* maneuver, the patient could easily assist the surgeon in identifying weak sites in the groin dissection along with ensuring that all weak areas were closed. *Early ambulation* and *exercise* on the next day were also features of his program. If the patients were overweight, Shouldice insisted on preoperative weight loss. This made good tissue easier to identify and permitted a more stable closure. Requiring weight loss significantly reduced the recurrence rate in his patients.

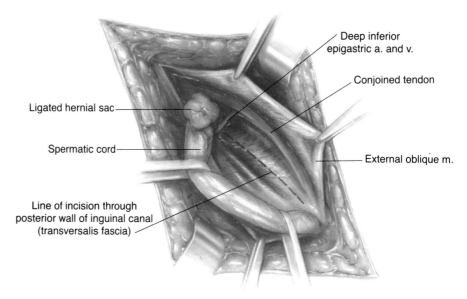

FIGURE 25–1. Groin anatomy is carefully dissected, and the indirect sac is ligated high.

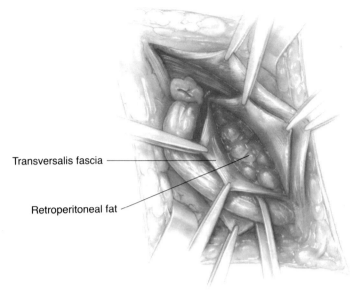

Transversalis fascia

Retroperitoneal fat

FIGURE 25–2. The transversalis fascia is fully opened, and the inferior epigastric vessels may be divided to facilitate opening the internal ring.

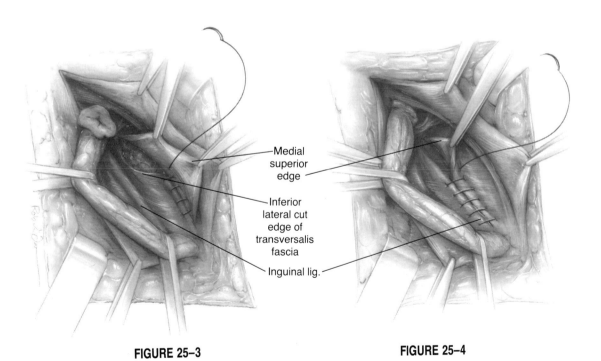

Medial superior edge

Inferior lateral cut edge of transversalis fascia

Inguinal lig.

FIGURE 25–3   **FIGURE 25–4**

FIGURE 25–3. The lateral (or inferior) cut edge of the transversalis fascia is sutured medially to the undersurface of the internal oblique muscle.

FIGURE 25–4. The medial superior edge is sutured to the inguinal ligament.

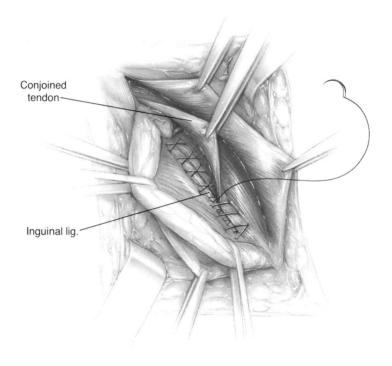

Conjoined
tendon

Inguinal lig.

FIGURE 25–5. The conjoined tendon is sutured to the inguinal ligament, providing a firm repair.

The external oblique aponeurosis is closed over the cord, leaving the external ring loose. Antibiotic solution is used to irrigate the incision, which is closed with a subcutaneous and subcuticular suture.

26

Laparoscopic Inguinal Hernia

THEODORE N. PAPPAS, M.D.
JOSEPH A. MOYLAN, M.D.

FIGURE 26–1. The trocar placement for a right laparoscopic inguinal hernia is depicted. The camera is placed at the umbilicus in a 10-mm. port, and a 12-mm. trocar is placed at the level of the umbilicus in the midclavicular line on the side of the hernia. Care is taken to avoid the epigastric vessels. A 5-mm. trocar is then placed no lower than the umbilical line directly over the right colon, and the final 5-mm. trocar is placed in the left lower quadrant. Alternate trocar placement would include only 3 trocars, a 10-mm. trocar in the umbilicus and 2 12-mm. trocars on either side of the umbilicus. Care is taken to place these trocars far enough away from the inguinal region to provide adequate visualization without "crowding" the field. Laparoscopic hernia repair requires a detailed knowledge of the intra-abdominal anatomy of this region.

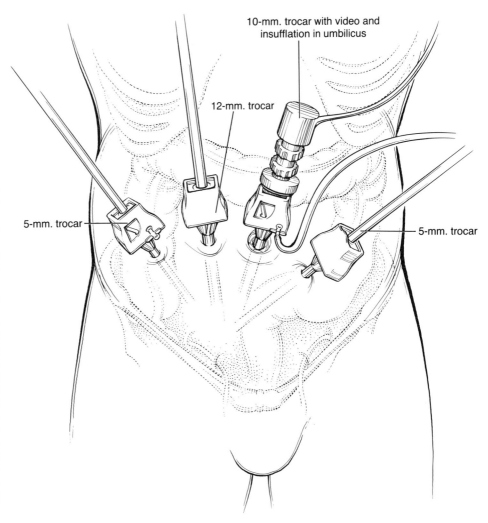

10-mm. trocar with video and insufflation in umbilicus

12-mm. trocar

5-mm. trocar

5-mm. trocar

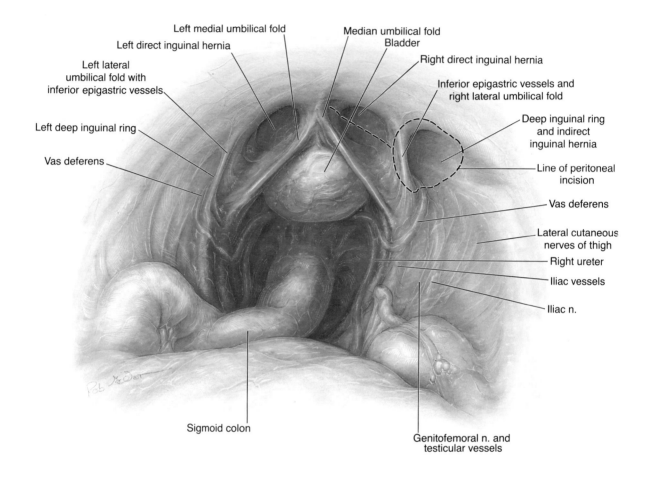

Left medial umbilical fold
Left direct inguinal hernia
Left lateral
umbilical fold with
inferior epigastric vessels
Left deep inguinal ring
Vas deferens
Median umbilical fold
Bladder
Right direct inguinal hernia
Inferior epigastric vessels and
right lateral umbilical fold
Deep inguinal ring
and indirect
inguinal hernia
Line of peritoneal
incision
Vas deferens
Lateral cutaneous
nerves of thigh
Right ureter
Iliac vessels
Iliac n.
Sigmoid colon
Genitofemoral n. and
testicular vessels

FIGURE 26–2. This illustration represents a right inguinal hernia, and the pertinent anatomy includes the inferior epigastric vessels, which course superiorly onto the anterior abdominal wall. The ability to expose Cooper's ligament is important. The medial umbilical fold has been demonstrated but is outside the field of most anatomic repairs. The vas deferens and the iliac neurovascular bundle course through the base of the indirect hernia and should be avoided during repair. The lateral femoral cutaneous nerve also can be injured and should be avoided when the mesh is stapled in place.

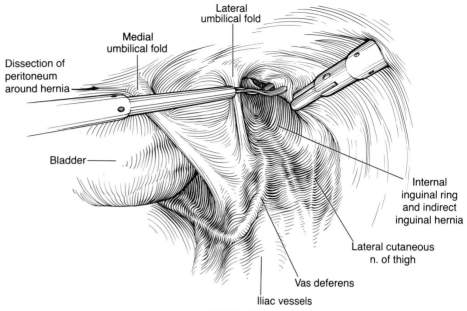

Dissection of
peritoneum
around hernia

Medial
umbilical fold

Lateral
umbilical fold

Bladder

Internal
inguinal ring
and indirect
inguinal hernia

Lateral cutaneous
n. of thigh

Vas deferens

Iliac vessels

FIGURE 26–3

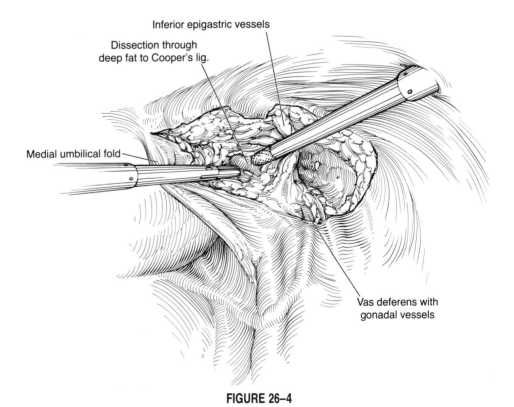

Inferior epigastric vessels

Dissection through
deep fat to Cooper's lig.

Medial umbilical fold

Vas deferens with
gonadal vessels

FIGURE 26–4

FIGURES 26–3 and 26–4. The peritoneum at the internal ring is incised. This allows transection of the sac and leads to mobilization of the peritoneum so that the mesh can be placed behind the peritoneum. Care is taken to incise only the peritoneal surface. Once the sac has been divided or reduced, blunt dissection is used to mobilize the peritoneum. Care is taken to avoid the epigastric vessels, and blunt dissection usually easily exposes Cooper's ligament. The peritoneum is mobilized superiorly up to the transversalis fascia, laterally to the anterior superior iliac crest, medially to the pubic tubercle, and inferiorly to the vas deferens.

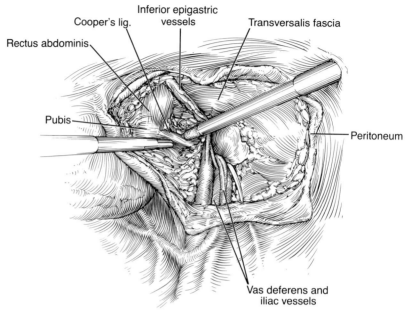

FIGURE 26-5

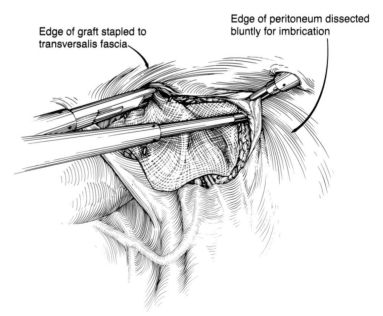

FIGURE 26-6

FIGURES 26-5 to 26-7. A 5 × 7 cm. patch of polypropylene mesh is then placed through the 12-mm. trocar and fixed with the hernia stapler. Hernia staples are used to fix the mesh to the pubic tubercle, transversalis fascia, and laterally to the anterior superior iliac crest. Care is taken not to place staples in the region of the neurovascular iliac bundle or the lateral femoral cutaneous nerve.

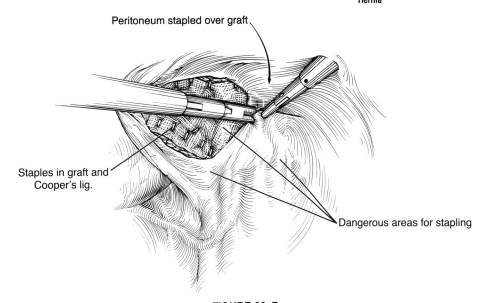

Peritoneum stapled over graft

Staples in graft and
Cooper's lig.

Dangerous areas for stapling

FIGURE 26–7

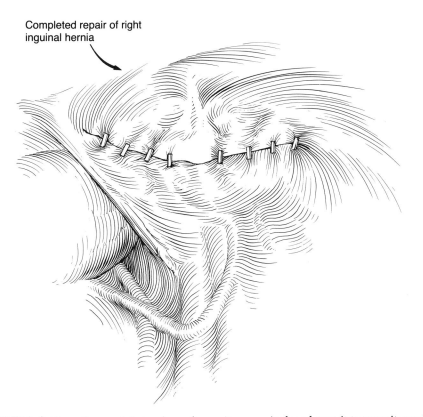

Completed repair of right
inguinal hernia

FIGURE 26–8. Once the mesh is in place, the peritoneum is closed over it to reperitonealize
the site.

27

Umbilical Hernia (CHILD)

NICHOLAS A. SHORTER, M.D.

An umbilical hernia in a child is not the same defect as in an adult. Although umbilical hernias in adults frequently incarcerate, this rarely occurs in childhood. Therefore, an expectant approach can be taken with umbilical hernias in infancy, and many will close spontaneously with time. A safe rule is that an umbilical hernia can be observed until the child reaches the age of 4 years, with the expectation that it will spontaneously close. If it remains open, the likelihood of spontaneous resolution is minimal and the defect should be repaired, preferably before the child reaches school age. Even if complete closure does not occur, the defect may decrease in size and make the surgical procedure less complex.

Umbilical hernia repairs in children should be performed under general anesthesia because complete muscular relaxation is necessary to prevent herniation of the bowel through the umbilical defect during the repair. If the anesthesia is too light and the bowel herniates, an otherwise simple procedure becomes aggravating.

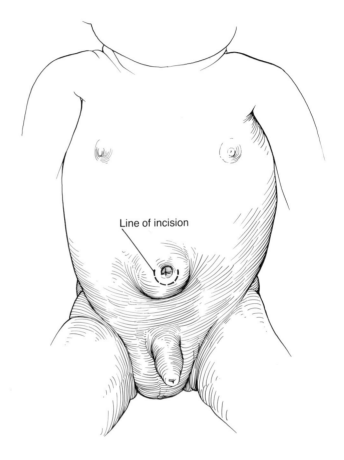

Line of incision

FIGURE 27–1. With the patient in the supine position, a small semicircular incision is made along the inferior edge of the umbilicus from 3 o'clock to 9 o'clock. The incision should not cross the umbilicus. The incision is deepened down to the fascial layer, and an adequate amount of the fascia is cleared in order to visualize good tissue.

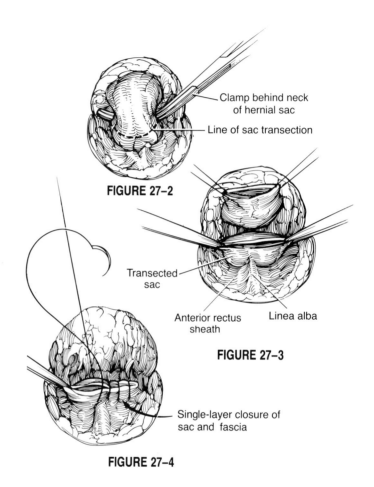

FIGURE 27-2

Clamp behind neck of hernial sac

Line of sac transection

FIGURE 27-3

Transected sac

Anterior rectus sheath

Linea alba

FIGURE 27-4

Single-layer closure of sac and fascia

FIGURE 27-2. With a Kelly clamp, both sides of the sac are dissected in order to completely encircle it. It is preferable to open the sac distally and to transect it completely after it is seen to be empty.

FIGURE 27-3. After the sac is completely transected, the small portion still attached to the umbilical skin can be left in place. The sac, which is still attached to the abdominal wall, should be excised back to solid fascial tissue. In some cases, the abdominal fascia is actually along the side of the sac. It is also important to remember that the umbilical hernia may occur in the setting of thinned-out and widened midline fascia; therefore, the tissues superior and inferior to the defect may not be particularly strong.

FIGURE 27-4. A number of quite intricate methods of closure have been described for umbilical hernia repair, but the author has found that simple interrupted closure is quite adequate. This can be done either transversely or vertically. Where the midline fascia is quite thin, a better repair is obtained with a vertical closure. In children, an absorbable suture such as Vicryl or Dexon is used and avoids the subsequent problems that may occur from the continued presence of nonabsorbable suture. However, in the occasional adolescent patient, it is wise to use nonabsorbable sutures such as Prolene because of the additional stress during healing. The back of the umbilicus is then tacked down to the fascia, and the incision is closed.

28

Umbilical Hernia (ADULT)

JOSEPH A. MOYLAN, M.D.

With large umbilical hernias, removal of the umbilicus should be discussed with the patient preoperatively. Depending on the size of the umbilical hernia, it may or may not be possible to save it.

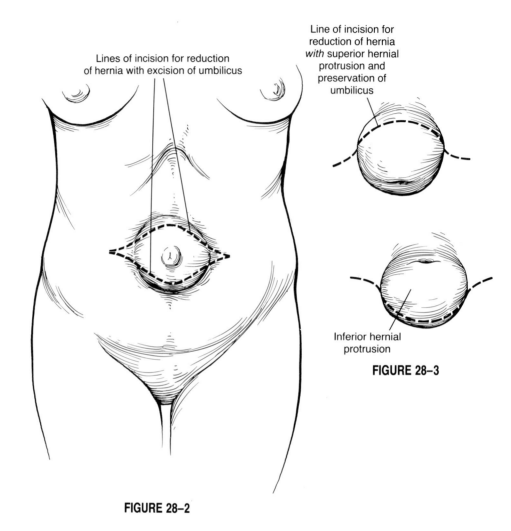

Lines of incision for reduction
of hernia with excision of umbilicus

Line of incision for
reduction of hernia
with superior hernial
protrusion and
preservation of
umbilicus

Inferior hernial
protrusion

FIGURE 28–3

FIGURE 28–2

FIGURE 28–1. To remove the umbilicus, an elliptical incision is made after the abdomen is prepared and draped in a sterile manner.

FIGURES 28–2 and 28–3. To preserve the umbilicus, the location of the semilunar incision is either above or below the umbilicus, depending on the location of the hernial protrusion.

Incision through neck
of hernial sac

Hernial ring

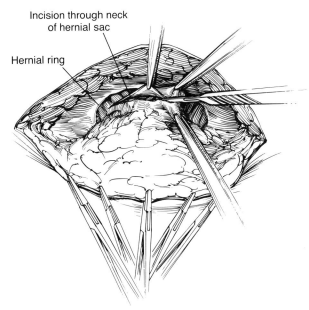

FIGURE 28–4. The dissection is then extended to the anterior abdominal fascia, raising flaps superiorly and inferiorly. The hernial sac is identified circumferentially, and the incision is carefully made through the sac itself. The intra-abdominal contents are reduced, if possible.

Ligation of omental vessels

Cut edge of hernial sac

Omental contents
of hernial sac
(divided)

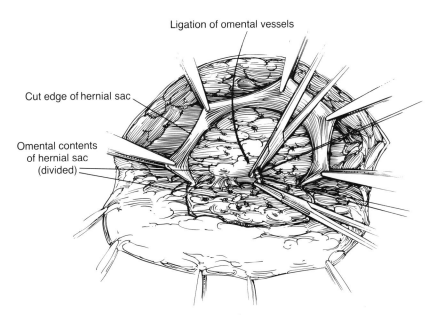

FIGURE 28–5. Occasionally, omentum may be incarcerated in the hernia, which may necessitate amputation with careful control of the omental vessels by individual ligatures.

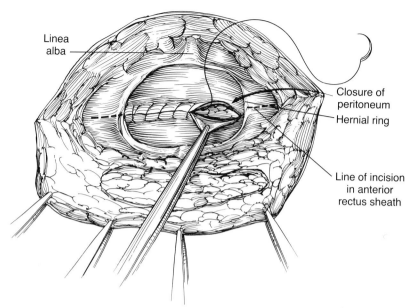

Linea
alba

Closure of
peritoneum

Hernial ring

Line of incision
in anterior
rectus sheath

FIGURE 28–6. The edges of the hernial sac are grasped, and the peritoneum is closed transversely with a continuous suture.

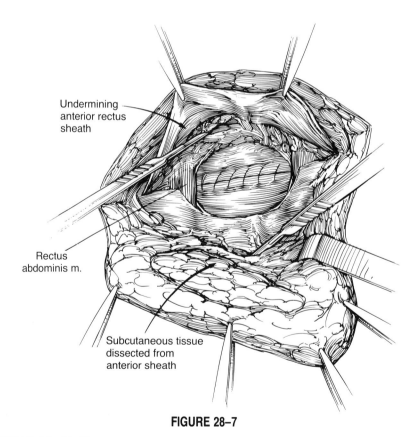

Undermining
anterior rectus
sheath

Rectus
abdominis m.

Subcutaneous tissue
dissected from
anterior sheath

FIGURE 28–7

FIGURES 28–7 to 28–10. Depending on the laxity of the anterior rectus sheath, it may be either imbricated transversely to reinforce the area or closed with figure-of-eight interrupted sutures in a single layer.

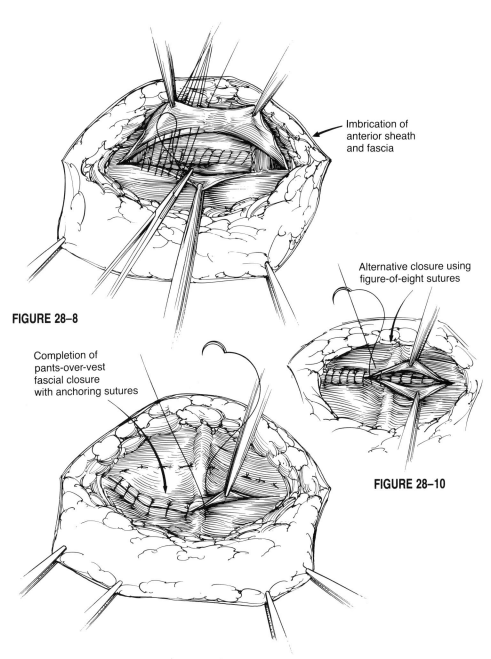

Imbrication of
anterior sheath
and fascia

FIGURE 28–8

Alternative closure using
figure-of-eight sutures

FIGURE 28–10

Completion of
pants-over-vest
fascial closure
with anchoring sutures

FIGURE 28–9

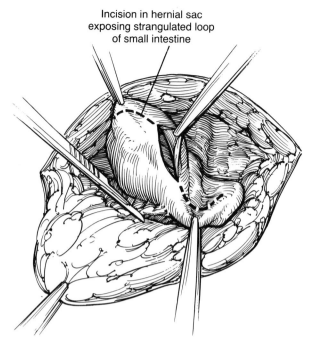

FIGURE 28–11. Occasionally, small intestine may be strangulated within the umbilical hernia. When the hernial sac is freed, the apex of the sac is incised and the strangulated bowel is identified.

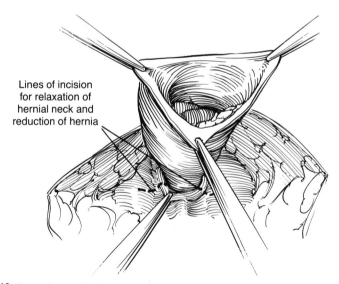

FIGURE 28–12. In order to facilitate small bowel resection through this approach, the hernial sac is enlarged transversely by dividing the fascia of the anterior abdominal wall, the posterior fascia, and the peritoneum with retraction of the rectus muscle laterally.

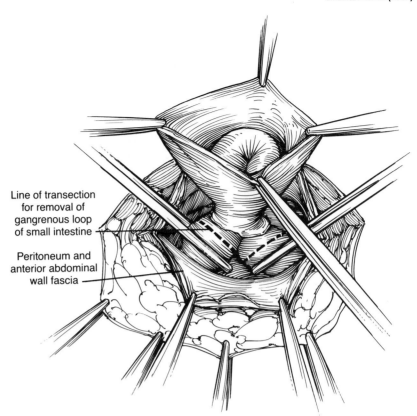

Line of transection
for removal of
gangrenous loop
of small intestine

Peritoneum and
anterior abdominal
wall fascia

FIGURE 28–13. A small bowel resection is performed in the usual manner as illustrated. The peritoneum and fascia are then closed in a two-layer transverse manner.

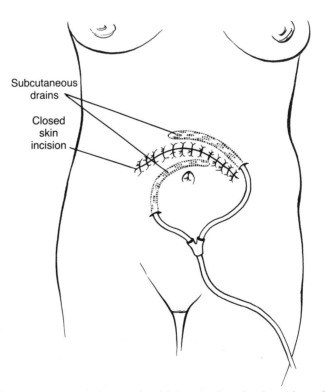

Subcutaneous
drains

Closed
skin
incision

FIGURE 28–14. Subcutaneous drains should be employed when there has been an extensive subcutaneous dissection and the risk of a seroma exists.

29

Inguinal Herniorrhaphy in Infants and Children

HOWARD C. FILSTON, M.D.

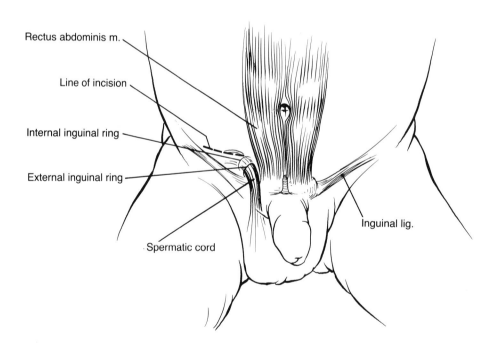

FIGURE 29–1. The placement of the incision is *crucial*. It should lie in a skin crease (transverse), and the medial end of the incision should be no more medial than the level of the pubic tubercle and should be placed approximately 1 cm. above it. In a small infant, the tubercle is best located by palpating the inguinal ligament and identifying the site at which it attaches to the bone, which is the pubic tubercle.

Placement of the incision too medially may cause entry into the rectus sheath. Inadvertent dissection of the rectus muscle, mistaking it for the cremaster, can lead to elevation of the bladder rather than of the hernial sac into the wound.

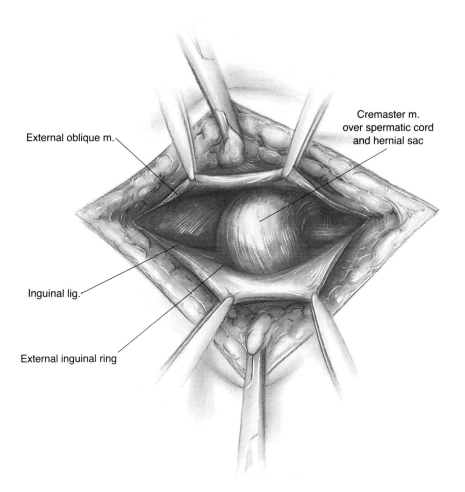

External oblique m.

Cremaster m.
over spermatic cord
and hernial sac

Inguinal lig.

External inguinal ring

FIGURE 29–2. The subcutaneous tissue is spread bluntly to Scarpa's fascia, which is incised and spread with scissors, exposing the external oblique aponeurosis. The aponeurosis is incised transversely and opened the full extent of the skin incision, carefully avoiding opening the external ring itself. Clamps are placed on each edge of the external oblique fascia for subsequent identification and for traction on the lower edge, and the dorsal surface of the external oblique aponeurosis is carefully dissected until the inguinal ligament is identified. The dissection is continued medially on the inguinal ligament until its attachment to the pubic tubercle is identified. This is the dorsal crus of the external ring. The lateral 180 degrees of the ring is then identified, along with the cremaster-covered spermatic cord and hernial sac. Positive identification of the external ring should be made by passing blunt-pointed scissors through the ring into the scrotum. The cremaster muscle is then split bluntly with a clamp at a point overlying the bony pubis to avoid injury to the direct wall, and the hernial sac is grasped gently and elevated into the wound.

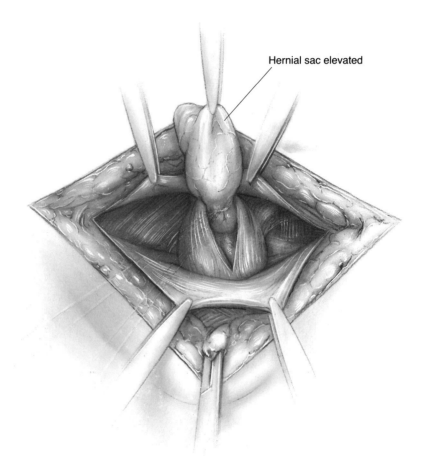

Hernial sac elevated

FIGURE 29–3. The cremasteric fibers are bluntly dissected from the hernial sac. The sac and spermatic cord are encircled at the level of the pubic tubercle; the entire cord and hernial sac are elevated into the wound. The sac is bluntly dissected from the cord, with careful identification of the vessels and the vas deferens.

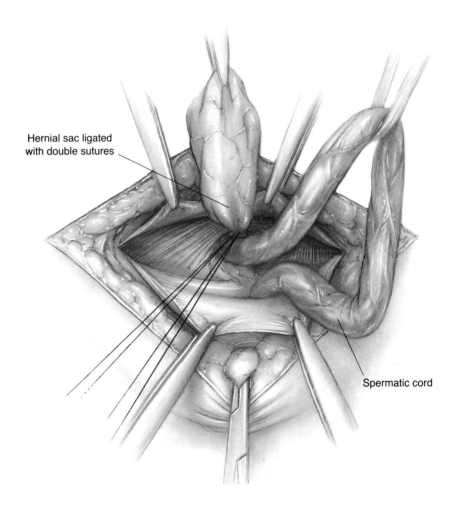

Hernial sac ligated
with double sutures

Spermatic cord

FIGURE 29–4. The sac is then divided and dissected to the internal ring. Frequently, there is a short "sleeve" of transversalis fascia and transversus abdominis aponeurosis encircling the cord and hernial sac, which should be incised to allow full dissection of the sac back to the internal ring. After palpation to be certain there is no sliding component or other contents, the sac is then twisted and doubly suture-ligated with 3–0 nonabsorbable sutures and the excess sac is excised. Unless there is a noncommunicating or poorly communicating hydrocele, no further dissection of the distal sac is needed. The testis is carefully returned to the scrotum and placed in the extended scrotum to ensure that the cord is placed well down into the scrotum and is not caught in the healing herniorrhaphy scar.

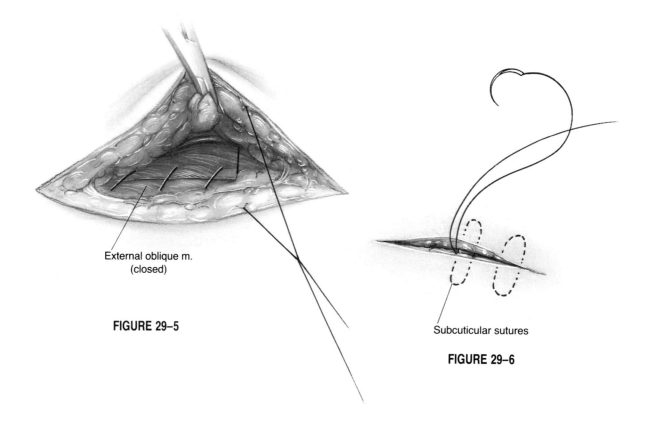

External oblique m.
(closed)

FIGURE 29–5

Subcuticular sutures

FIGURE 29–6

FIGURES 29–5 and 29–6. No attention need be given to the external ring because it was not opened, and the external oblique aponeurosis can be closed with a fine running absorbable suture. The subcutaneous tissue is reapproximated with a plain catgut suture, and the skin is closed with subcuticular sutures of absorbable material such as fine chromic catgut. Collodion is usually placed over the wound as a dressing.

30

Hydrocelectomy

NICHOLAS A. SHORTER, M.D.

Only rarely does a primary (i.e., not due to a patent processus vaginalis) scrotal hydrocele occur in the pediatric age group. Hydroceles occasionally occur following an inguinal hernia repair but usually resolve spontaneously within about 6 months. In the rare patient in whom hydrocele does not resolve spontaneously or respond to needle aspiration, and in the even rarer situation in which the surgeon is convinced, after thorough exploration, that no patent processus vaginalis is present, a primary hydrocelectomy should be performed.

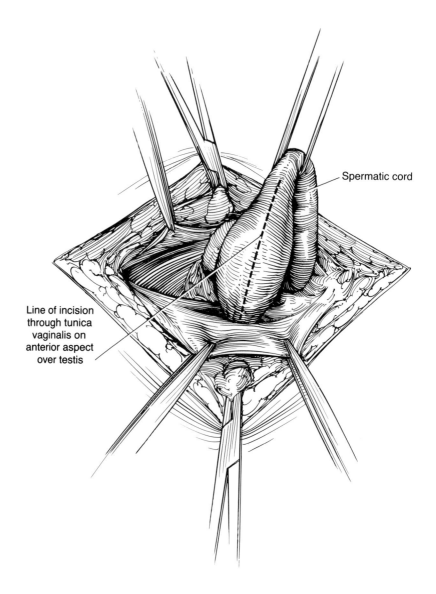

Spermatic cord

Line of incision
through tunica
vaginalis on
anterior aspect
over testis

FIGURE 30–1. Hydrocelectomy can be accomplished through an inguinal or a scrotal incision. The tunica vaginalis is mobilized from the scrotum and is opened anteriorly, exposing the testis. Care should be taken to preserve the most distal scrotal attachments to ensure that the testis remains fixed to the scrotum securely.

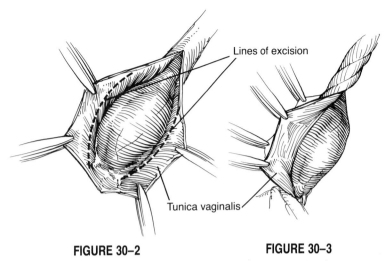

Lines of excision

Tunica vaginalis

FIGURE 30–2   **FIGURE 30–3**

FIGURES 30–2 and 30–3. After mobilization of the tunica vaginalis, the excess is excised, the remainder is folded back behind the testicle and spermatic cord, and the two sides are sutured together in the posterior midline using an absorbable suture.

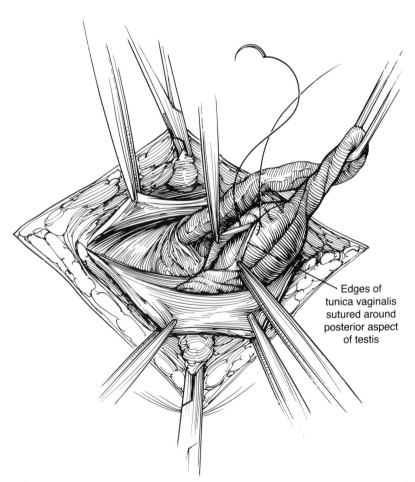

Edges of tunica vaginalis sutured around posterior aspect of testis

FIGURE 30–4. The testis is returned to the scrotum, and the incision is closed in a standard manner.

31

Hydrocelectomy: Bottle Procedure

LOWELL R. KING, M.D.

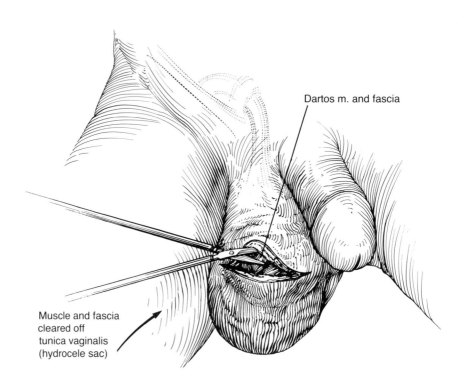

Dartos m. and fascia

Muscle and fascia
cleared off
tunica vaginalis
(hydrocele sac)

FIGURE 31–1. Whenever possible, the scrotum is opened transversely. Because the rugae and blood vessels in the scrotal skin course horizontally, less bleeding is encountered. The scar is usually invisible when healing is complete.

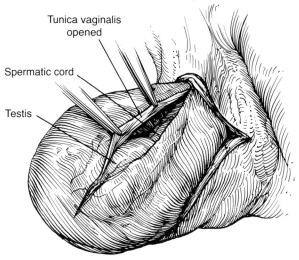

Tunica vaginalis
opened

Spermatic cord

Testis

FIGURE 31–2. The wall of the hydrocele, the tunica vaginalis, is opened longitudinally and ventrally, away from the cord structures. This exposes the testis, the epididymis, and the lower spermatic cord.

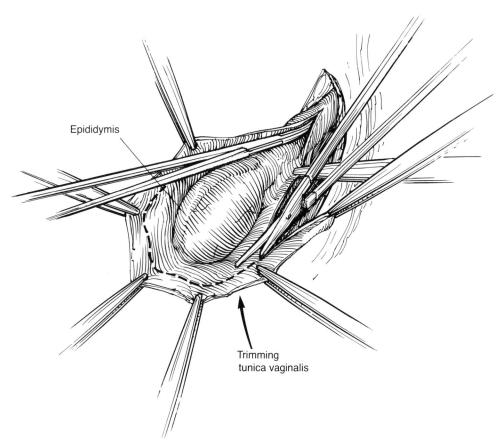

Epididymis

Trimming
tunica vaginalis

FIGURE 31–3. Excess tunica vaginalis is resected, leaving a cuff 1.5 to 2 cm. wide attached to the testis. A blunt clamp is passed along the cord within the tunica vaginalis. If it enters the peritoneal cavity, the hydrocele is termed *communicating*. In other words, an indirect inguinal hernia is present and can be repaired through a second inguinal incision.

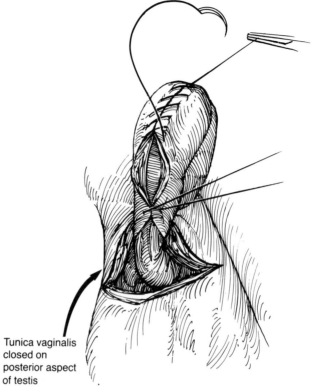

Tunica vaginalis
closed on
posterior aspect
of testis

FIGURE 31–4. The tunica vaginalis is inverted so that the serosal surface now faces the dartos muscle. The edges are approximated with a running suture. Care is taken not to close the proximal end tightly around the cord.

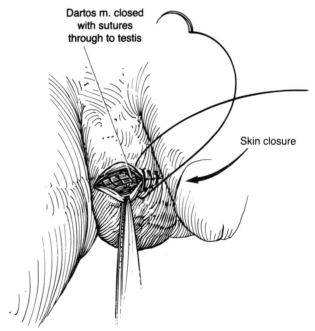

Dartos m. closed
with sutures
through to testis

Skin closure

FIGURE 31–5. The testis is sewn to the dartos muscle with absorbable sutures at two or three points to prevent torsion or retraction. The dartos muscle and skin are closed in separate layers. Meticulous hemostasis is essential to prevent a hematoma. A pressure dressing is also recommended for at least an hour or two postoperatively.

32

Preperitoneal Herniorrhaphy

JOSEPH A. MOYLAN, M.D.

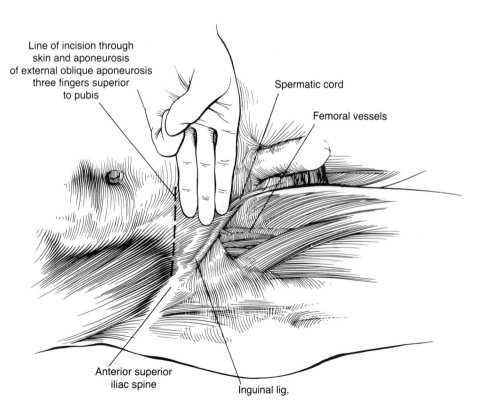

Line of incision through
skin and aponeurosis
of external oblique aponeurosis
three fingers superior
to pubis

Spermatic cord

Femoral vessels

Anterior superior
iliac spine

Inguinal lig.

FIGURE 32–1. The topical anatomy of the inguinal area is shown. An incision through the skin and the external aponeurosis fascia is made approximately three finger-breadths above the pubic symphysis.

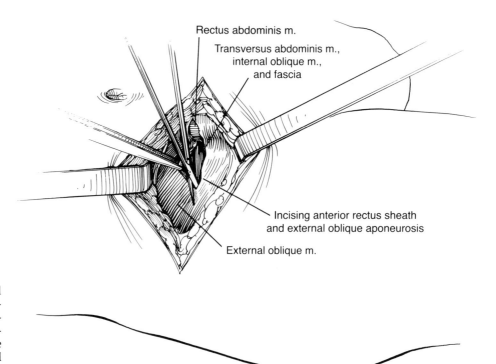

Rectus abdominis m.

Transversus abdominis m.,
internal oblique m.,
and fascia

Incising anterior rectus sheath
and external oblique aponeurosis

External oblique m.

FIGURE 32–2. The external oblique aponeurosis and anterior rectus sheath are incised, exposing the transversus abdominis muscle, the external oblique muscle, and the rectus muscle.

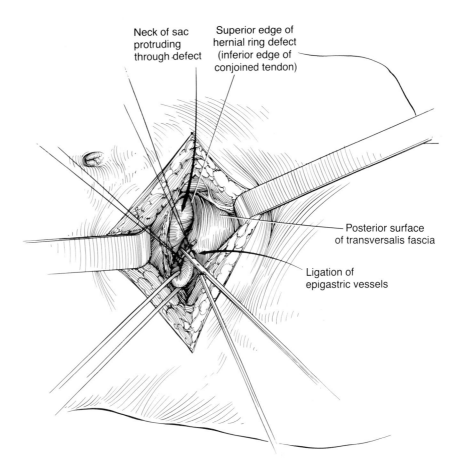

Neck of sac
protruding
through defect

Superior edge of
hernial ring defect
(inferior edge of
conjoined tendon)

Posterior surface
of transversalis fascia

Ligation of
epigastric vessels

FIGURE 32–3. The rectus muscle is retracted medially, and the transversus abdominis muscle, the internal oblique muscle, and the transversalis fascia are incised laterally, exposing the preperitoneal space. The gastric vessels are identified and can be divided for additional exposure. The cord is encircled at the internal ring, exposing both the direct and the indirect area. A direct hernia is present medial to the inferior epigastric vessels.

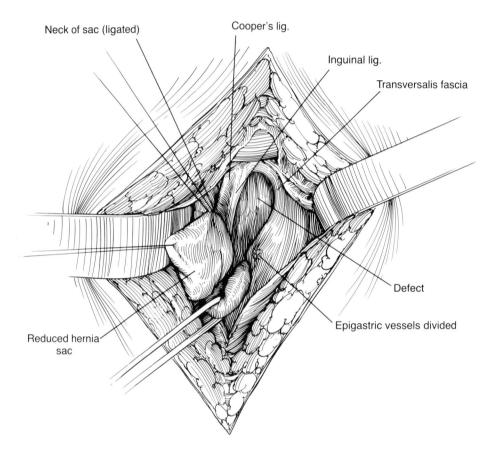

Neck of sac (ligated)

Cooper's lig.

Inguinal lig.

Transversalis fascia

Defect

Epigastric vessels divided

Reduced hernia
sac

FIGURE 32–4. The hernial sac is then dissected free and retracted into the preperitoneal space so that the hernial sac can be opened and the neck of the sac ligated with a tie. The direct defect is shown bound superiorly by the transversalis fascia and inferiorly by the shelving portion of the ilioinguinal ligament.

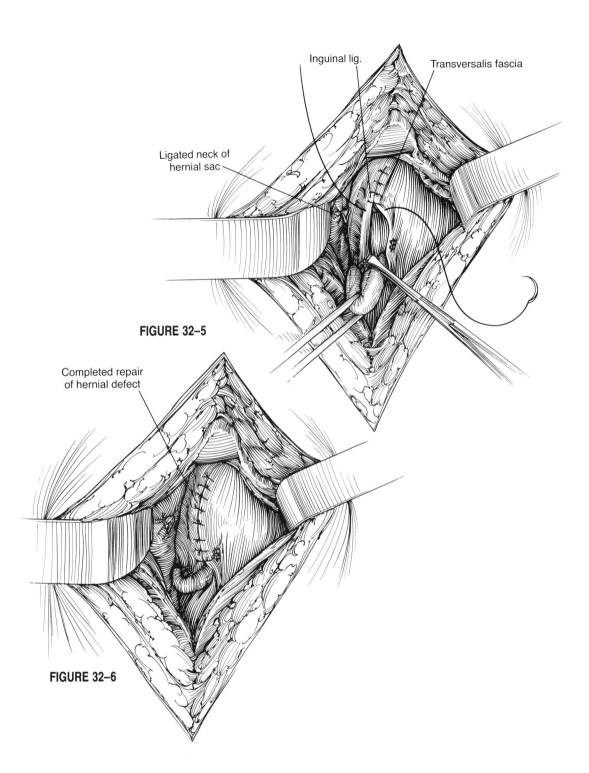

Inguinal lig.

Transversalis fascia

Ligated neck of
hernial sac

FIGURE 32–5

Completed repair
of hernial defect

FIGURE 32–6

FIGURE 32–5. The transversalis fascia is approximated with interrupted sutures to the iliopubic tract (shelving portion of the inguinal ligament), beginning medially and extending laterally, obliterating the direct area.

FIGURE 32–6. The herniorrhaphy is completed by approximating the fascia and muscular fibers of the internal transversus abdominis muscle and the external oblique fascia. The skin is closed in the usual manner with interrupted sutures.

33

Repair of Incisional Hernia

JOHN P. GRANT, M.D.

SMALL INCISIONAL HERNIAS

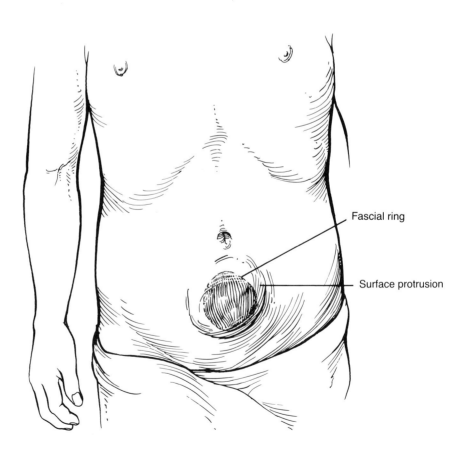

Fascial ring

Surface protrusion

FIGURE 33–1. The previous scar is excised, and the incision is extended to the hernial sac, care being taken not to damage any contents of the sac.

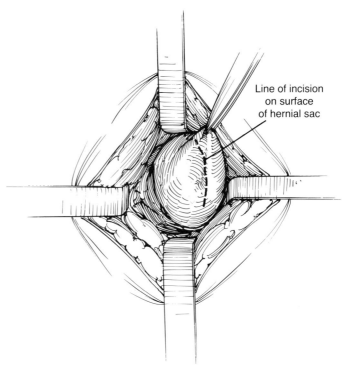

FIGURE 33–2. The hernial sac is freed from surrounding tissues by blunt and sharp dissection.

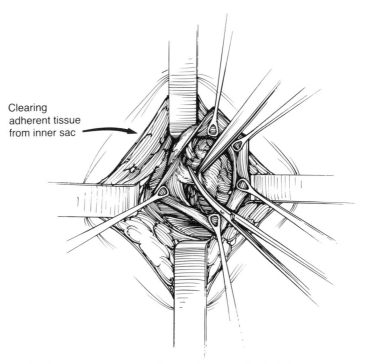

FIGURE 33–3. The sac is opened, and adhesions are divided from the inner wall.

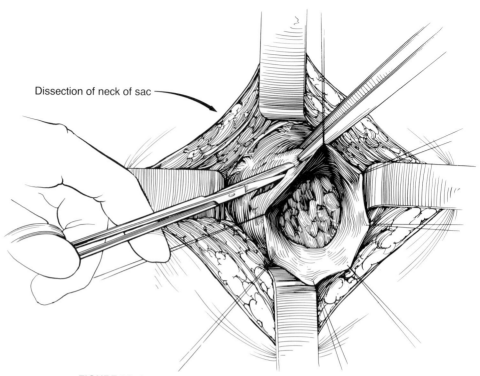

FIGURE 33–4. The sac is removed by incising around its neck.

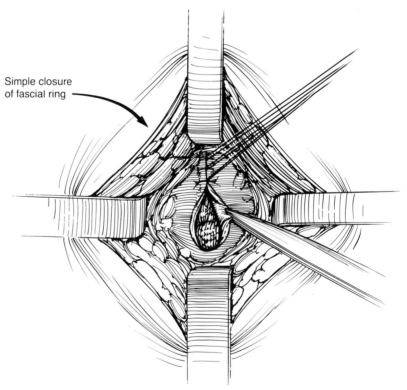

FIGURE 33–5. After hemostasis is ensured, the fascial ring is closed with interrupted heavy permanent sutures (1–0 nylon). The subcutaneous tissues are allowed to fall together, and the skin is approximated with fine sutures or skin clips. Any excess skin is trimmed away.

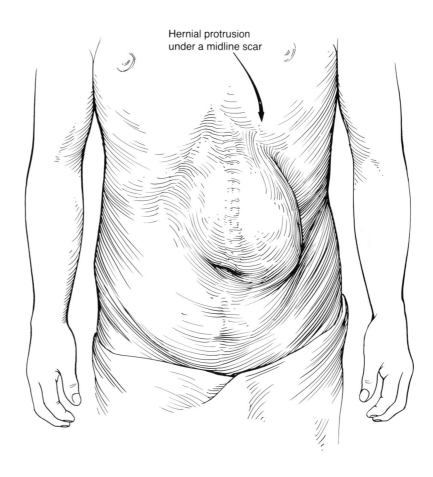

Hernial protrusion
under a midline scar

FIGURE 33–6. The skin is opened, excising the previous scar as in repair of a small incisional hernia.

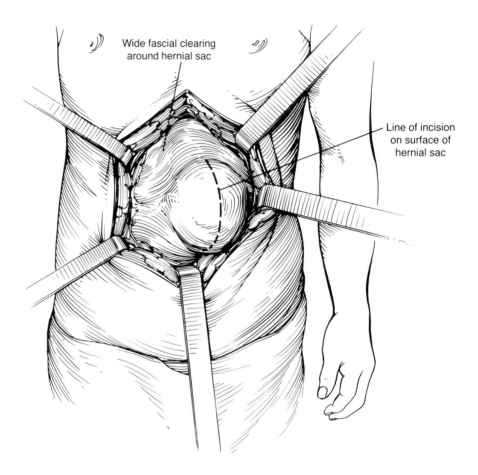

Wide fascial clearing
around hernial sac

Line of incision
on surface of
hernial sac

FIGURE 33–7. The hernial sac is opened vertically.

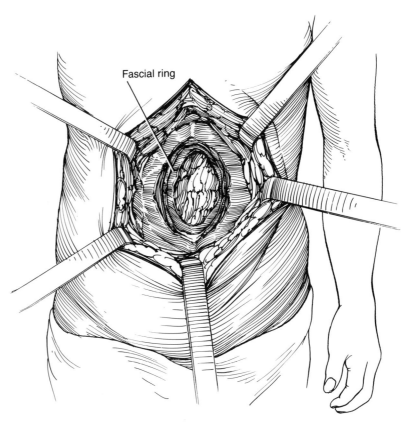

Fascial ring

FIGURE 33–8. Adhesions are divided from the outer and inner walls, extending the dissection for several centimeters beyond the fascial ring. The omentum is carefully placed over the bowel to protect it from injury. The fascial defect is then approximated by simple closure as in the small incisional hernia or, preferably, especially with a recurrent hernia, in a pants-over-vest manner.

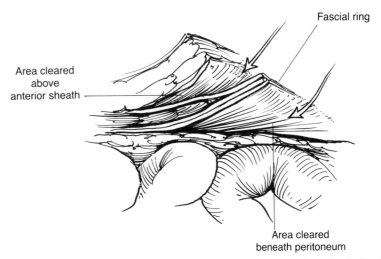

Fascial ring

Area cleared
above
anterior sheath

Area cleared
beneath peritoneum

FIGURE 33–9. In the pants-over-vest repair, the fascial ring is cleared of all adhesions, both inside and outside, for 5 to 6 cm. from its edge.

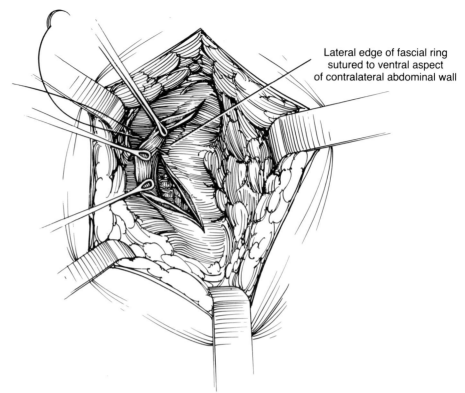

FIGURE 33–10. One side of the fascial ring is sutured to the underside of the opposite side using a mattress-type suture of heavy permanent material (e.g., 1–0 nylon).

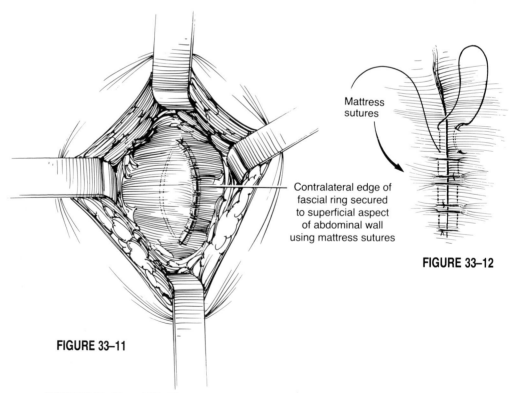

FIGURES 33–11 and 33–12. The remaining free edge is sutured to the underlying fascia with another series of mattress sutures. This method prevents a raised edge, which might be misinterpreted later as a recurrent hernia.

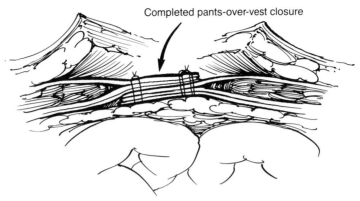

Completed pants-over-vest closure

FIGURE 33–13. The completed suture line produces a double thickness of fascia with two suture lines to distribute tension.

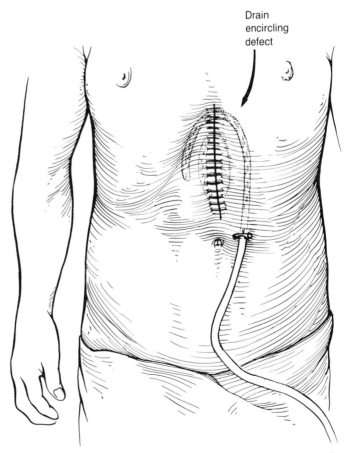

Drain
encircling
defect

FIGURE 33–14. Owing to the wide dissection, it is preferable to place a large Hemovac drain to prevent fluid collection. The drain is left in place until drainage is less than 30 ml. per day for two days. Excess skin is trimmed, and the skin edges approximated with fine sutures or with skin clips.

LARGE INCISIONAL HERNIA WITH DEFECT THAT CANNOT BE APPROXIMATED

If after dissection and removal of the hernial sac the fascial ring is of such size that it cannot be approximated without excessive tension, graft material can be used to accomplish closure.

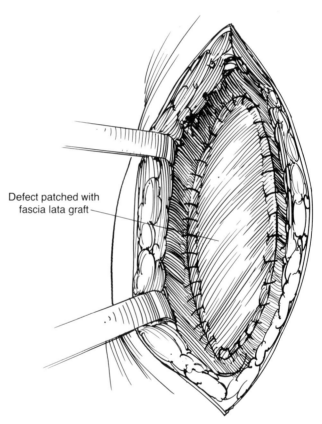

Defect patched with fascia lata graft

FIGURE 33–15. Fascia lata obtained from the leg can be sutured to the edges of the hernia defect.

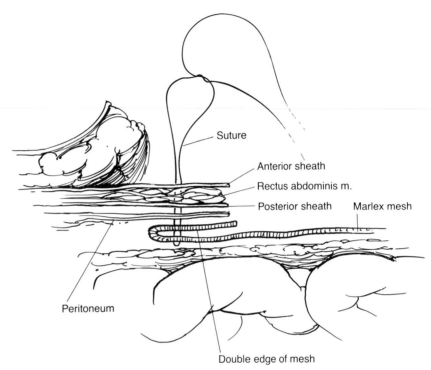

Suture

Anterior sheath

Rectus abdominis m.

Posterior sheath   Marlex mesh

Peritoneum

Double edge of mesh

FIGURE 33–16

FIGURES 33–16 to 33–18. Other materials that have been found useful include Marlex mesh and Gore-Tex. Marlex mesh is best sutured to the edges of the fascial ring by doubling back the edge and placing a ring of mattress sutures. The doubling prevents any sharp edges of the mesh from damaging the bowel and may reduce adhesion formation. Gore-Tex can be sewn directly to the edges of the fascial ring or doubled back as with Marlex mesh.

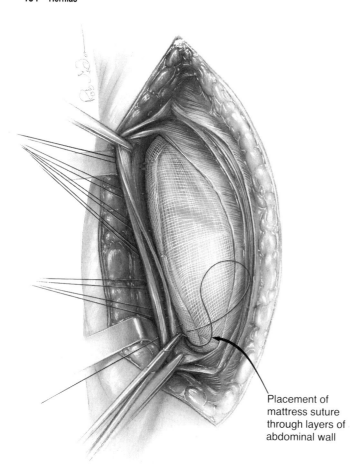

Placement of
mattress suture
through layers of
abdominal wall

FIGURE 33–17

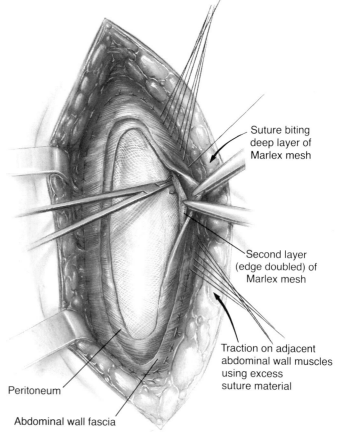

Suture biting
deep layer of
Marlex mesh

Second layer
(edge doubled) of
Marlex mesh

Traction on adjacent
abdominal wall muscles
using excess
suture material

Peritoneum

Abdominal wall fascia

FIGURE 33–18

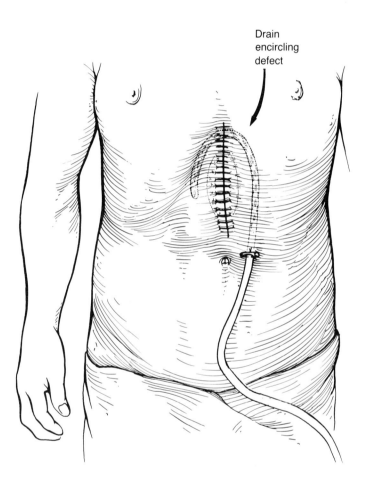

Drain
encircling
defect

FIGURE 33–19. A large Hemovac drain is placed in the subcutaneous space. The skin edges are approximated with fine sutures or with skin clips. The drain is left in place until drainage is less than 30 ml. per day for two days.

34

Repair of Petit's Hernia

JOHN P. GRANT, M.D.

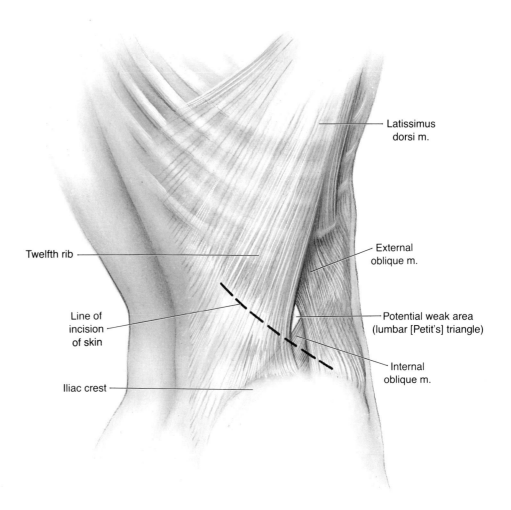

Latissimus
dorsi m.

External
oblique m.

Potential weak area
(lumbar [Petit's] triangle)

Internal
oblique m.

Twelfth rib

Line of
incision
of skin

Iliac crest

FIGURE 34–1. The inferior lumbar triangle is bounded by the external oblique muscle anteriorly, the anterior border of the latissimus dorsi muscle posteriorly, and the crest of the ilium inferiorly. The floor is the deep lumbar fascia that covers the internal oblique muscle.

For repair of a lumbar hernia, the patient should be placed in an oblique or true lateral position. The true lateral position is for small hernias. In the true lateral position, the lower leg should be bent 45 degrees at the knee, and the upper leg should be straight and overlie the lower leg. Extension of the kidney elevator helps increase the distance between the twelfth rib and the iliac crest. The entire flank should be cleansed, as well as the upper leg, if a fascia lata graft is needed.

An oblique incision is preferable following the neurovascular and dermatome distributions, beginning just below the twelfth rib and extending over the hernia to the anterior iliac crest. Alternatively, a vertical incision may be used, passing over the hernia from the twelfth rib down to the iliac crest. The oblique incision provides the best exposure, especially for larger hernias.

A hernial sac is usually not present but, if found, should be opened with examination and reduction of any contents and closure of the neck. Common contents of a sac include large and small intestine, omentum, preperitoneal fat, mesentery, appendix, cecum, stomach, ovary, spleen, and, rarely, the kidney. If a sliding component is present, it should be carefully inverted and plicated, avoiding injury to the viscera and its blood supply.

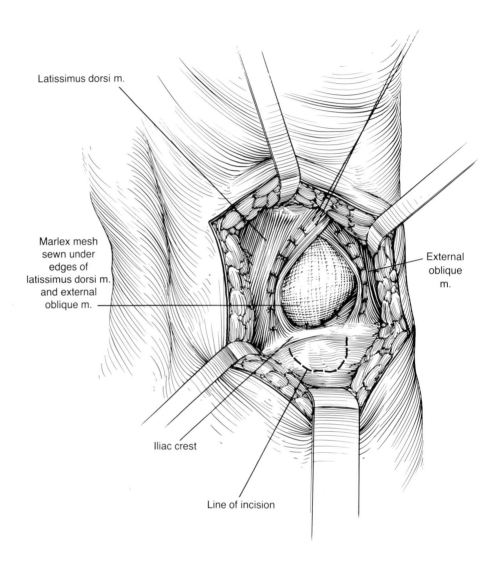

Latissimus dorsi m.

Marlex mesh
sewn under
edges of
latissimus dorsi m.
and external
oblique m.

External
oblique
m.

Iliac crest

Line of incision

FIGURE 34–2. The tranversalis fascia is imbricated to reduce the hernia. A piece of synthetic mesh is placed over the transversalis fascia, suturing its edges to the underside of the surrounding latissimus dorsi muscle, external and internal oblique muscles, and periosteum of the iliac crest.

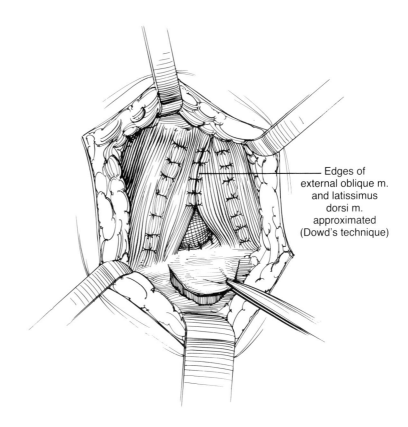

Edges of
external oblique m.
and latissimus
dorsi m.
approximated
(Dowd's technique)

FIGURE 34–3. A second layer is constructed by sewing the edges of the latissimus dorsi and external oblique muscles together until tension prevents further approximation.

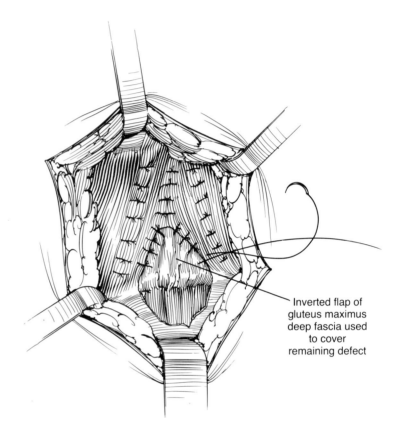

Inverted flap of
gluteus maximus
deep fascia used
to cover
remaining defect

FIGURE 34–4. At this point, a flap of fascia from the gluteus maximus and medius muscles is raised and flipped upward to close the remaining defect. The repair can be reinforced with a free fascia lata graft or by swinging the fascia of the latissimus dorsi muscle anteriorly.

If the inferior lumbar hernia is of moderate size, it can usually be closed without the use of synthetic mesh. The transversalis fascia is imbricated, and the next layer begins with approximation of the external oblique muscle to the edge of the latissimus dorsi muscle, beginning at the superior end of the hernia defect and continuing inferiorly to the iliac crest. If the defect is not completely closed owing to excessive tension, a flap of fascia from the gluteus maximus and medius muscles is raised and reflected superiorly to close the remaining defect. The repair can again be reinforced with a free fascia lata graft or by swinging the fascia of the latissimus dorsi muscle anteriorly.

Small inferior lumbar hernias can usually be repaired with a two-layer closure using nonabsorbable sutures. The transversalis fascia is imbricated for the first layer. The second layer is constructed by suturing the edge of the external oblique muscle to the edge of the latissimus dorsi muscle, continuing down to the iliac crest (see Fig. 34–3). The repair can be reinforced with a piece of fascia lata or by swinging a flap of the latissimus dorsi muscle fascia anteriorly.

35

Repair of Spigelian Hernia

JOSEPH A. MOYLAN, M.D.

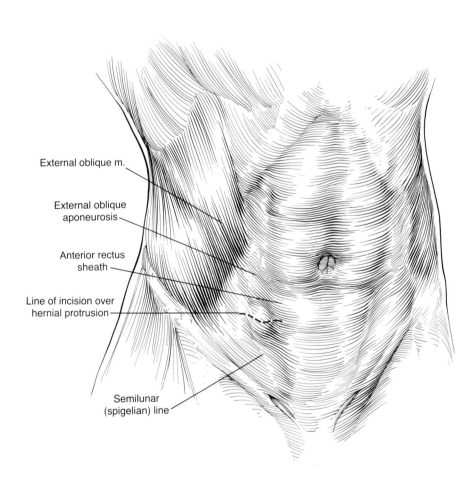

External oblique m.

External oblique
aponeurosis

Anterior rectus
sheath

Line of incision over
hernial protrusion

Semilunar
(spigelian) line

FIGURE 35–1. The topical anatomy of the abdominal wall is illustrated. In the spigelian line, the abdominal wall consists of only two layers of fascia. These are the transversalis fascia and the joined fascial layers of the internal and external oblique muscles. The strength of the latter layer is compromised where the anterior intercostal nerves perforate it as they course between the internal and external oblique muscles toward the rectus abdominis muscle. These weak areas are susceptible to herniation.

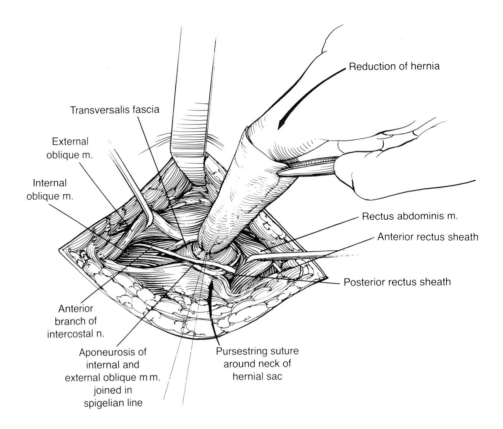

Transversalis fascia

External
oblique m.

Internal
oblique m.

Anterior
branch of
intercostal n.

Aponeurosis of
internal and
external oblique m m.
joined in
spigelian line

Pursestring suture
around neck of
hernial sac

Reduction of hernia

Rectus abdominis m.

Anterior rectus sheath

Posterior rectus sheath

FIGURE 35–2. Through a transverse incision over the hernia, dissection is extended to the external oblique fascia. With a transverse incision through the fascia, beginning at the lateral border of the rectus and extending over the external oblique fascia, the rectus muscle is exposed and retracted medially. The sac is identified perforating the internal oblique muscle, which is then separated. The hernial sac is dissected down to the transversalis fascia. The sac is opened, and the contents are reduced.

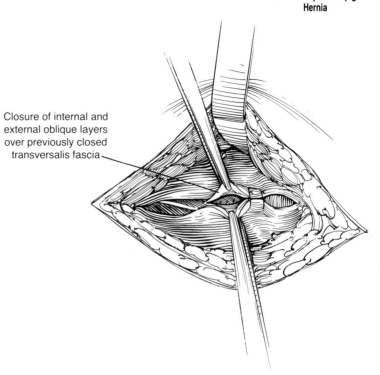

Closure of internal and
external oblique layers
over previously closed
transversalis fascia

FIGURE 35–3. The base of the neck of the sac is ligated, and the internal oblique and transverse abdominal muscles are closed with interrupted sutures in a linear manner.

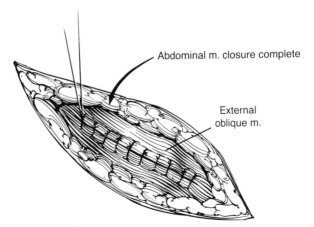

Abdominal m. closure complete

External
oblique m.

FIGURE 35–4. The external oblique muscle, subcutaneous tissue, and skin are closed in the usual manner.

The Breast

36

Excision of Benign Tumor

J. DIRK IGLEHART, M.D.

The most common benign tumor in the female breast is a *simple cyst*. Simple cysts rarely necessitate biopsy. The diagnosis is suggested if a smooth, round density is felt in the breast of a young menstruating female or a woman on estrogen replacement therapy after menopause. Cysts, which are fluid-filled cavities lined by epithelium, are easily diagnosed by either aspiration or ultrasonography. Aspiration is performed using a 22-gauge needle fixed to an appropriate syringe. A biopsy is performed if the cysts recur multiple times following aspiration, if a residual mass is palpated in the breast after aspiration, or if an atraumatic aspiration reveals bloody fluid. Under these circumstances, the biopsy should be conducted with the assumption that the lesion is malignant, necessitating a procedure different from that described for excision of benign tumors.

The second most common tumor in the female breast is a *fibroadenoma*. Physical examination reveals a firm, smooth, and mobile mass. The patient is usually in her teens or twenties and is menstruating normally. These lesions are hormonally sensitive and can grow to large size in the breast of a young woman (giant fibroadenoma). They are entirely benign but should be examined pathologically to exclude the rare and related tumor *cystosarcoma phylloides*, which can be malignant. Fibroadenomas are distinguished from cysts by ultrasound examination that shows a solid lesion or by needle aspiration that fails to produce fluid. A solid, mobile mass with a smooth contour in the breast of a young woman is usually a fibroadenoma. A procedure to excise fibroadenomas is illustrated in Figure 36–2. If there is doubt about the nature of a breast mass, it should be assumed to be malignant, and a biopsy should be performed.

A consideration when planning the surgical incision is the final cosmetic result. In the biopsy of indeterminate masses, when malignancy is possible, the principal consideration is complete excision. The surgical incision must be placed in a location that will not compromise a future mastectomy if required.

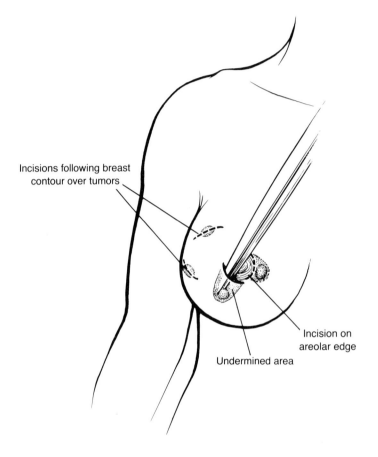

Incisions following breast
contour over tumors

Incision on
areolar edge

Undermined area

FIGURE 36–1. The incisions that can be used to excise benign breast masses are shown. The lines of skin tension described by Langer are concentric and follow the contour of the areola. However, tension on the skin of the breast is influenced by gravity and varies with the position of the patient. Tension on the skin of the breast, although curved around the breast, becomes more horizontal as one moves farther from the nipple and areola to more peripheral locations. For centrally located tumors, incisions placed in the junction of the darker skin of the areola and the lighter skin of the breast will be hidden after healing. Tumors that are close to the areola can be excised through a circumferential periareolar incision by undermining breast tissue for a short distance. Tumors that are located in the periphery of the breast are best excised through more horizontally placed incisions over the lesions. Tumors below the areola and in the lower quadrants of the breast can be approached with incisions placed in the inframammary crease, which are hidden from view.

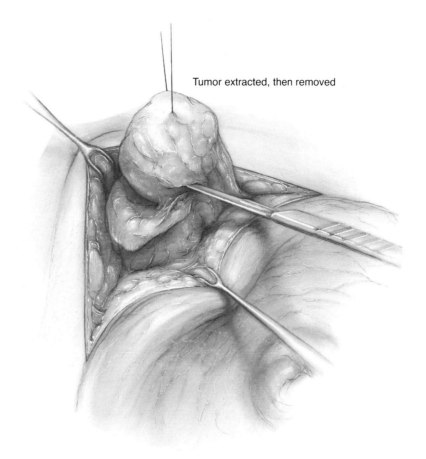

Tumor extracted, then removed

FIGURE 36–2. The skin incision is deepened by sharp dissection into the subcutaneous tissue and through the breast parenchyma. The choice of instruments is dictated by the level of anesthesia and the density of the breast tissue. Very dense tissue in young patients is difficult to separate with scissors, and use of cutting cautery or a scalpel is preferred. Under local anesthesia, pain may be more intense using cautery, and a scalpel may be a better choice. With the appropriate instrument, the breast tissue is incised directly down to the tumor without undermining other tissues. Fibroadenomas are usually quite firm and well circumscribed, and in fatty tissues, the tumor separates easily from the surrounding parenchyma. When present in denser breast tissue, the tumor is more difficult to separate from the surrounding breast and its borders are less defined.

When the outer shell of the tumor is reached, the overlying tissue can be separated bluntly by spreading the blades of the scissors. The tumor is transfixed with a suture (1–0 silk) on a sharp needle. This suture is then used to elevate the tumor out of the wound. The surrounding breast tissue is delivered with the tumor. With the scalpel or sharp scissors, the tumor can be precisely separated from the investing normal breast tissue. By using this technique, the least amount of normal breast tissue is removed or traumatized. This is important in young patients with a tumor close to the nipple and areola. Minimizing dissection of normal tissue lessens the chance of hematoma and may decrease the potential for distortion of the breast by scarring.

It is important to obtain complete hemostasis within the biopsy cavity. During dissection of the tumor, bleeding points should be electrocoagulated; it is important to avoid damaging the skin edges during this step. Following removal of the lesion, the cavity should be meticulously inspected and bleeding points again coagulated. Larger arteries may be controlled best by fine absorbable transfixing sutures. The cavity is thoroughly irrigated with saline and again inspected prior to closure. No attempt is made to approximate the underlying breast tissue. A hematoma is an avoidable complication, prevented by meticulous hemostasis. Moreover, it is cosmetically unacceptable and may lead to disfiguring scarring.

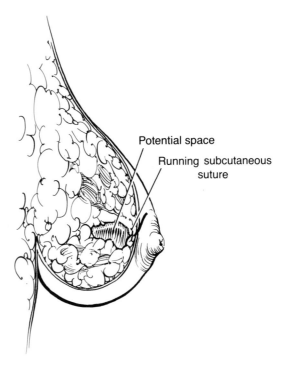

Potential space
Running subcutaneous
        suture

FIGURE 36–3. The subcutaneous tissue just under the dermis is approximated with a 4–0 absorbable suture, bringing the skin edges together. The dermis is closed using a running suture, which can be a 4–0 monofilament, leaving the ends external to be removed 5 to 7 days later. Alternatively, a 4–0 absorbable suture can be buried under the epidermis. Adhesive tapes (Steri-Strips) can be applied to further support the closure of the skin incision.

37

Wide Local Excision Breast Biopsy—
Segmentectomy, Tylectomy, or Lumpectomy

J. DIRK IGLEHART, M.D.

Conservative excision of breast cancer is a procedure in which the primary tumor is removed, leaving the majority of the breast and usually leaving the nipple and areola undisturbed. The procedure is also termed *segmentectomy, tylectomy,* or *lumpectomy* and is a *wide* local excision. Implied in any of these definitions is *total excision* of the primary tumor, achieving at least grossly negative margins as confirmed pathologically. The intention to excise a tumor totally and to document surgical margins distinguishes wide local excision from the less precise *excisional biopsy*. These procedures are usually combined with an axillary dissection either simultaneously or later, particularly if the operation is performed for invasive breast cancer.

The indications for conservative excision of breast cancer are generally the same as those for standard mastectomy. The patient and the surgeon may include consideration of tumor size, breast size, tumor location, histologic features, and other factors in making a decision to conserve the breast. Grossly or histologically positive margins are usually an indication for mastectomy.

A wide local excision is usually performed after a cytologic or core biopsy diagnosis of breast cancer. However, lesions that are clinically or mammographically suspicious should be approached with careful planning. A wide local excision may be performed under local anesthesia, but the addition of sedation increases the surgeon's ability to provide a complete excision. General anesthesia should be considered for larger masses or tumors that are deep within the breast.

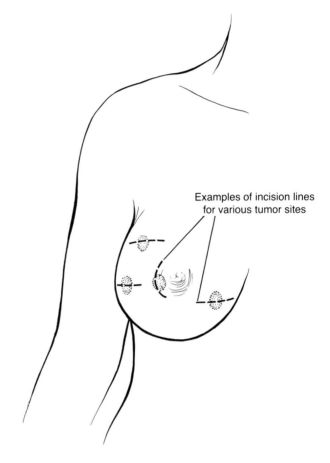

Examples of incision lines
for various tumor sites

FIGURE 37–1. Incisions should be *transverse* and placed *directly over* the underlying mass. Transverse incisions do not compromise subsequent mastectomy incisions, and placing the skin incision directly over the tumor permits precise planning of postexcision portals for radiotherapy.

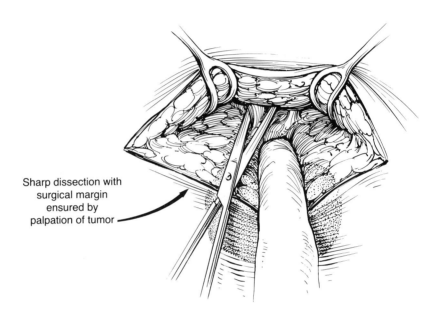

Sharp dissection with
surgical margin
ensured by
palpation of tumor

FIGURE 37–2. Elevation of skin flaps around the circumference of the wound for a short distance (1 to 2 cm.) assists the surgeon in avoiding incising the tumor itself and in achieving a complete gross excision. With the palpable mass behind the index finger, the surgeon avoids dissection near the tumor. After elevating the skin flaps and incising widely around the tumor, the surgeon can transfix the mass with a suture for upward retraction away from the field. It is wise to avoid crushing the tumor by application of instruments such as Allis clamps.

Dissection of tumor and
surrounding tissue
nearly complete

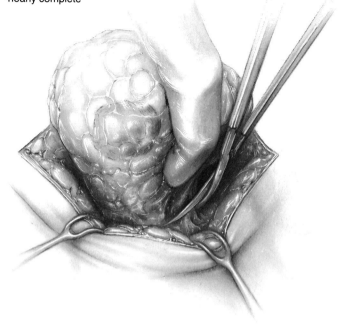

FIGURE 37–3

Portion frozen for
hormone receptor studies

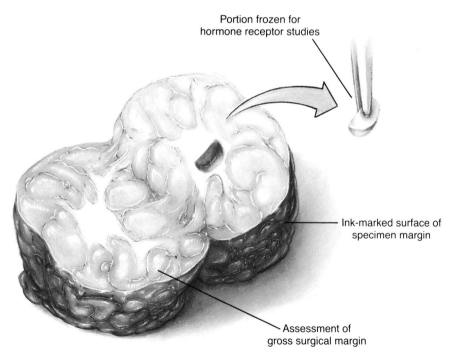

Ink-marked surface of
specimen margin

Assessment of
gross surgical margin

FIGURE 37–4

FIGURES 37–3 and 37–4. It is the surgeon's responsibility to inspect and document the gross surgical margins. This inspection should be performed prior to bisecting the specimen. Preferably, the specimen should be marked with ink (alcian blue) to identify the margins histologically before cutting into it. It is not necessary to obtain frozen sections of the margins unless there is a question concerning a particular surface or its corresponding position at the site of the biopsy. After the specimen is marked, it can be incised, the tumor measured, and samples taken for hormone receptor assay. It is necessary to retrieve at least 200 mg. for biochemical determination of estrogen and progesterone receptor contents. Because breast conservation depends on disease-free surgical margins, the surgeon must document the completeness of the excision and request the pathologist to be certain that information is not lost. Furthermore, because adjunctive treatment of breast cancer may depend on tumor size and hormone receptor content, the surgeon must be certain that the specimens are managed to ensure that these measurements are made.

Complete hemostasis is essential in the biopsy cavity and is best achieved by retraction of the skin edges sequentially in all directions while using forceps and electrocautery to secure all bleeding points. This sequence of steps should be repeated several times along all surfaces of the cavity. A hematoma can cause delay in treatment and occasionally lead to disqualification for breast conservation. No attempt should be made to oppose the walls of the cavity, nor should drains be used because they do not prevent a hematoma and are unnecessary if there is no bleeding. The cavity fills with serous fluid, which serves to restore lost volume to the breast with gradual retraction of the cavity, resulting in minimal deformity. The subcutaneous tissue is approximated with interrupted absorbable sutures, and the skin is closed with an absorbable subcuticular or subcuticular pull-out suture.

38

Breast Biopsy After Needle Localization

J. DIRK IGLEHART, M.D.

Following a decision to perform a biopsy, a thin needle is inserted into the breast under mammographic control. A fine wire with a hooked end is inserted through the needle and secured within or next to the abnormality. This procedure is generally performed by an experienced radiologist in a mammography unit. After wire localization, the patient is ready for biopsy. Success in localizing the lesion surgically depends on accurate placement of the guide wire, which should be assessed by the surgeon prior to biopsy.

The biopsy should be performed in an operating room but is commonly done as an outpatient procedure. For superficial abnormalities, local anesthesia is adequate, particularly when supplemented by light sedation. For deeper lesions in large-breasted patients, general anesthesia may be required.

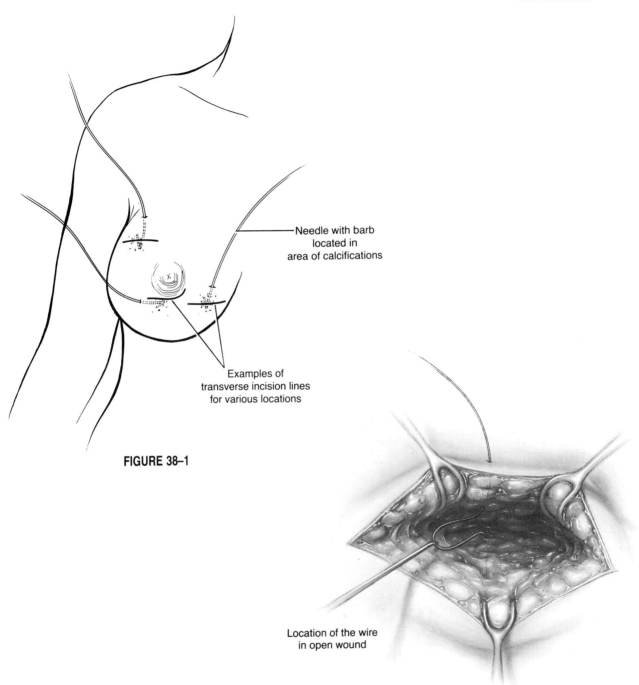

Needle with barb
located in
area of calcifications

Examples of
transverse incision lines
for various locations

FIGURE 38–1

Location of the wire
in open wound

FIGURE 38–2

FIGURES 38–1 and 38–2. Current techniques for wire placement involve a grid system for
peripheral entry of the wire, which extends a variable distance within the breast. The
surgeon must determine the position of the abnormality and estimate the course of the
wire by inspecting two views of the mammogram after needle placement. Transverse
incisions are always safely employed. When the abnormality is centrally located, an
incision at the margin of the areola may be used. Generally, the incisions are placed
along the predicted course of the wire and dissection is made to locate the wire. If the
abnormality is located at a distance from the wire entrance, dissection is made to the
wire, which can be pulled into the wound from under the skin flap. The surgeon can
then follow the wire into the substance of the breast, bearing in mind the location of
the abnormality, its distance down the wire, and its position in space relative to the
wire. This requires the ability to visualize the lesion and the wire in three dimensions
and to plan the dissection to include the entire abnormality.

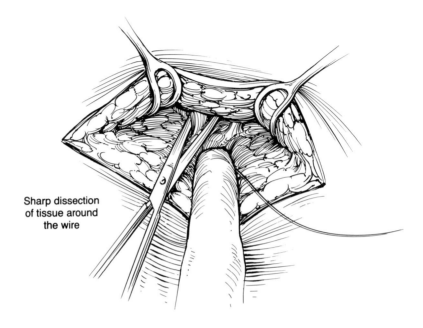

Sharp dissection
of tissue around
the wire

FIGURE 38–3. Keeping the wire and the lesion behind the index finger ensures that the course of the dissection includes the abnormality in the specimen. As with dissection of benign and malignant tumors, the use of a sturdy transfixing suture allows retraction of the tissue into the wound and avoids the use of crushing clamps, which can distort the tissue.

It is imperative to obtain a radiograph of the specimen to be certain that the lesion is included in the resected tissue. The specimen and the wire should be placed on a disposable paper x-ray cassette containing the film and should be photographed without disturbing the orientation of the wire and specimen. It is not enough to document that the abnormality is included in the specimen because the pathologist must know the *exact* location of the abnormality in the specimen. The specimen sent to the pathologist should include the undisturbed tissue containing the wire and the corresponding x-ray film showing the location of the abnormality. Prior to bisecting the specimen, the tissue margins should be indicated with ink (alcian blue) so that the status of the surgical margin can be assessed histologically. Furthermore, if the biopsy is done for microcalcifications, there must be a comment in the pathology report that calcifications were seen histologically. The findings on the radiograph of the specimen should be documented in the operative note, and the radiograph becomes part of the patient's permanent file. Because these abnormalities are frequently small *in situ* cancers, a frozen section is rarely obtained for fear of jeopardizing permanent pathology.

Meticulous hemostasis should be achieved in closing the incision. A breast hematoma should be viewed as an avoidable and compromising complication and should rarely occur. As with biopsy of lesions, no attempt is made to approximate the walls of the deep cavity, and drains are rarely, if ever, used. The volume loss and resulting deformity are avoided if the cavity is allowed to fill with serous fluid. The fluid is slowly absorbed, the cavity closes concentrically, and the breast parenchyma are allowed to mold gradually. The subcutaneous tissue may be approximated with interrupted absorbable suture, and the skin is closed with a subcuticular absorbable or pull-out suture.

39

Modified Radical Mastectomy

H. KIM LYERLY, M.D.

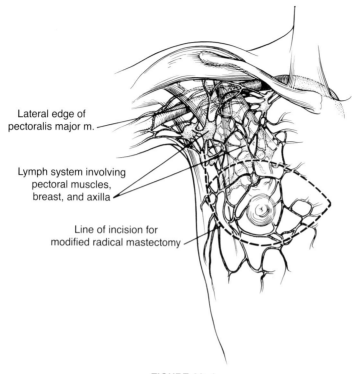

Lateral edge of
pectoralis major m.

Lymph system involving
pectoral muscles,
breast, and axilla

Line of incision for
modified radical mastectomy

FIGURE 39–1

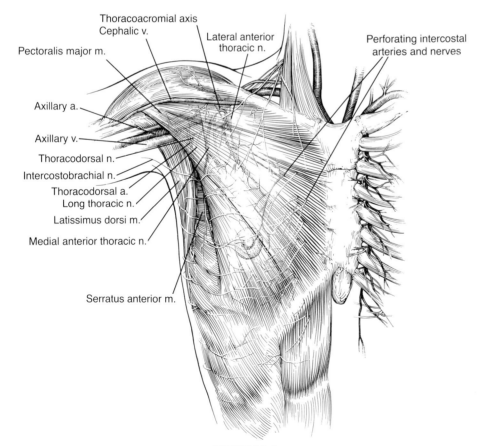

Thoracoacromial axis
Cephalic v.

Lateral anterior
thoracic n.

Perforating intercostal
arteries and nerves

Pectoralis major m.

Axillary a.

Axillary v.

Thoracodorsal n.

Intercostobrachial n.

Thoracodorsal a.

Long thoracic n.

Latissimus dorsi m.

Medial anterior thoracic n.

Serratus anterior m.

FIGURE 39–2

FIGURES 39–1 and 39–2. The patient is placed in the supine position with the arm on the affected side extended at a right angle. The entire chest, axilla, and upper arm on the side of the cancer are prepared and draped. Although modified radical mastectomy may be performed through many incisions, the objectives of the incision are to allow removal of a wide margin of tissue at the level of the tumor, exposure of the axillary and supraclavicular regions, and extension downward to permit exposure of the upper part of the anterior sheath of the rectus muscle. A transverse or slightly oblique skin incision is used to attain a less restrictive scar and an improved cosmetic result. However, the primary consideration is to make a circumferential incision that includes the previous biopsy or needle puncture as well as the nipple and areola with a surrounding margin. The incision, with the major vessels and lymphatics of the breast and axilla, is illustrated.

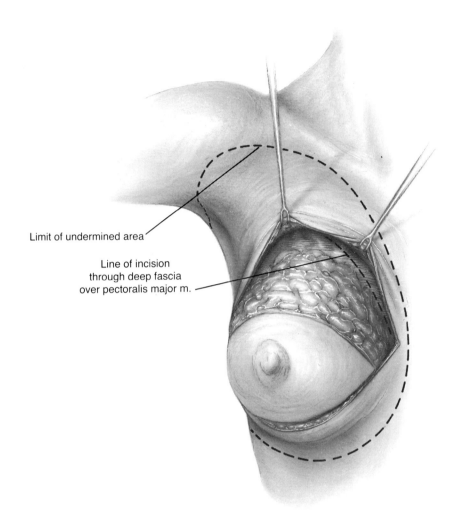

Limit of undermined area

Line of incision
through deep fascia
over pectoralis major m.

FIGURE 39–3. The initial skin incision is extended to the level of the superficial fascia. The skin flap is retracted anteriorly with skin hooks while countertraction on the breast tissue is provided. The flaps are retracted anteriorly and perpendicularly to the chest wall to avoid buttonholes. Superior and inferior skin flaps are developed in a plane above the superficial fascia to the midsternum medially, to the clavicle superiorly, to the latissimus dorsi muscle laterally, and to the costal margin inferiorly. Care must be taken that the skin flaps remain thin. This is especially important as the axilla is approached because the breast tissue often lies immediately beneath the superficial fascia and may be inadvertently incised. The completed skin flaps are usually 1 to 2 mm. thick at the skin edge and not more than 6 mm. thick at the base.

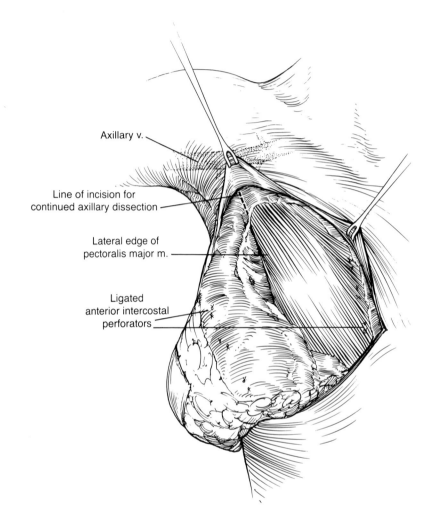

Axillary v.

Line of incision for
continued axillary dissection

Lateral edge of
pectoralis major m.

Ligated
anterior intercostal
perforators

FIGURE 39–4. The fasciae overlying the pectoralis major muscle and the breast are removed by subfascial dissection, starting near the midportion of the sternum and proceeding medially to laterally. The perforating intercostal arteries and veins near the sternal margins must be carefully clamped and ligated. The fascia is meticulously dissected from the pectoralis major without leaving any muscle in the gross specimen. If the cancer has penetrated this fascia and invaded the pectoralis major, excision of the entire pectoralis major muscle may be considered. A wide excision of the muscle at the site of penetration must be performed. The dissection of the pectoralis fascia is continued laterally (limited superiorly by the clavicle and inferiorly by the costal margin) until the lateral margin of the pectoralis major is reached.

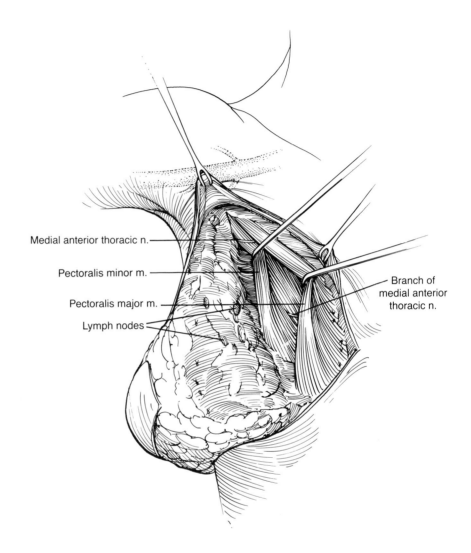

Medial anterior thoracic n.

Pectoralis minor m.

Pectoralis major m.

Lymph nodes

Branch of
medial anterior
thoracic n.

FIGURE 39–5. The lateral margin of the pectoralis major muscle is retracted medially and anteriorly, exposing the clavipectoral fascia, the interpectoral lymph nodes, and the pectoralis minor muscle. The subfascial dissection of the pectoralis major is extended to the lateral border of the pectoralis major and the fascia beneath. The interpectoral lymph nodes and the fascia of the pectoralis minor are freed to the lateral border of the pectoralis minor. Precautions are taken to avoid the medial and lateral anterior thoracic nerves to the pectoralis major. The medial anterior thoracic nerve arises from the medial cord of the brachial plexus and then passes through the pectoralis minor in about 60 per cent of patients, or passes laterally around the pectoralis minor in 40 per cent, innervating the lower region of the pectoralis major. The dominant lateral anterior thoracic nerve to the pectoralis major arises from the lateral cord, passes medially to the pectoralis minor near its insertion, and is closely associated with the thoracoacromial artery.

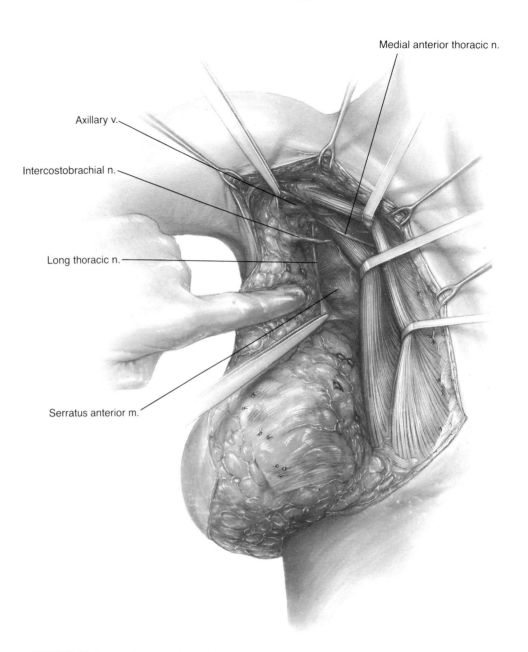

Medial anterior thoracic n.

Axillary v.

Intercostobrachial n.

Long thoracic n.

Serratus anterior m.

FIGURE 39–6. The lateral edge of the pectoralis minor muscle is cleared of fascia, and several veins are ligated as they arise from the axillary vein. A careful search is made for the medial anterior thoracic nerve to the pectoralis major muscle, which is preserved. A sensory nerve that may be sacrificed is the more transverse intercostobrachial nerve, which appears beneath the second rib and provides sensory innervation to the upper aspect of the inner arm. The pectoralis major and minor are then retracted anteriorly and medially, exposing the uppermost tissue to be divided over the axillary vein. The axillary vessels lie beneath a thin layer of fascia. Beginning medially in the apex of the axilla, the sheath of the axillary vein is incised on its cephalic portion and is extended laterally as far as possible. The fatty tissue and lymph nodes that are immediately inferior to the axillary vein are dissected free of the vein, and the several small arteries that traverse the vein anteriorly are ligated and cut. The axillary artery and portions of the brachial plexus lie superior to the vein. The axillary contents, including the lymph nodes, should be dissected beneath the axillary vessels after identification of the long thoracic and thoracodorsal nerves.

The long thoracic nerve is identified deep to the axillary artery. It lies within the loose fascia over the serratus anterior muscle. It must be carefully dissected from the axillary contents and maintained against the serratus anterior muscle. The identity and integrity of the nerve can be verified by a brisk but gentle pinch that causes a twitch of the serratus anterior muscle. If the long thoracic nerve is divided, a winged scapula will result, owing to the loss of the serratus anterior. The remaining fascia over the serratus anterior is dissected free, and the axillary fat and lymph nodes are mobilized from the chest wall.

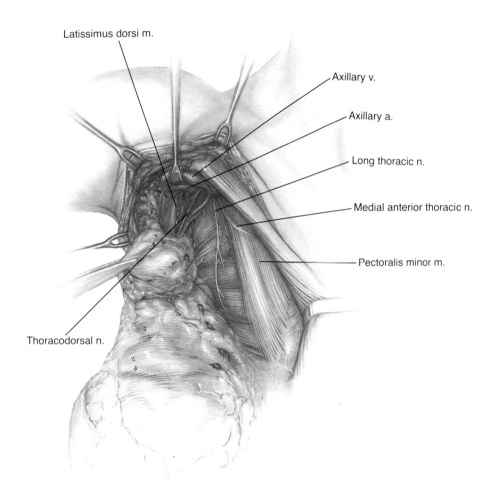

Latissimus dorsi m.

Axillary v.

Axillary a.

Long thoracic n.

Medial anterior thoracic n.

Pectoralis minor m.

Thoracodorsal n.

FIGURE 39–7. The thoracodorsal nerve is characteristically located adjacent to the deep subscapular vein and artery. This is in a slightly deeper plane than is the axillary vein. Division of the thoracodorsal nerve is avoided unless it is involved with tumor because it innervates the latissimus dorsi muscle. The specimen is freed from the latissimus dorsi and finally from the suspensory ligaments of the axilla, where large veins and lymphatics are carefully ligated. The operative field is repeatedly inspected for any bleeding points. The two major nerves are identified to be certain their course is free of ligatures.

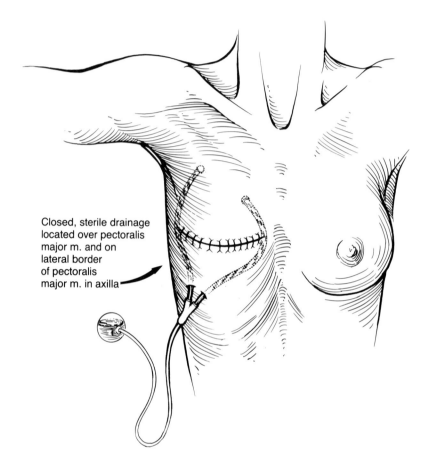

Closed, sterile drainage located over pectoralis major m. and on lateral border of pectoralis major m. in axilla

FIGURE 39–8. The wound is irrigated with saline, and a final inspection is made for hemostasis prior to closure. Two closed-system perforated suction catheters are inserted for sterile drainage. They are usually introduced posteriorly through separate stab wounds made in the lower flap. One is placed in the axilla, and the other is directed anteriorly over the pectoralis major muscle to drain the space beneath the skin flaps.

The skin flaps are compressed into place in the axilla and elsewhere as the skin is finally closed. If a moderate amount of subcutaneous fat remains, a few interrupted absorbable sutures should be placed in the subcutaneous tissue. The skin is then closed with sutures or staples.

40

Insertion of Breast Prosthesis

DONALD SERAFIN, M.D.

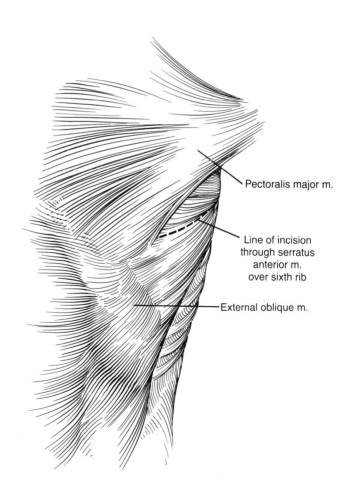

FIGURE 40–1. Following completion of the mastectomy, an incision is made approximately 5 to 6 cm. in length overlying the sixth rib and serratus anterior muscle.

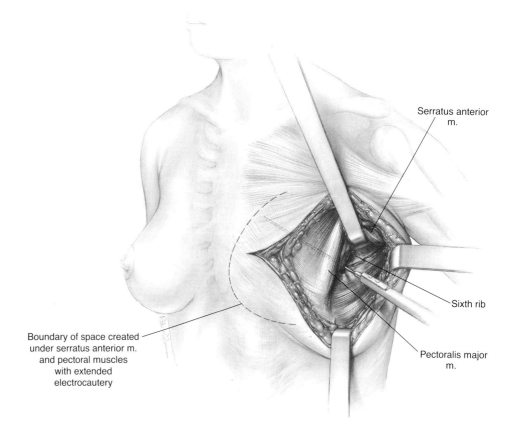

Serratus anterior
m.

Sixth rib

Pectoralis major
m.

Boundary of space created
under serratus anterior m.
and pectoral muscles
with extended
electrocautery

FIGURE 40–2. The incision is made with electrocautery down to the periosteum overlying the sixth rib. The diameter of the tissue expander, approximately 13.1 to 13.4 cm., is outlined on the skin. This area dictates the limits of undermining. With the cutting current of the electrocautery, a pocket is created beneath the serratus anterior and pectoralis major muscles, with care taken not to enter the intercostal space and cause a pneumothorax. A common error in dissection is the failure to extend the dissection sufficiently inferior and medial to the rectus fascia. Minimal dissection is conducted superiorly beneath the pectoralis major muscle. The dissecting plane is between the pectoralis major muscle anteriorly and the pectoralis minor muscle posteriorly and is continued laterally to the anterior axillary fold. Lateral dissection must be limited at this point to provide adequate anterior projection of the prosthesis. Excessive dissection laterally produces a flattened appearance of the prosthesis with excessive lateral projection. Medial dissection is conducted to the point of emergence of the anterior perforating branches of the intercostal artery and nerves. As indicated previously, the diameter of the pocket should be slightly greater than the diameter of the expanding prosthesis.

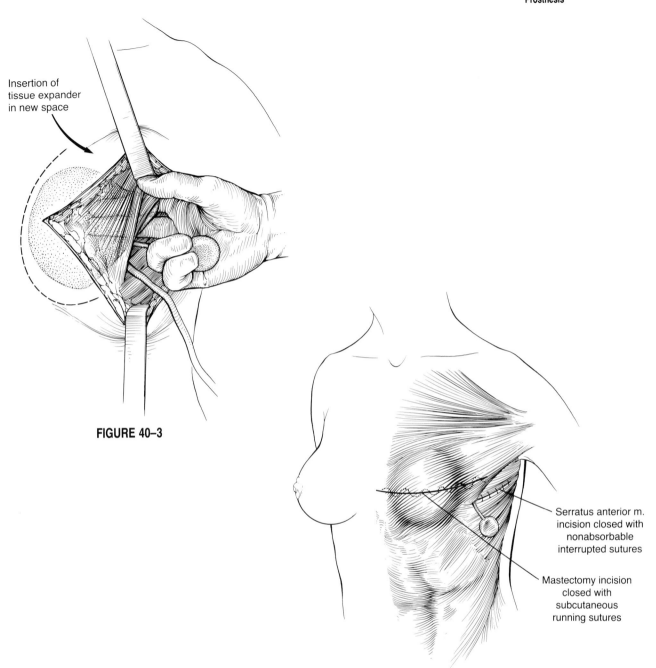

Insertion of
tissue expander
in new space

FIGURE 40–3

Serratus anterior m.
incision closed with
nonabsorbable
interrupted sutures

Mastectomy incision
closed with
subcutaneous
running sutures

FIGURE 40–4

FIGURES 40–3 and 40–4. The wound is irrigated with copious amounts of bacitracin and
saline solution and meticulously inspected for bleeding points. A single round drain is
placed in the submuscular pocket. The deflated tissue expander is then placed in the
new submuscular pocket. It is very important to avoid wrinkling of the prosthesis. The
Silastic stem of the prosthesis is placed in an inferior lateral position. Next, the incision
is closed with interrupted 2–0 absorbable Vicryl sutures. Following closure, 100 to 150
ml. of normal saline is instilled to expand the prosthesis. The receptacle is then attached
to the stem of the prosthesis and placed in a subcutaneous position overlying the lower
lateral ribs. The pocket must be adequate for the receptacle but not large enough to
allow turning. Great care must be taken in placement of the receptacle to avoid later
rotation. The skin incision is closed appropriately with interrupted 2–0 Vicryl sutures.
Closure is begun medially to avoid a medial dog ear. Lateral closure is then undertaken
to avoid a lateral dog ear. Finally, the middle third of the incision is closed. A 4–0 Vicryl
suture is placed in the dermis, and a continuous 3–0 subcuticular Prolene suture is used
to close the skin.

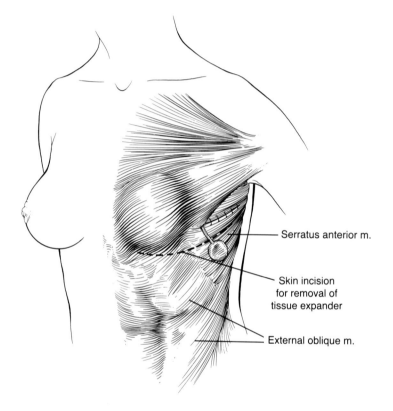

Serratus anterior m.

Skin incision
for removal of
tissue expander

External oblique m.

FIGURE 40–5. During the series of inflations over the next 6 weeks to 3 months, volume is added to the submuscular prosthesis. The injections are made using a 22-gauge needle into the receptacle overlying the anterior lateral thoracic wall. Approximately 50 to 60 ml. of saline is injected at approximately 2-week intervals. During the serial expansions, the final appropriate volume is obtained for a cosmetically pleasing size for the breast. This is recorded in the patient's chart. This volume will be the size of the new silicone prosthesis to be placed later. Expansion continues until the pocket is overexpanded by approximately 75 to 100 ml. At a second stage, 2 to 3 months later, a 5- to 6-cm. inframammary skin incision is made at the approximate level of the inframammary fold.

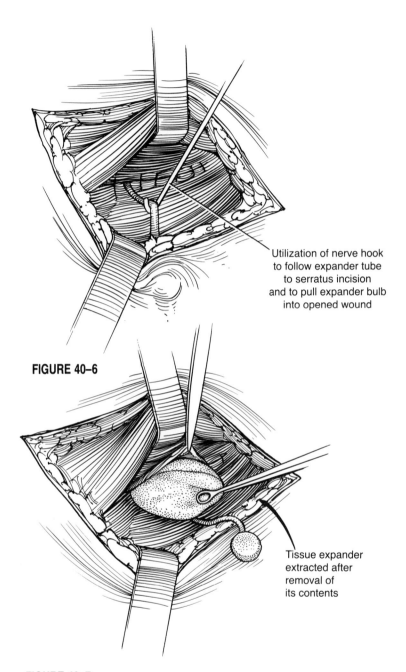

Utilization of nerve hook
to follow expander tube
to serratus incision
and to pull expander bulb
into opened wound

FIGURE 40–6

Tissue expander
extracted after
removal of
its contents

FIGURE 40–7

FIGURE 40–6. The Silastic conduit is identified. Traction is applied, and, with blunt and sharp dissection, the receptacle is removed from its subcutaneous pocket. The juncture site in the conduit is identified, the previously placed silk sutures are cut, and the expander is deflated.

FIGURE 40–7. The previous serratus incision is identified by following the course of the conduit through the previous incision. The incision is opened, and the tissue expander is extracted.

Insertion of silicone prosthesis

Serratus anterior m.

Pectoralis major m.

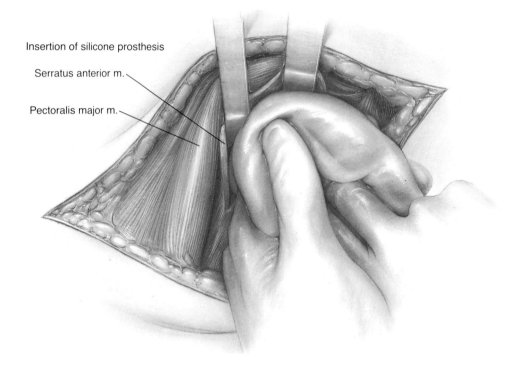

FIGURE 40–8. The pocket is irrigated copiously with saline. Any discrepancies in contour resulting from an inadequate dissection of the pocket during the initial operative procedure are corrected. The expander is replaced with a permanent silicone prosthesis, the volume of which is determined during the course of the serial inflations. The incision is then closed in layers with 2–0 Vicryl for the muscular layer, 2–0 Vicryl for the subcutaneous and deep dermis, 4–0 Vicryl for the dermis, and a continuous 3–0 subcuticular Prolene suture.

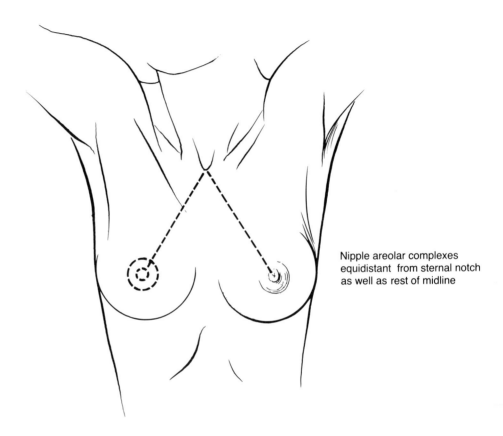

Nipple areolar complexes
equidistant from sternal notch
as well as rest of midline

FIGURE 40–9. The nipple-areolar complex can be reconstructed during the second stage when the permanent prosthesis is inserted, or it may be deferred for a third stage after maximal settling has occurred. With the patient in the sitting position, the diameter and position of the nipple-areolar complex on the contralateral side are marked using a line drawn from the suprasternal notch to the contralateral nipple.

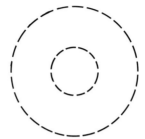

Outline drawn using template of areola
and nipple of other breast

FIGURE 40–10. The area of the reconstructed breast is similarly marked, with the diameter equal to the contralateral side. A nipple circumference also is marked.

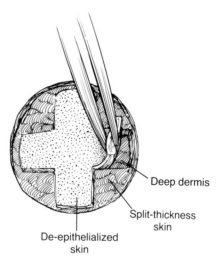

Deep dermis

Split-thickness
skin

De-epithelialized
skin

FIGURE 40–11. A cruciate pattern is marked within the circumference of the previously outlined areola. The width of each limb is equal to the diameter of the nipple. A quadrant of de-epithelialized skin, including part of the dermis, is removed from each of the four quadrants. The cruciate portion of the pattern and the future nipple are tattooed with the appropriate pigment. Next, each limb of the cruciate pattern is elevated from the dermis in a somewhat deeper plane than that of the quadrant portion. The dermis will support the viability of the overlying epithelium.

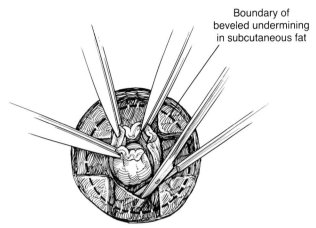

Boundary of
beveled undermining
in subcutaneous fat

FIGURE 40–12. After elevating all four segments of the cruciate pattern, a circumferential incision is made at the base of the nipple through the dermis to the underlying fat. Dissection then continues sharply beneath the dermis toward the circumference of the areola. The dissection should not be directed posteriorly (deep), as this disrupts too much of the subcutaneous blood supply. During the course of the dissection, the reconstructed nipple gains projection. The degree of undermining determines the extent of the projection.

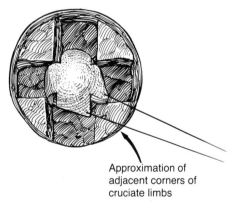

Approximation of
adjacent corners of
cruciate limbs

FIGURE 40–13. With gentle traction on the projecting nipple, the limbs of the cruciate pattern are sutured to each other with interrupted 6–0 Vicryl sutures, very much like the projecting portion of a top hat.

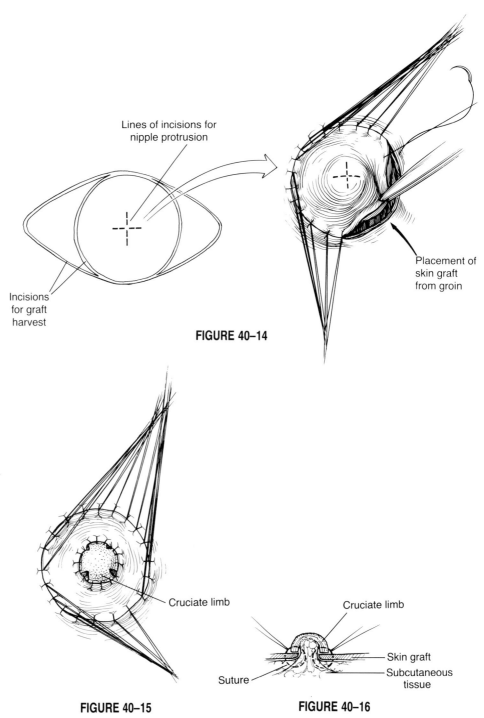

Lines of incisions for
nipple protrusion

Incisions
for graft
harvest

Placement of
skin graft
from groin

FIGURE 40–14

Cruciate limb

FIGURE 40–15

Cruciate limb

Skin graft

Subcutaneous
tissue

Suture

FIGURE 40–16

FIGURES 40–14 to 40–16. With a template employed for marking the areola and the nipple, a similar pattern is made in the region of the groin crease away from the hair-bearing area. After the circular template is marked, an elliptical portion is added so that, upon final closure, the line of closure will be parallel to or within the groin crease. A full-thickness graft is taken from the inguinal region. The diameter of the graft is equal to the diameter of the reconstructed areola. An opening for the nipple is not made at this time. The full-thickness graft is then sutured to the circumference of the recipient areolar defect with interrupted 6–0 Duralon sutures. After suturing is complete, a tiny cruciate incision is made over the nipple, permitting extrusion of the nipple through the full-thickness graft. A portion of the skin graft lies posterior, or deep, to the cruciate limbs of the projecting nipple, maintaining adequate projection. This is not possible if the aperture for the nipple is made too large. As a result, later retraction and loss of projection occur. The full-thickness graft is sutured to the deep dermis with interrupted 6–0 Vicryl sutures. A foam rubber stent is placed like a doughnut over the projecting nipple; and previously placed Duralon sutures, which were left long, are tied as a bolus dressing over the full-thickness graft, avoiding compression of the nipple.

Abdominal Operations

41

Stamm Gastrostomy

JOHN P. GRANT, M.D.

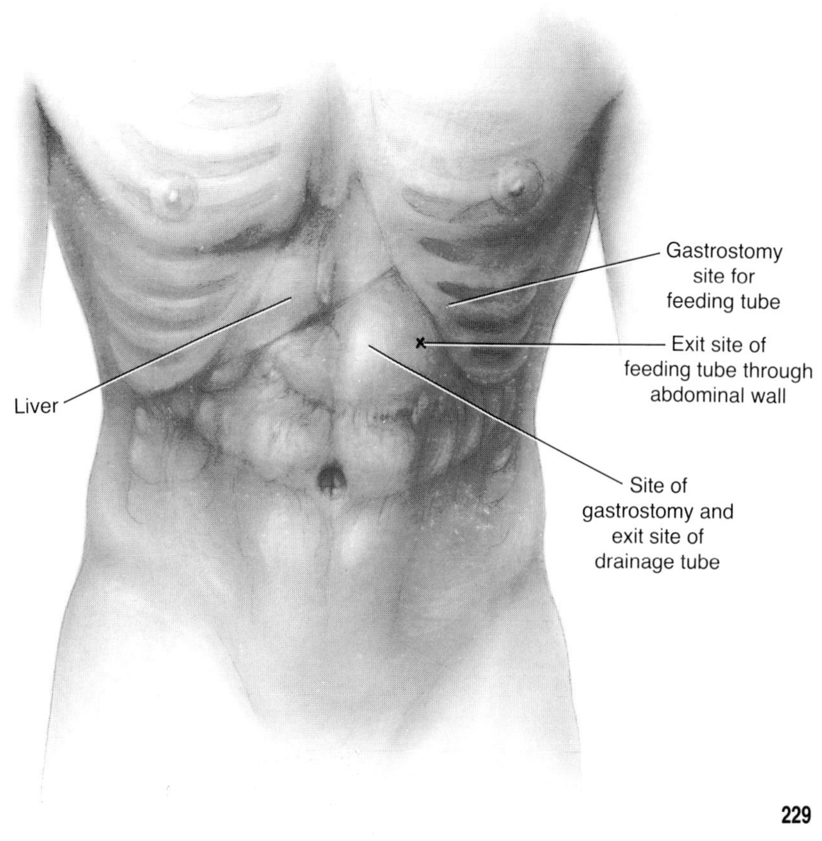

FIGURE 41–1. For feeding purposes, a Stamm gastrostomy should be placed high in the fundus of the stomach on the anterior gastric wall. For drainage purposes, the tube should be placed low in the antrum. The skin exit site should be one-third the distance from the midclavicular line at the rib margin to the umbilicus on the left side.

Liver

Gastrostomy site for feeding tube

Exit site of feeding tube through abdominal wall

Site of gastrostomy and exit site of drainage tube

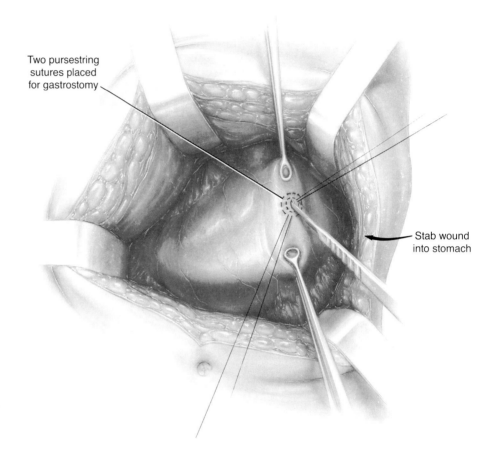

Two pursestring
sutures placed
for gastrostomy

Stab wound
into stomach

FIGURE 41–2. A 6- to 8-cm. upper midline skin incision is made, and the linea alba is divided. The transverse colon is displaced downward, and the stomach is grasped with Babcock clamps. With gentle traction and repositioning of the clamps, the stomach can be drawn down and the site for the catheter exposed.

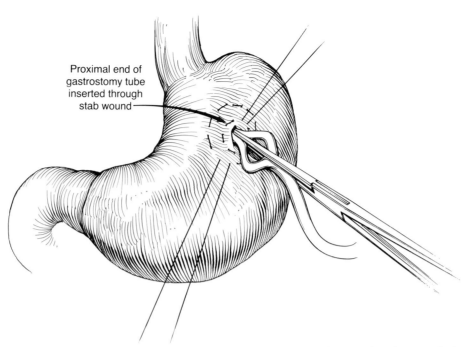

Proximal end of
gastrostomy tube
inserted through
stab wound

FIGURE 41–3. Two or three pursestring sutures of 2–0 silk are placed around the proposed entrance site on the anterior surface of the stomach at least 2 cm. apart. A stab wound is placed into the stomach through the center of the inner pursestring suture, and a Malecot or mushroom gastrostomy tube is inserted into the stomach.

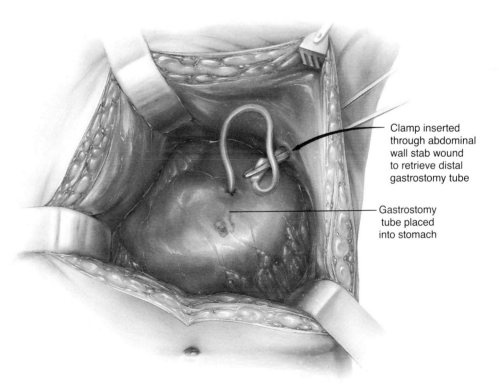

Clamp inserted
through abdominal
wall stab wound
to retrieve distal
gastrostomy tube

Gastrostomy
tube placed
into stomach

FIGURE 41–4. The end of the gastrostomy tube is drawn through the abdominal wall through a stab wound at a selected site for exit.

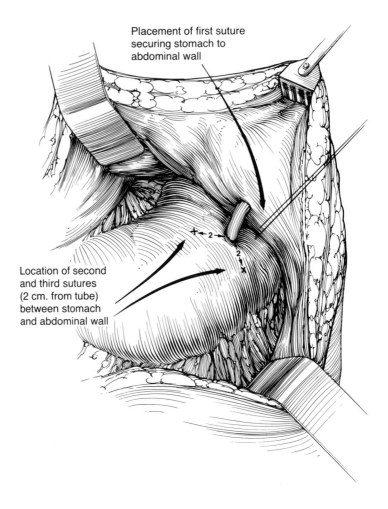

Placement of first suture
securing stomach to
abdominal wall

Location of second
and third sutures
(2 cm. from tube)
between stomach
and abdominal wall

FIGURE 41–5. Three tacking sutures of 2–0 silk are placed in the stomach around the gastrostomy tube and then through the anterior abdominal wall near the exit site of the tube. When these sutures are tied, the stomach is fixed to the abdominal wall and risk of leakage is minimized.

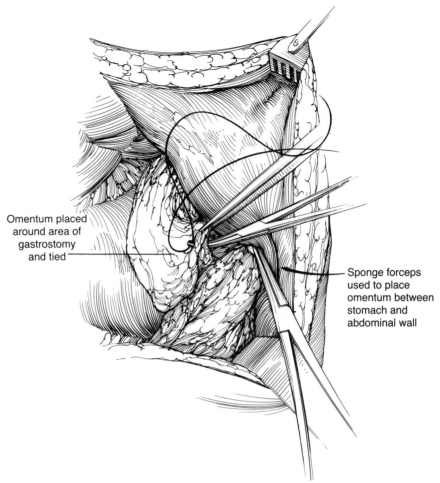

Omentum placed
around area of
gastrostomy
and tied

Sponge forceps
used to place
omentum between
stomach and
abdominal wall

FIGURE 41–6. (Optional) Further security against leaks can be achieved by wrapping greater omentum around the gastrostomy site.

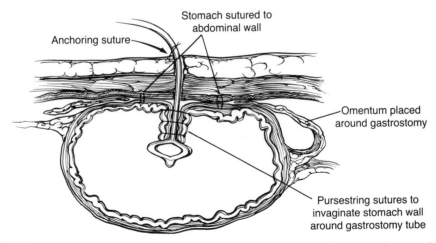

Stomach sutured to
abdominal wall

Anchoring suture

Omentum placed
around gastrostomy

Pursestring sutures to
invaginate stomach wall
around gastrostomy tube

FIGURE 41–7. The pursestring sutures are secured, invaginating the stomach around the feeding tube.

A 2–0 silk suture is placed in the skin at the exit site of the tube and secured around the gastrostomy tube to fix it in place. A sterile dressing is placed, and the gastrostomy tube is connected to straight drainage. Feedings can be initiated when normal gastric emptying is restored.

42

Witzel Gastrostomy

JOHN P. GRANT, M.D.

With this procedure, the abdominal incision, placement of the feeding tube in the stomach, and location of the tube exit site on the skin are the same as for the Stamm gastrostomy.

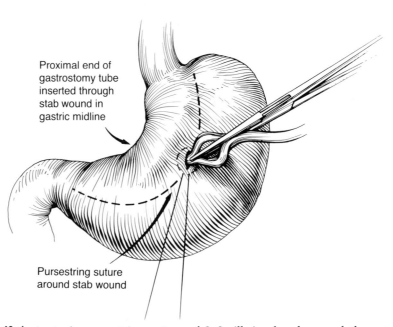

Proximal end of gastrostomy tube inserted through stab wound in gastric midline

Pursestring suture around stab wound

FIGURE 42–1. A single pursestring suture of 2–0 silk is placed around the proposed entrance site on the anterior surface of the stomach. A stab wound is made into the stomach through the center of the pursestring suture, and a Malecot or mushroom gastrostomy tube is inserted into the stomach. The pursestring suture is secured, invaginating the stomach around the feeding tube.

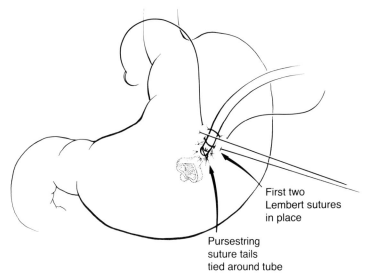

First two
Lembert sutures
in place

Pursestring
suture tails
tied around tube

FIGURE 42–2

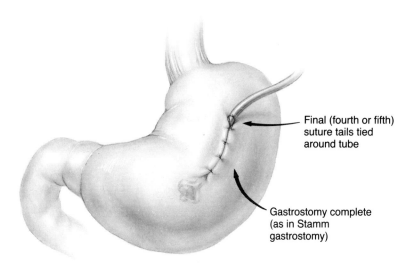

Final (fourth or fifth)
suture tails tied
around tube

Gastrostomy complete
(as in Stamm
gastrostomy)

FIGURE 42–3

FIGURES 42–2 and 42–3. A serosal tunnel is created by suturing the wall of the stomach over the tube for a distance of 4 to 5 cm. The last suture is tied around the feeding tube to secure it in place.

The end of the gastrostomy tube is then drawn through the abdominal wall from a stab wound at the selected exit site, and the stomach is sutured to the abdominal wall as in the Stamm gastrostomy. A 2–0 silk suture is placed in the skin at the tube exit site and secured around the gastrostomy tube to anchor it in place. A sterile dressing is applied, and the gastrostomy tube is connected to straight drainage. Feedings can be initiated when normal gastric emptying is restored.

43

Percutaneous Endoscopic Gastrostomy

JOHN P. GRANT, M.D.

Several percutaneous gastrostomy kits are available, and selection depends on the surgeon's preference. Essential criteria, however, are that the tube have a broad inner retention device (a simple crossbar is inadequate) and markings at centimeter intervals at the end to aid in positioning.

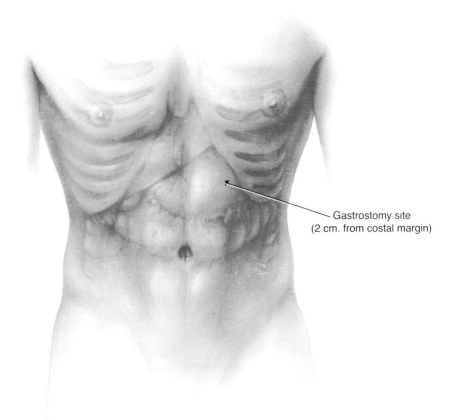

Gastrostomy site
(2 cm. from costal margin)

FIGURE 43–1. The optimal position for placement of a percutaneous gastrostomy is through the midportion of the stomach. The skin exit site is usually one third the distance from the midclavicular line at the rib margin to the umbilicus, although this point can vary from a midline position to the axillary line, depending on the position of the stomach. The exit site should not be next to the rib margin because rubbing by the tube can be quite painful for the patient. It is mandatory that placement be at least 2 cm. from the rib edge.

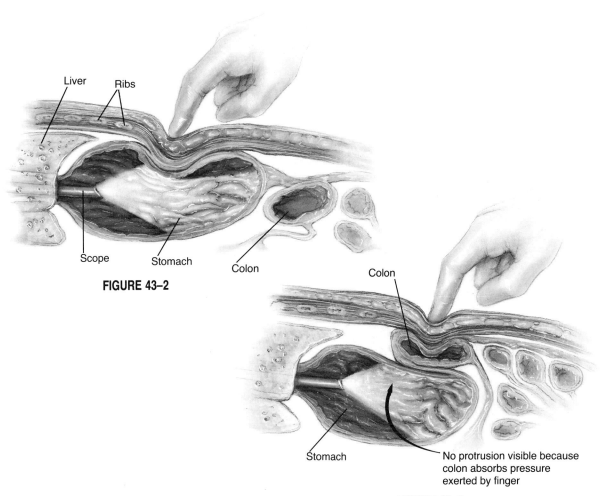

Liver   Ribs

Scope   Stomach   Colon

FIGURE 43–2

Colon

Stomach   No protrusion visible because
colon absorbs pressure
exerted by finger

FIGURE 43–3

FIGURES 43–2 and 43–3. Minimal topical anesthesia of the oropharynx is used to avoid aspiration following tube placement. A pediatric gastroscope is introduced, and air is insufflated to distend the stomach. During insufflation, the stomach and pylorus should be examined for any abnormalities, especially gastric outlet obstruction. When the stomach is fully distended, a finger is pressed into the abdominal wall at the proposed site of puncture. A clear indentation of the stomach seen through the endoscope ensures that the stomach is adjacent to the abdominal wall and that neither colon nor small bowel is interposed. A second method for confirming satisfactory anatomy is to direct the endoscope anteriorly while darkening the room. A clear, well-defined transillumination of light through the wall should be present. If the light is obscure or diffuse, the stomach is probably not directly under the abdominal wall.

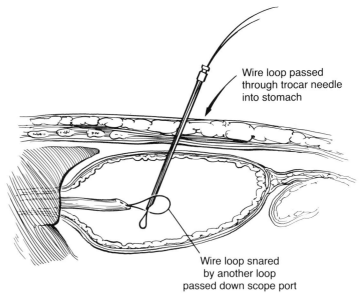

Wire loop passed
through trocar needle
into stomach

Wire loop snared
by another loop
passed down scope port

FIGURE 43–4. After induction of local anesthesia, an incision 0.5 cm. larger than the diameter of the gastrostomy tube is placed at the selected exit site and a trocar needle is passed into the stomach. Passage of the needle into the stomach is confirmed visually through the endoscope over the needle, and the trocar is removed. A braided wire (or heavy nylon suture) is passed through the needle and snared.

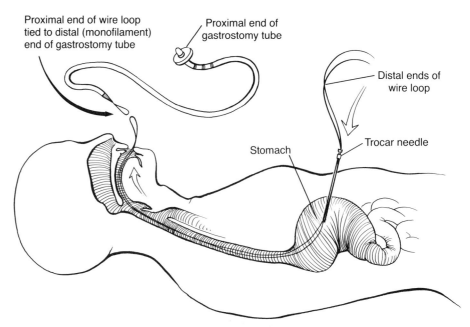

Proximal end of wire loop
tied to distal (monofilament)
end of gastrostomy tube

Proximal end of
gastrostomy tube

Distal ends of
wire loop

Stomach

Trocar needle

FIGURE 43–5. The gastroscope and snare are withdrawn, drawing the wire out of the mouth.

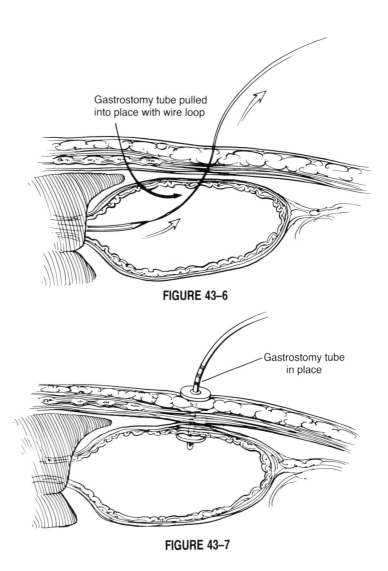

Gastrostomy tube pulled
into place with wire loop

FIGURE 43–6

Gastrostomy tube
in place

FIGURE 43–7

FIGURES 43–6 and 43–7. The end of the wire is attached to the percutaneous gastrostomy tube, and the wire is withdrawn from the exit site on the stomach, drawing the gastrostomy tube down the esophagus and out the abdominal wall. Proper location of the tube is indicated by the dots placed on the tube near the end disc. Usually, the abdominal wall is 2 to 4 cm. thick. It is unnecessary to perform a second endoscopy to confirm proper placement. A disc retainer is passed over the end of the tube and firmly drawn against the abdominal wall to draw the stomach to the anterior abdominal wall tightly. The discs should be kept tight for 48 hours. After 48 hours, the discs should be loosened to prevent erosion into the gastric wall or abdominal skin. The gastrostomy tube is connected to straight drainage for 24 hours, after which feedings can begin.

44

Witzel Jejunostomy

JOHN P. GRANT, M.D.

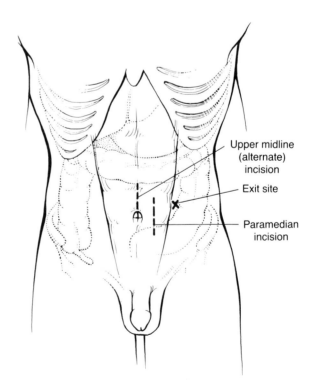

FIGURE 44–1. Under local or general anesthesia, a 6- to 8-cm. paramedian incision is placed just to the left of and centered slightly above the umbilicus (a midline incision is also acceptable). The incision is extended to the anterior rectus sheath, which is incised. The rectus muscle is mobilized laterally, and the posterior rectus sheath and peritoneum are incised.

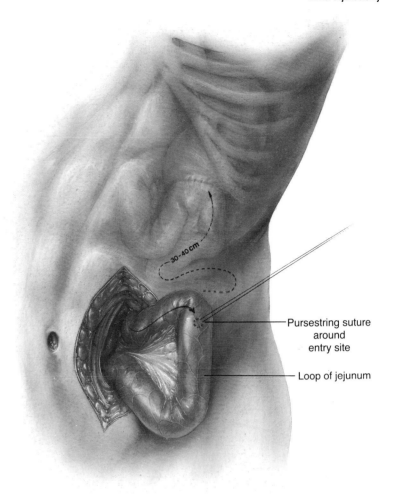

FIGURE 44–2. A point on the jejunum 30 to 40 cm. from the ligament of Treitz is identified, and a pursestring suture of 3–0 chromic catgut is placed.

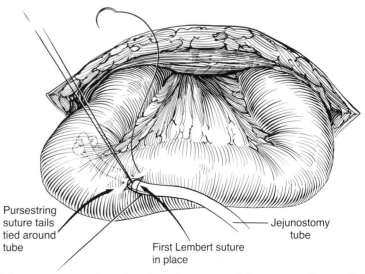

FIGURE 44–3. A stab wound is placed in the center of the pursestring, and a feeding jejunostomy tube (8 to 16 French) is passed distally into the bowel. The pursestring suture is secured around the tube.

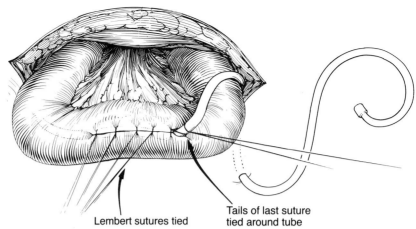

Lembert sutures tied

Tails of last suture
tied around tube

FIGURE 44–4. Four to six vertical mattress sutures of 4–0 silk are placed, beginning at the entrance site of the tube and extending proximally on the jejunum to create a serosal tunnel over the tube. The tails of the last suture are tied around the tube to secure it in place. A stab wound is made in the left upper quadrant of the abdomen, and the feeding tube is drawn through the stab wound with a Kelly clamp.

Jejunal loop sutured to
abdominal wall to prevent twisting

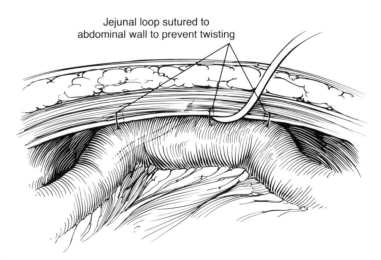

FIGURE 44–5. The jejunum is sutured to the anterior abdominal wall with three 3–0 silk sutures. One suture is placed at the tube exit site, one just proximal to it, and another just distal to it. These sutures prevent torsion. The tube is secured to the abdominal wall and flushed with saline to ensure patency. The posterior rectus sheath and peritoneum are closed with 1–0 chromic catgut suture, and the anterior rectus sheath is closed with 1–0 or 2–0 permanent suture. Sterile dressings are applied. The jejunostomy may be used as soon as bowel sounds return.

45

Feeding (Needle Tube) Jejunostomy

JOHN P. GRANT, M.D.

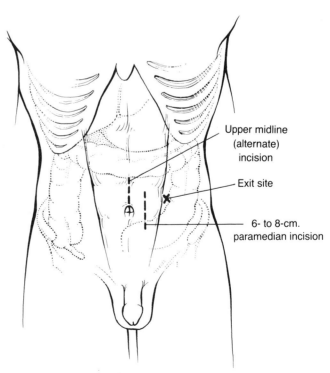

FIGURE 45–1. The abdominal incision is identical to that for the Witzel jejunostomy. A midline incision is also acceptable.

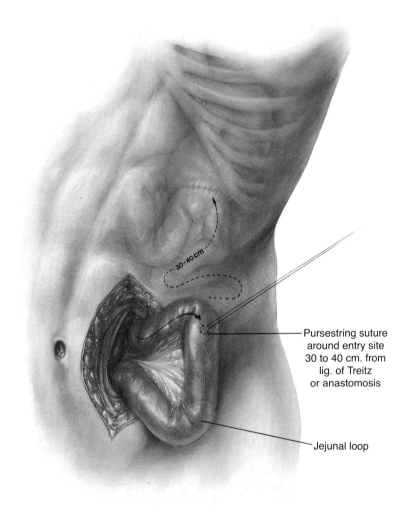

Pursestring suture
around entry site
30 to 40 cm. from
lig. of Treitz
or anastomosis

Jejunal loop

FIGURE 45–2. A point on the proximal jejunum 30 to 40 cm. distal to the ligament of Treitz is identified.

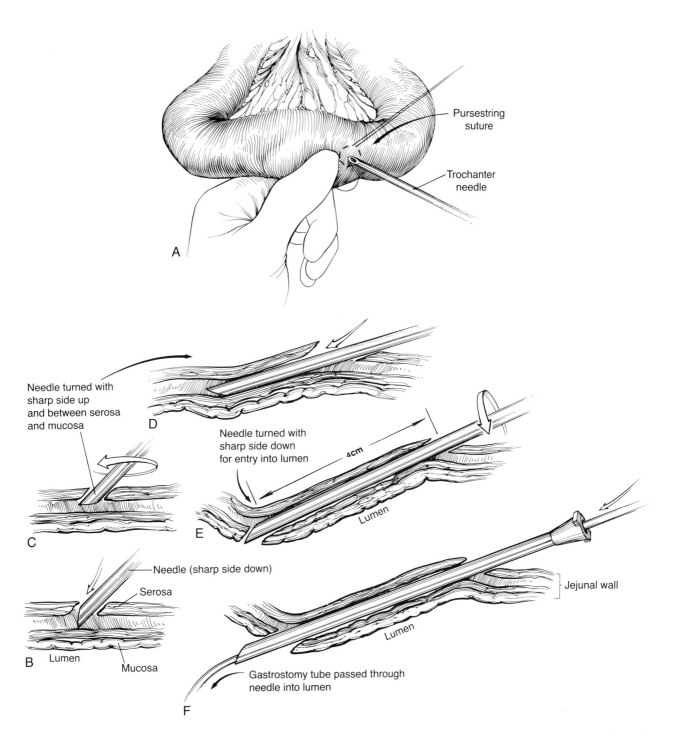

FIGURE 45–3. *A* and *B*, A pursestring suture of 3–0 absorbable material is placed at the selected site, and a 14-gauge needle is advanced through the pursestring with the bevel up.

    C and *D*, The bevel is then rotated down, and the needle is advanced distally between the serosa and mucosa of the bowel wall for a distance of about 4 cm.

    E and *F*, An 18-gauge jejunostomy feeding tube is passed through the needle into the jejunum for a distance of 30 to 40 cm., and the needle is removed.

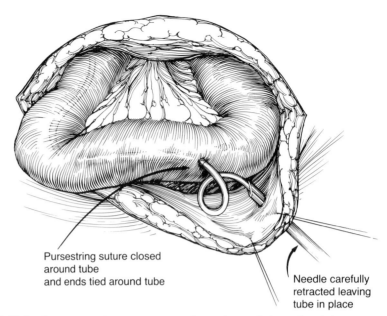

Pursestring suture closed
around tube
and ends tied around tube

Needle carefully
retracted leaving
tube in place

FIGURE 45–4. The pursestring suture is tied snugly, and the tails of the suture are tied around the catheter to secure it in place. Another 14-gauge needle is passed through the abdominal wall, directing it from the left upper quadrant toward the umbilicus. The feeding catheter is passed through the needle, and the needle is withdrawn.

Jejunal loop sutured to
abdominal wall to prevent twisting

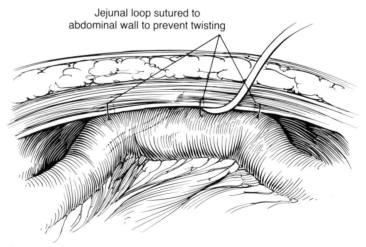

FIGURE 45–5. The bowel is sutured to the abdominal wall with three 3–0 silk sutures, one at the exit site of the catheter, one proximal to it, and one distal to it to prevent torsion of the bowel. The tube is secured to the abdominal wall and flushed with saline to ensure patency. The posterior rectus sheath and peritoneum are closed with a 1–0 chromic catgut suture, and the anterior rectus sheath is closed with a 1–0 or 2–0 permanent suture. Sterile dressings are applied. The jejunostomy may be used as soon as bowel sounds return.

46

Laparoscopic Jejunostomy

JOHN P. GRANT, M.D.

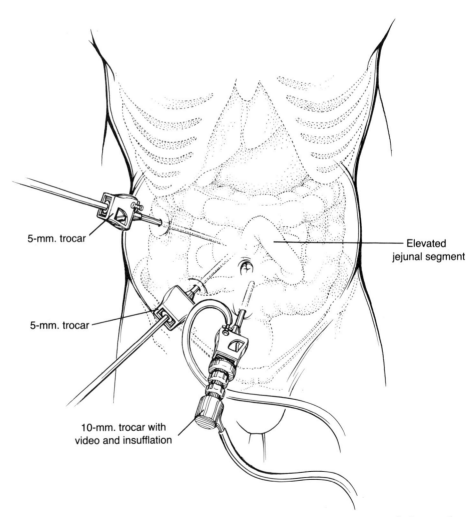

FIGURE 46–1. Under either general anesthesia or generous intravenous sedation, carbon dioxide is insufflated into the abdomen to 15 mm. Hg via an insufflator needle inserted just below the umbilicus by means of standard techniques. A 10-mm. trocar is passed into the abdomen, and the camera is inserted. Two 5-mm. trocars are inserted under direct vision, one through the right midabdomen and one through the right lower quadrant.

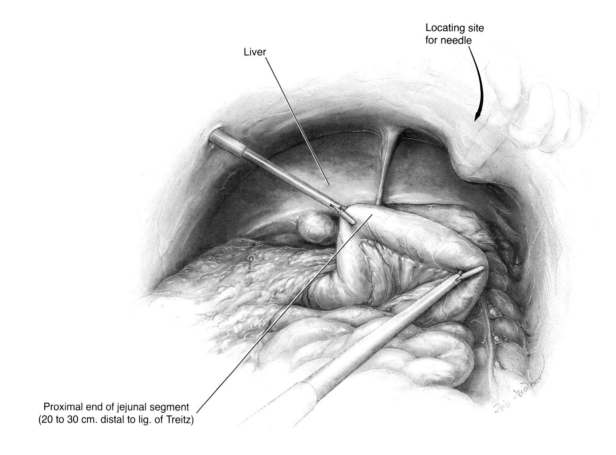

Locating site
for needle

Liver

Proximal end of jejunal segment
(20 to 30 cm. distal to lig. of Treitz)

FIGURE 46–2. With atraumatic graspers, the bowel is run proximally to the ligament of Treitz. A site for jejunostomy placement is identified approximately 20 to 30 cm. from the ligament of Treitz.

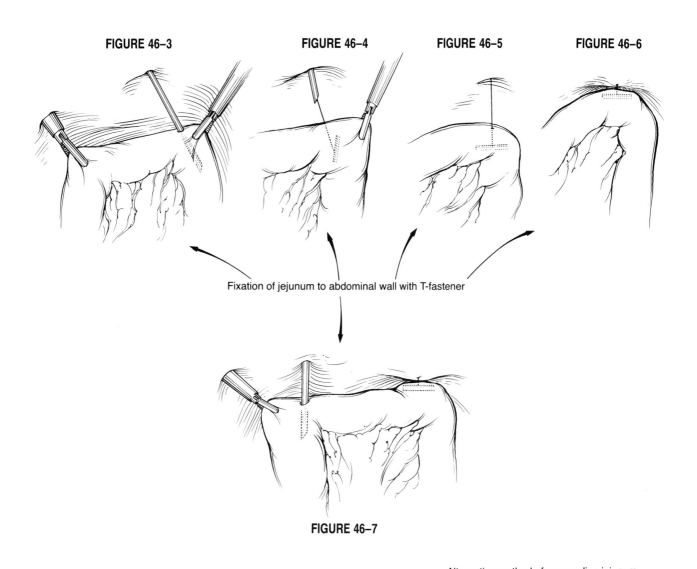

FIGURE 46–3   **FIGURE 46–4**   **FIGURE 46–5**   **FIGURE 46–6**

Fixation of jejunum to abdominal wall with T-fastener

FIGURE 46–7

Placement of fourth T-fastener

Alternative method of suspending jejunum
with Keith needles

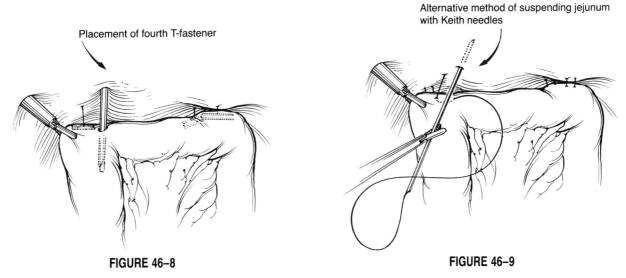

FIGURE 46–8   **FIGURE 46–9**

FIGURES 46–3 to 46–9. Four retraction sutures are placed with either T-fasteners or 3–0 nylon sutures on Keith needles.

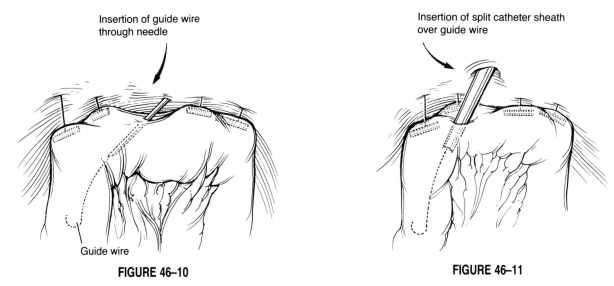

Insertion of guide wire
through needle

Insertion of split catheter sheath
over guide wire

Guide wire

FIGURE 46–10

FIGURE 46–11

FIGURE 46–10. A 14-gauge needle is passed through the abdominal wall and into the jejunum in the center of the four retention sutures. A guide wire is passed through the needle and directed distally into the bowel. The needle is removed.

FIGURE 46–11. A 16 French split catheter sheath and dilator are passed over the guide wire and advanced into the small bowel.

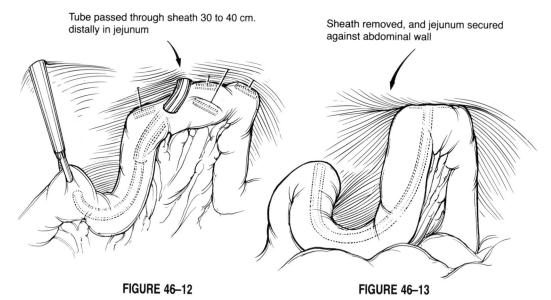

Tube passed through sheath 30 to 40 cm.
distally in jejunum

Sheath removed, and jejunum secured
against abdominal wall

FIGURE 46–12

FIGURE 46–13

FIGURE 46–12. The guide wire and introducer are removed, and a 14 French jejunostomy tube is passed through the sheath into the small bowel.

FIGURE 46–13. The sheath is removed. Gas is allowed to escape, reducing the intra-abdominal pressure to 8 to 10 mm. Hg, and the small bowel is drawn up and secured against the abdominal wall under minimal tension with the four retention sutures. The jejunostomy tube is anchored to the skin at the exit site with a 3–0 nylon suture. The tube is tested for patency by injection of a saline solution. All of the gas is then allowed to exit from the abdomen, the trocars are removed, the fascia at the 10-mm. trocar site is approximated with an absorbable suture, and sterile dressings are applied.

The jejunostomy can be used immediately. The retention sutures are left in place for 3 to 4 weeks and then removed.

47

Heineke-Mikulicz Pyloroplasty

WILLIAM C. MEYERS, M.D.

Of the three types of pyloroplasty used for interruption of vagus innervation of the stomach, the Heineke-Mikulicz is by far the most common.

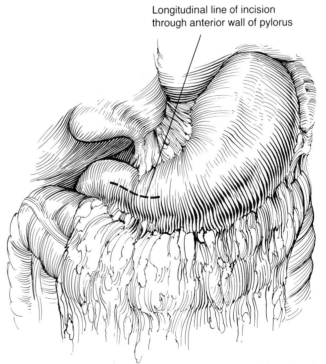

Longitudinal line of incision through anterior wall of pylorus

FIGURE 47–1. After performance of a Kocher maneuver to mobilize the duodenum, a 2- to 3-cm. longitudinal (vertical) incision is made through the pylorus wall anteriorly through all layers. Bleeding from the edges of the bowel during this procedure is usually controlled with electrocautery.

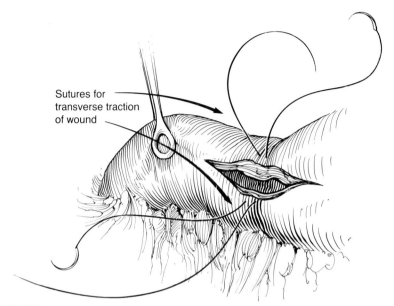

FIGURE 47–2. Silk sutures are placed for anatomic orientation and traction.

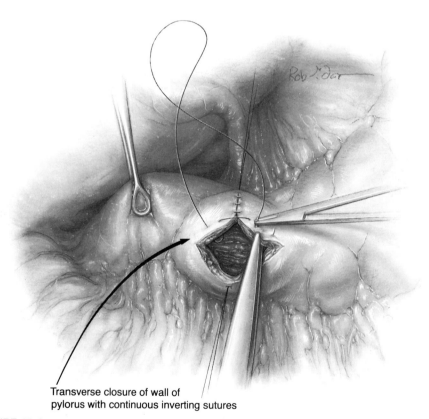

FIGURE 47–3. The defect is closed in a perpendicular (horizontal) manner. Full-thickness sutures are placed through all layers of the bowel using a double-layer technique. Traction sutures of silk are usually placed at the ends of the transverse closure prior to placement of the inner layer, which is formed by continuous 3–0 chromic Connell sutures.

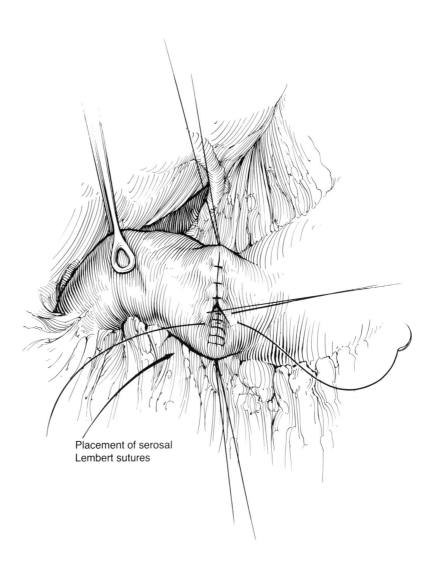

Placement of serosal
Lembert sutures

FIGURE 47–4. Interrupted seromuscular Lembert sutures form the outer layer.

48

Heineke-Mikulicz Pyloroplasty (STAPLER)

HILLIARD F. SEIGLER, M.D.

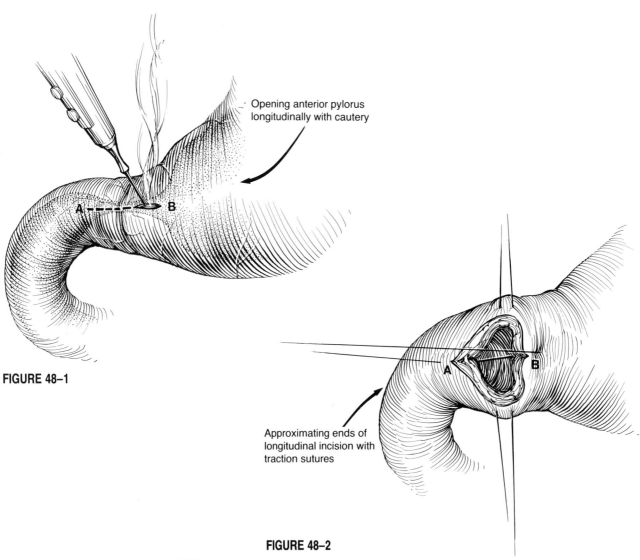

Opening anterior pylorus
longitudinally with cautery

FIGURE 48–1

Approximating ends of
longitudinal incision with
traction sutures

FIGURE 48–2

FIGURE 48–1. A longitudinal incision is made across the pyloric muscle approximately 1 to 2 cm. in each direction. With careful use of the cautery, hemostasis should be accomplished. A traction suture is placed on each side of the incision at the level of the pyloric muscle.

FIGURE 48–2. An additional traction suture is placed at the midpoint, and this now permits redirecting the longitudinal incision to a transverse orientation.

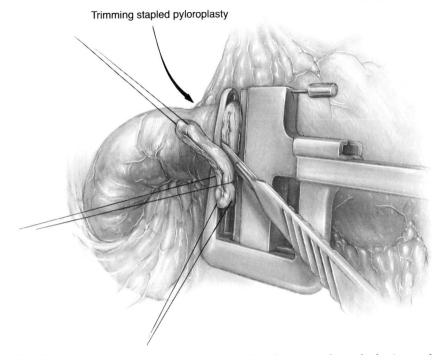

Trimming stapled pyloroplasty

FIGURE 48–3. The traction sutures are used to align the tissue through the jaws of a PI 55 stapler. It is recommended that the 4.8-mm. staple cartridge be used. Care should be taken to include the entire thickness of the stomach and duodenum prior to firing the stapler. After the instrument is fired, the excess tissue should be excised using a scalpel. Hemostasis should be obtained with the cautery prior to release of the instrument.

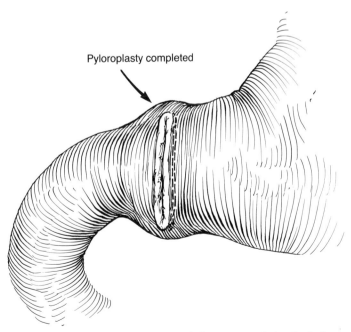

Pyloroplasty completed

FIGURE 48–4. The staple line should be carefully inspected for both hemostasis and integrity.

49

Finney Pyloroplasty

WILLIAM C. MEYERS, M.D.

The Finney pyloroplasty involves an extensive Kocher maneuver of the duodenum and a U-shaped, side-to-side gastroduodenostomy to include the pyloric muscle. Classically, as in the Heineke-Mikulicz pyloroplasty, the closure is also performed with a double-layer technique. However, the anastomosis is less complex using the GIA stapler, a single stab incision through the pylorus, and the TA-55 suture for closure of the defect with appropriate retraction sutures.

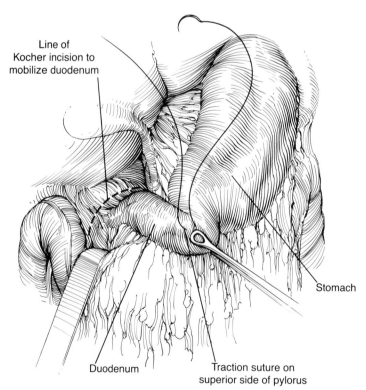

Line of
Kocher incision to
mobilize duodenum

Stomach

Duodenum

Traction suture on
superior side of pylorus

FIGURE 49–1. The Kocher maneuver is performed to mobilize the pyloric end of the stomach, the pylorus, and the first and second sections of the duodenum.

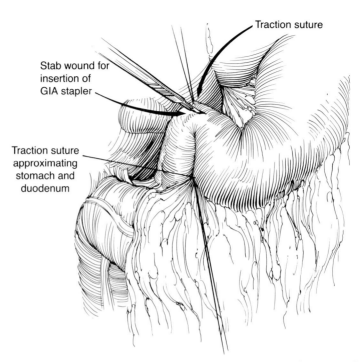

Traction suture

Stab wound for insertion of GIA stapler

Traction suture approximating stomach and duodenum

FIGURE 49–2. After traction sutures are placed approximating the stomach and duodenum, a stab incision is made into the stomach from just above the traction suture through the pylorus and into the duodenal wall.

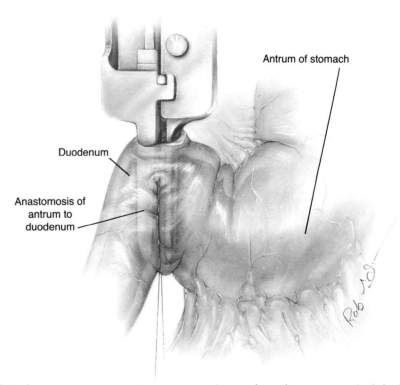

Antrum of stomach

Duodenum

Anastomosis of antrum to duodenum

FIGURE 49–3. After the GIA stapler is positioned to perform the anastomosis, it is closed and fired.

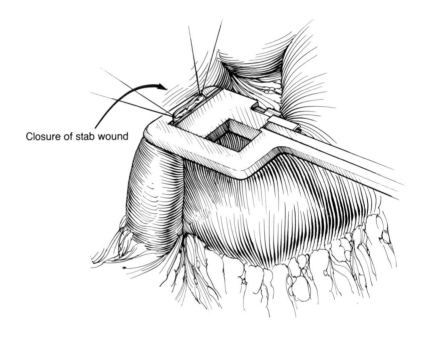

Closure of stab wound

FIGURE 49–4. It is quite important to inspect the mucosa for hemostasis prior to TA-55 closure. This is best done by using Army-Navy–type retractors and figure-of-eight 4–0 silk sutures as necessary.

50

Jaboulay Pyloroplasty

WILLIAM C. MEYERS, M.D.

The Jaboulay operation is actually not a pyloroplasty but rather a side-to-side gastroduodenostomy, usually used in the presence of marked inflammatory reaction or severe scarring and deformity of the duodenal side of the gastric outlet. An extensive Kocher maneuver is performed down to the third portion of the duodenum. The Jaboulay pyloroplasty can be performed with either the stapler or the hand-sewn technique. The hand-sewn technique is similar to that for other gastrointestinal anastomoses. Depicted is a two-layer technique with interrupted outer-layer silk sutures and running inner-layer chromic sutures. In this procedure, the pyloric wall is actually not incised.

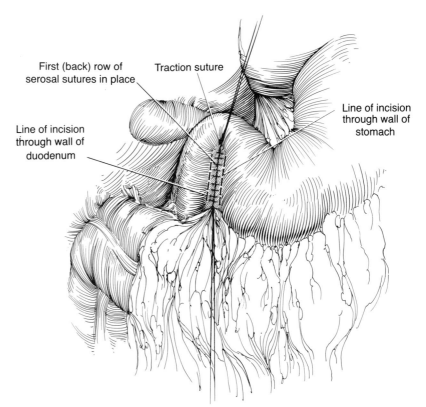

First (back) row of
serosal sutures in place

Traction suture

Line of incision
through wall of
stomach

Line of incision
through wall of
duodenum

FIGURE 50–1. After performance of a Kocher maneuver and placement of silk traction sutures, sutures should be placed approximating 6 to 8 cm. of duodenum and gastric wall. Incisions are made in the gastric wall and duodenal wall, leaving the pylorus intact.

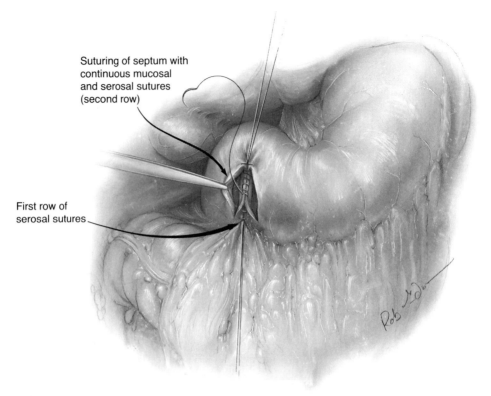

Suturing of septum with
continuous mucosal
and serosal sutures
(second row)

First row of
serosal sutures

FIGURE 50–2. The septum is sutured with an interrupted row of serosal silk sutures and a second row of continuous mucosal sutures.

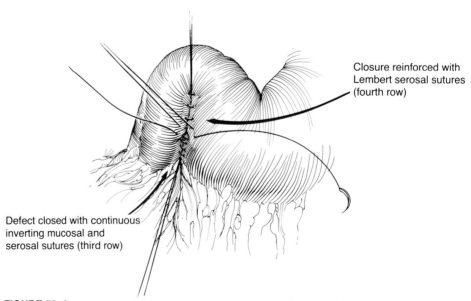

Closure reinforced with
Lembert serosal sutures
(fourth row)

Defect closed with continuous
inverting mucosal and
serosal sutures (third row)

FIGURE 50–3. The defect is closed with continuous inverting full-thickness sutures (third row) and reinforced with a fourth row of Lembert serosal sutures.

51

Gastric Resection: Billroth I Anastomosis

R. SCOTT JONES, M.D.

Either an upper abdominal midline or a bilateral subcostal incision provides good exposure for gastrectomy. Because of greater convenience, less trauma, reduced blood loss, and ease of closure, a midline incision extending from the xiphoid process to the umbilicus or to a point 2 to 3 cm. inferior to the umbilicus is preferred. After the abdomen has been entered, its contents should be examined carefully, with special attention given to the stomach and duodenum. The pylorus and duodenum must be assessed for evidence of edema and scarring, and complete circumferential evaluation of the first part of the duodenum should follow mobilization of the distal stomach. Duodenal edema, shortening, or deformity may prevent use of the duodenum for an anastomosis. When severe duodenal disease is present, a procedure other than gastrectomy should be used.

Splenic injury is a preventable complication during any upper abdominal operation, including gastrectomy. Particular attention should be given to the spleen and its relationship to the stomach to avoid splenic injury.

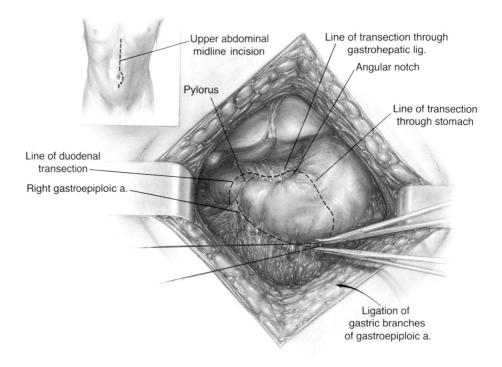

Upper abdominal midline incision

Line of transection through gastrohepatic lig.

Angular notch

Pylorus

Line of transection through stomach

Line of duodenal transection

Right gastroepiploic a.

Ligation of gastric branches of gastroepiploic a.

FIGURE 51–1. The gastrocolic ligament is detached from the greater curvature of the stomach. Beginning this step in the vicinity of the area selected for gastric transection allows easier entry into the lesser peritoneal sac. With dissection proceeding from left to right, hemostats are used to dissect and clamp the branches of the gastroepiploic vessels between their origin and their point of entry into the stomach. After the gastroepiploic branches to the stomach are transected, they are ligated with nonabsorbable material, taking care to avoid injury to the stomach, transverse colon, and transverse mesocolon.

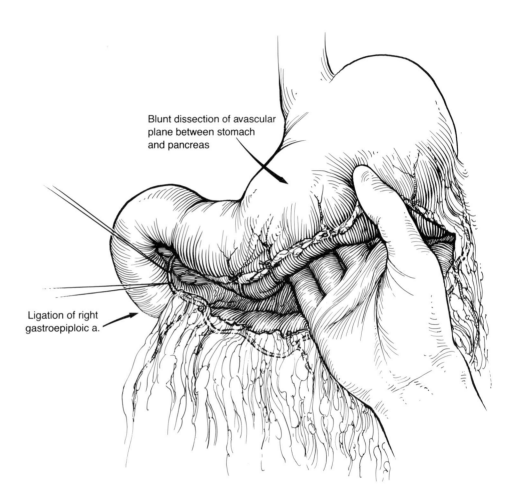

Blunt dissection of avascular
plane between stomach
and pancreas

Ligation of right
gastroepiploic a.

FIGURE 51–2. As this dissection proceeds, the posterior wall of the gastric antrum is separated from the anterior surface of the neck of the pancreas and from the base of the transverse mesocolon. After initial division of peritoneal attachments, an areolar plane permits a bloodless and easy mobilization of the distal stomach. During mobilization of the inferior portion of the distal stomach, the right gastroepiploic vessels are identified, dissected, and transected between clamps; their ends are secured with ligatures and suture ligatures.

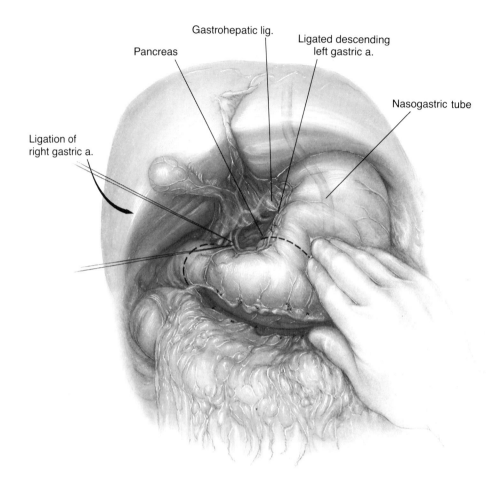

Gastrohepatic lig.

Pancreas

Ligated descending
left gastric a.

Nasogastric tube

Ligation of
right gastric a.

FIGURE 51–3. The stomach is gently retracted inferiorly and to the patient's left, and the lateral segment of the left lobe of the liver is lifted anteriorly and superiorly to expose the gastrohepatic ligament. Even obese patients have a relatively avascular and accessible area in the gastrohepatic ligament that may be divided easily to permit mobilization of the lesser curvature of the stomach. The hepatic branches of the right vagus nerve may be seen coursing through the gastrohepatic ligament anterior to the caudate lobe (segment I) of the liver. The gastrocolic ligament can be divided inferiorly to a point opposite the pylorus and proximally to a point to the right of the cardia. About 15 per cent of patients have either a replaced or an accessory left hepatic artery arising from the left gastric artery that passes into the liver through the gastrohepatic ligament. These vessels can remain undisturbed during an antrectomy. During an antrectomy for duodenal ulcer, the left gastric artery does not need to be divided; however, its descending branch must be dissected for transection along the lesser curvature of the stomach. The pyloric gland area of the stomach, or the antrum containing the mucosa which secretes gastrin, composes about 25 per cent of the distalmost gastric mucosa. The pyloric gland area usually extends a few centimeters more proximal on the lesser curvature than on the greater curvature. The objective in performing an antrectomy is to remove the gastrin-secreting mucosa. A 50 per cent distal gastrectomy usually accomplishes this goal from the practical or therapeutic standpoint. Therefore, the stomach should be transected at, or slightly proximal to, the incisura angularis. Hemostats are used to dissect, divide, and ligate the descending branches of the left gastric vessels along the lesser curvature at a point to permit removal of the antrum. This dissection should expose enough of the serosal surface of the lesser curvature (2 to 3 cm.) to allow easy closure of the distal stomach.

By retracting the distal stomach slightly inferiorly, the area in which the right gastric artery approaches the stomach can be examined. The right gastric artery is now dissected, ligated, and divided.

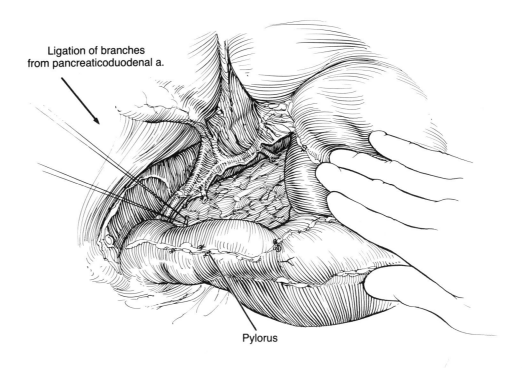

Ligation of branches
from pancreaticoduodenal a.

Pylorus

FIGURE 51–4. The first portion of the duodenum is inspected circumferentially to evaluate the degree of edema or scarring. Severe edema, shortening, and deformity are indications to avoid gastrectomy, particularly a Billroth I, and to choose another procedure, such as a vagotomy and pyloroplasty or a vagotomy and gastroenterostomy. If the decision is to proceed with a gastrectomy, about 3 cm. of duodenum is mobilized. The distance on the posterior medial wall of the duodenum between the pylorus and the pancreas determines the amount of duodenum available for constructing the gastroduodenostomy. A small hemostat is used to dissect the several small vessels going into the duodenum for ligation and transection, avoiding injury to the pancreas.

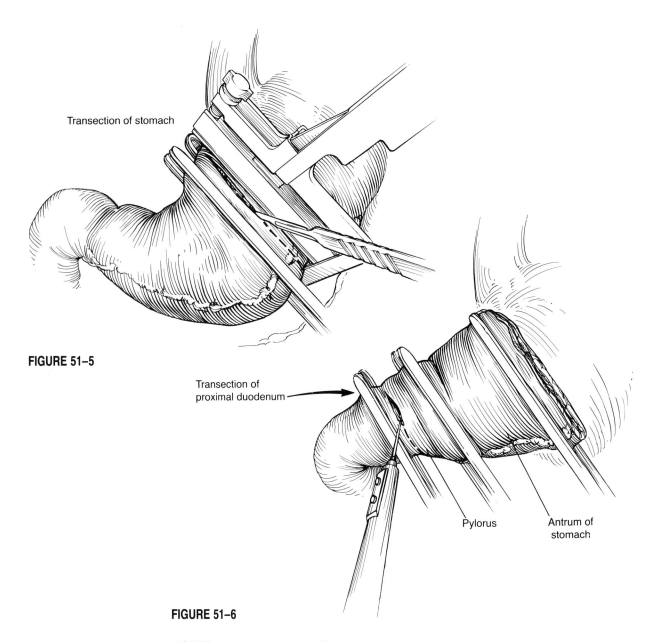

Transection of stomach

FIGURE 51–5

Transection of
proximal duodenum →

Pylorus   Antrum of
                 stomach

FIGURE 51–6

FIGURE 51–5. A 90-mm. stapler is placed on the stomach at the site selected for transection. This should allow removal of all of the antrum by including the incisura angularis. Before applying the stapler, position of the nasogastric tube is verified to avoid including it in the closure. The stapler is closed on the stomach, and staples are applied. The stomach is clamped with a Payr clamp distal to the stapler, and a scalpel is used to transect the stomach by cutting the stomach as close as possible to the stapler. The stapler is loosened from the stomach and removed from the field.

FIGURE 51–6. The distal portion of the transected stomach is held anteriorly to position the duodenum for clamping and transection, and a clamp is placed on the duodenum immediately distal to the pylorus. A small Payr clamp is then placed on, or just proximal to, the pylorus. The duodenum is divided as close as possible to the proximal side of the distal clamp, and the gastric specimen is removed from the field. Division of the duodenum immediately distal to the pylorus using electrocoagulation provides an alternative method for preparing the duodenum for anastomosis.

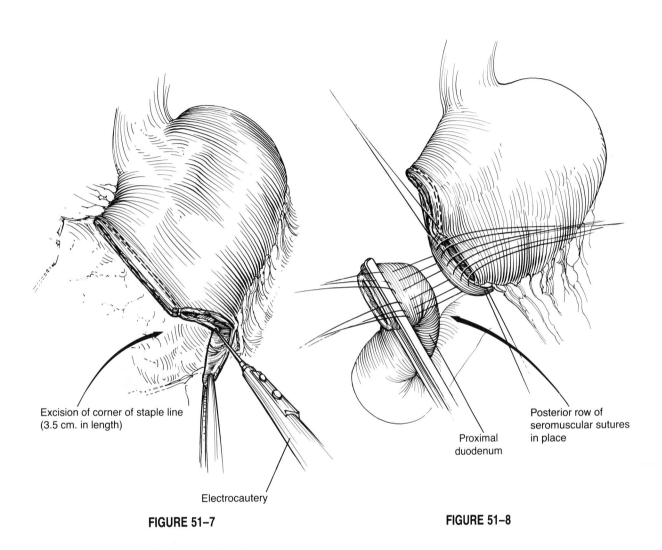

Excision of corner of staple line
(3.5 cm. in length)

Electrocautery

FIGURE 51–7

Proximal
duodenum

Posterior row of
seromuscular sutures
in place

FIGURE 51–8

FIGURE 51–7. With electrocoagulation, approximately 3.5 cm. of the staple line is excised from the greater curvature side of the distal stomach.

FIGURE 51–8. A posterior row of interrupted 4–0 nonabsorbable seromuscular sutures is placed to approximate the opened portion of the stomach to the duodenum. The sutures should be 3 to 4 mm. distal to the duodenal clamp and 3 to 4 mm. proximal to the edge of the opened stomach. The duodenal clamp is removed before tying the sutures.

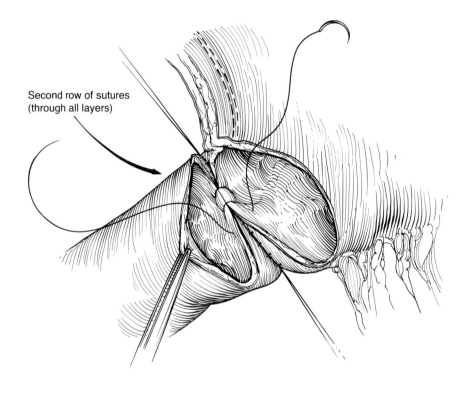

Second row of sutures
(through all layers)

FIGURE 51–9. Beginning at the midpoint, a back row of interrupted nonabsorbable sutures is placed through all layers of the stomach and duodenum.

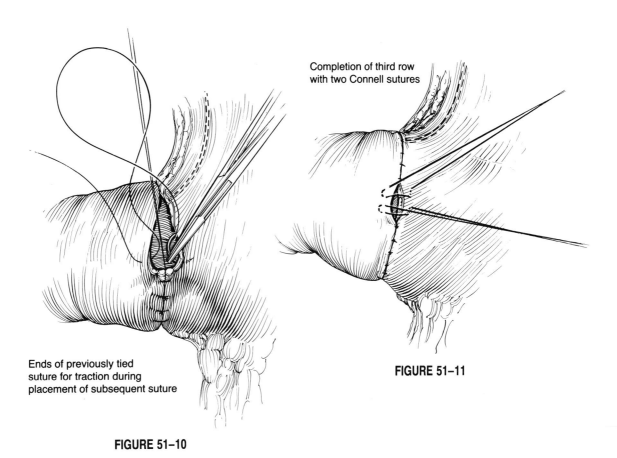

Completion of third row
with two Connell sutures

Ends of previously tied
suture for traction during
placement of subsequent suture

FIGURE 51–11

FIGURE 51–10

FIGURE 51–10. The suture line is continued around each corner of the anastomosis and is placed so that the knots remain on the luminal side.

FIGURE 51–11. The anterior layer of the anastomosis is completed by placing two interrupted Connell sutures, but they are not tied until both sutures have been placed.

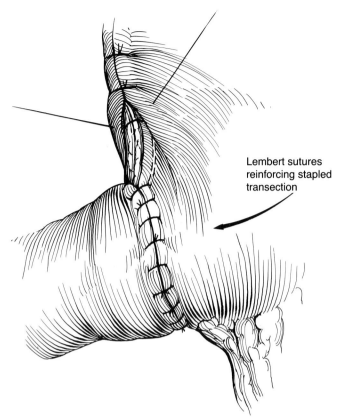

Lembert sutures
reinforcing stapled
transection

FIGURE 51–12. The closure of the lesser curvature of the stomach is completed with a layer of interrupted seromuscular Lembert sutures.

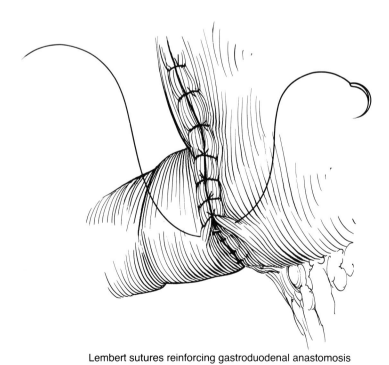

Lembert sutures reinforcing gastroduodenal anastomosis

FIGURE 51–13. Placement of an anterior layer of interrupted seromuscular sutures of nonabsorbable material completes the gastroduodenostomy.

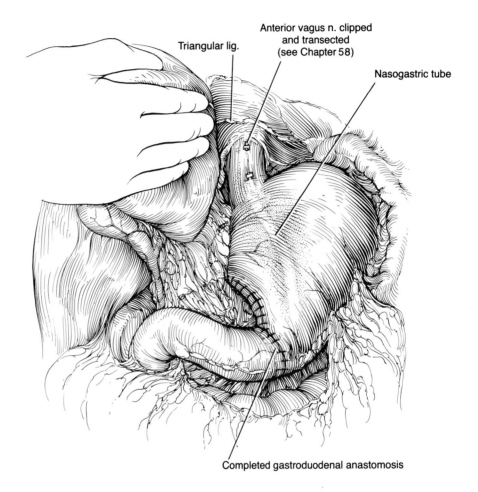

Triangular lig.

Anterior vagus n. clipped
and transected
(see Chapter 58)

Nasogastric tube

Completed gastroduodenal anastomosis

FIGURE 51–14. After completion of the gastrectomy, the nasogastric tube is positioned with the tip 2 cm. proximal to the anastomosis. In operations for duodenal ulcer, a vagotomy is performed. In this situation, a truncal vagotomy usually accompanies the gastrectomy. In a truncal vagotomy, the triangular ligament is incised to permit retraction of the lateral segment of the left lobe of the liver toward the patient's right. The peritoneum is incised over the abdominal esophagus at the level of the esophageal hiatus, and the esophagus is dissected and encircled with fingers in the inferior portion of the posterior mediastinum. A Penrose drain is passed around the esophagus for traction, and the anterior and posterior vagal trunks are identified by palpation. The anterior vagal trunk is then dissected. With the use of an index finger, the anterior vagus nerve is clamped; a 1- to 2-cm. portion of the nerve from between the silver clips applied to the nerve trunk is excised. The posterior vagus nerve is then dissected and held with a clamp to apply the silver clips. The 1- to 2-cm. portion between the clips is then excised.

The operative site is inspected for bleeding, and all laparotomy pads and instruments are removed from the abdomen before the incision is closed.

52

Gastric Resection: Billroth I Anastomosis

(STAPLER)

HILLIARD F. SEIGLER, M.D.

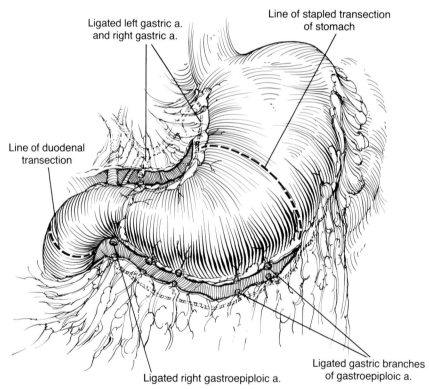

Ligated left gastric a.
and right gastric a.

Line of stapled transection
of stomach

Line of duodenal
transection

Ligated gastric branches
of gastroepiploic a.

Ligated right gastroepiploic a.

FIGURE 52–1. The portion of stomach to be removed is isolated by initially dividing the branches of the right and left gastroepiploic vessels using either a clamping and tying technique or the LDS stapler. The vessels and soft tissues selected for division are placed within the jaws of the LDS, and the instrument is fired. Careful observation must be used to be certain that hemostasis is complete. This permits entry into the lesser sac, and the avascular plane between the stomach, duodenum, and pancreas can be sharply dissected. The lesser omentum can be divided using the same technique. Care must be taken to preserve the middle colic artery and its branches. A standard Kocher maneuver should be performed, and this permits adequate exposure of the first portion of the duodenum. The line for gastric and duodenal division is selected.

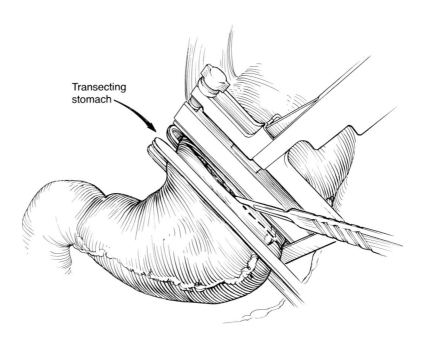

Transecting
stomach

FIGURE 52–2. Division of the stomach should be accomplished first by placing and firing the 90-mm. stapler loaded with 4.5-mm. staples. The distal stomach should be clamped with a Kocher clamp.

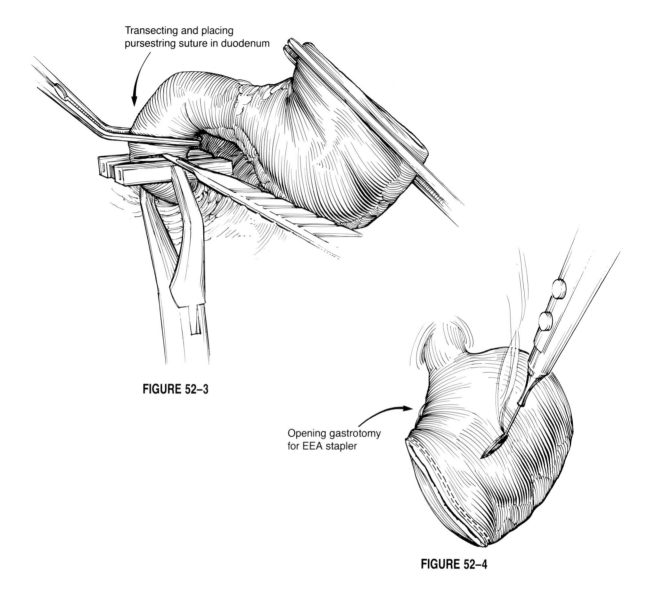

Transecting and placing pursestring suture in duodenum

FIGURE 52–3

Opening gastrotomy for EEA stapler

FIGURE 52–4

FIGURE 52–3. A Dennis clamp can be placed across the proximal duodenum, and the pursestring device can be placed at the selected site of duodenal division.

FIGURE 52–4. A gastrotomy is made with the cautery on the anterior surface of the stomach, carefully avoiding large vascular arcades. This should be done at least 3 cm. proximal to the row of staples. The gastrotomy should be large enough to accommodate the end-to-end stapling device easily.

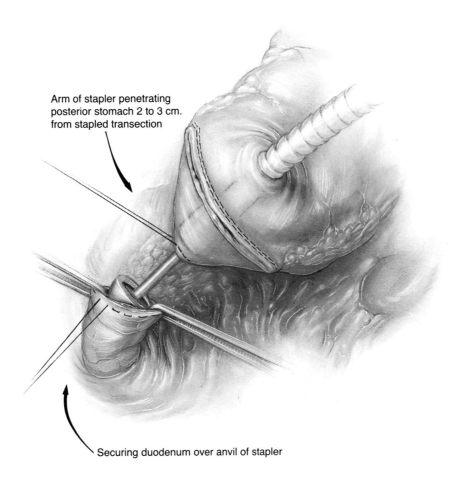

Arm of stapler penetrating
posterior stomach 2 to 3 cm.
from stapled transection

Securing duodenum over anvil of stapler

FIGURE 52–5. The gastrotomy edges should be grasped with two Babcock clamps; and the end-to-end stapling device, minus the anvil, should be passed into the lumen of the stomach. The center rod should be gently pressed against the posterior wall of the stomach approximately 4 cm. from the gastric staple line, and cautery should be used to permit passage of the rod through the posterior wall of the stomach. A pursestring suture will ensure that the stomach does not tear at the site of center rod penetration. The selected anvil size should be applied, and the open end of the duodenum should be grasped with Allis clamps. The duodenal wall should be gently pulled over the anvil, and the pursestring suture should be snugly tied around the center rod.

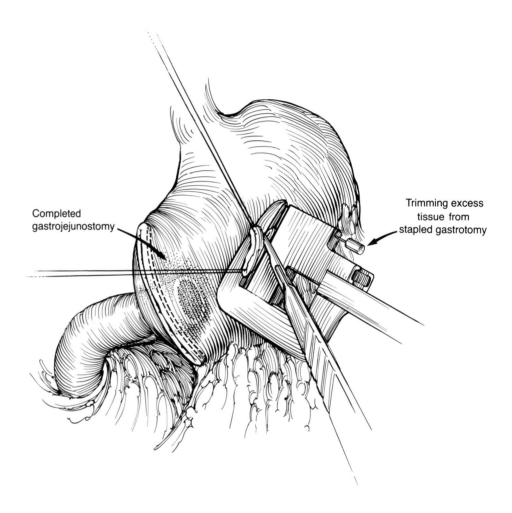

Completed
gastrojejunostomy

Trimming excess
tissue from
stapled gastrotomy

FIGURE 52–6. The cartridge and the anvil should then be approximated, being certain that no extraneous tissues are caught between the anvil and the circular cartridge. The instrument should be fired, and the anastomosis should then be carefully observed by direct visualization to ensure that hemostasis is adequate. The surgeon should then remove the anvil and check the circular tissue from both the duodenum and the stomach to be certain that the tissue doughnuts are intact. If the doughnuts are defective, external Lembert sutures will need to be applied to secure a complete anastomosis. The gastrotomy is closed by grasping each end with Allis clamps and incorporating the entire thickness of the stomach wall through the jaws of the 55-mm. stapler.

53

Gastric Resection: Billroth II

R. SCOTT JONES, M.D.

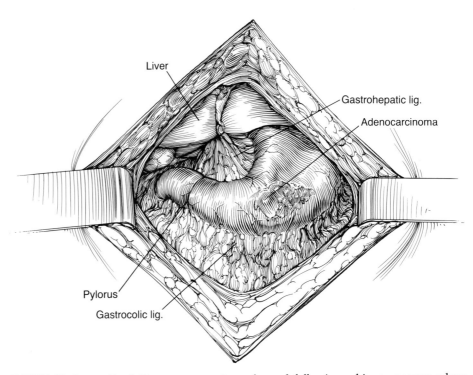

Liver

Gastrohepatic lig.

Adenocarcinoma

Pylorus

Gastrocolic lig.

FIGURE 53–1. A Billroth II gastrectomy is performed following a biopsy-proven adenocarcinoma located in the midportion of the stomach that is confined to the stomach and has no associated palpable cancer in the lymph nodes. After the peritoneal cavity is opened and entered, the abdominal contents and especially the stomach are examined carefully.

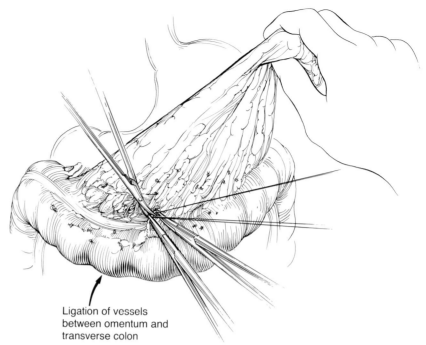

Ligation of vessels
between omentum and
transverse colon

FIGURE 53–2. The greater omentum is identified and retracted anteriorly and superiorly to expose the transverse colon. The transverse colon is retracted inferiorly, and the site where the omentum approximates the colon is identified. Electrocoagulation is used to detach the greater omentum from the transverse colon, allowing access to the lesser peritoneal cavity. The omentum is left attached to the stomach and removed as part of the specimen.

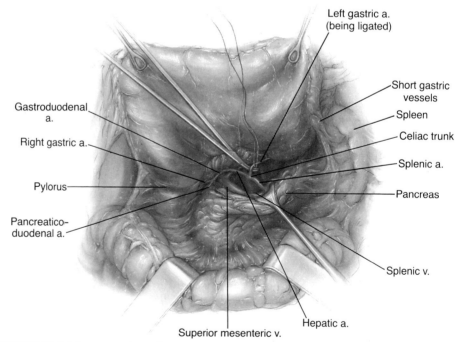

Left gastric a.
(being ligated)

Short gastric
vessels

Spleen

Celiac trunk

Splenic a.

Pancreas

Gastroduodenal
a.

Right gastric a.

Pylorus

Pancreatico-
duodenal a.

Splenic v.

Hepatic a.

Superior mesenteric v.

FIGURE 53–3. The stomach is lifted anteriorly to expose the peritoneum over the pancreas, and the peritoneum is incised over the superior aspect of the pancreas. Maximal exposure is gained for this step by placing the patient in a slight reversed Trendelenburg position. The pancreas is retracted inferiorly, and the celiac axis is dissected. The lymph nodes are then mobilized for inclusion in the specimen. The left gastric artery and its origin from the celiac are identified, and the artery is doubly ligated, suture-ligated, and divided. The left gastric vein is also ligated and divided. This permits removal of the left gastric vessels and associated lymph nodes.

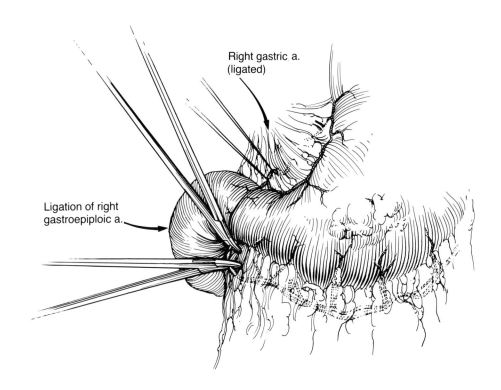

Right gastric a.
(ligated)

Ligation of right
gastroepiploic a.

FIGURE 53–4. The filmy gastrohepatic ligament is divided to facilitate mobilization of the lesser curvature. The stomach is retracted inferiorly and to the right to approach the right gastric artery. The right gastric artery is dissected, ligated, and divided. Attention is then returned to the inferior aspect of the antrum to identify the right gastroepiploic vessels, which are dissected, divided between clamps, and ligated.

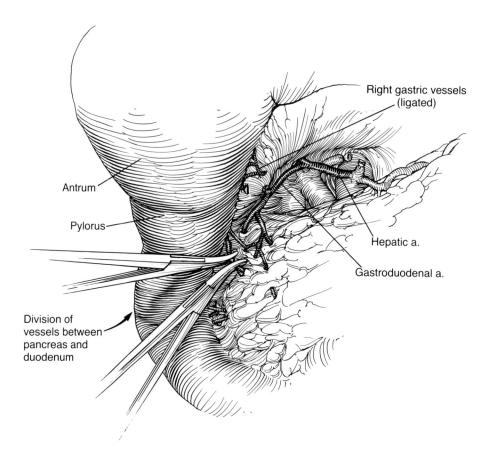

Right gastric vessels
(ligated)

Antrum

Pylorus

Hepatic a.

Gastroduodenal a.

Division of
vessels between
pancreas and
duodenum

FIGURE 53–5. The stomach is lifted anteriorly to expose the dorsal wall of the duodenum. The areolar tissue is divided, and a hemostat is used to dissect several of the small vessels between the duodenum and the pancreas. To facilitate safe closure of the duodenum, approximately 3 cm. of the first portion of the duodenum distal to the pylorus should be obtained. Care should be taken during this dissection to avoid injury to the pancreas.

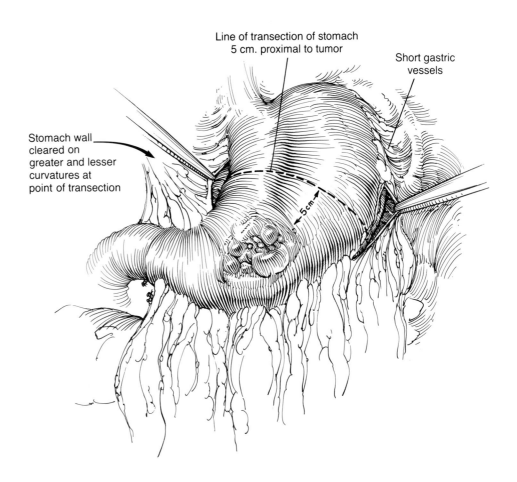

Line of transection of stomach
5 cm. proximal to tumor

Short gastric
vessels

Stomach wall
cleared on
greater and lesser
curvatures at
point of transection

5 cm

FIGURE 53–6. With attention returned to the greater curvature of the stomach, tumor location needs to be assessed in order to select a site for transecting the stomach. For a midgastric tumor, a 75 per cent gastrectomy is performed to provide at least a 5-cm. margin proximal to the gross tumor. This usually requires dissection up to a point just distal to the most inferior short gastric vessels. A site is prepared on the greater and lesser curvatures for transection of the stomach by freeing 1 to 2 cm. of the stomach wall.

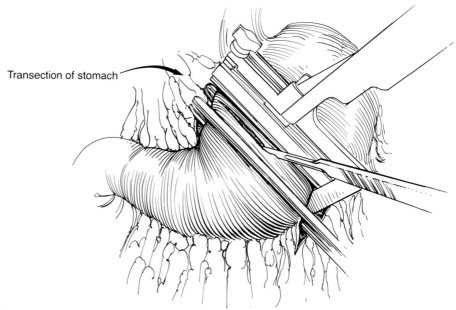

Transection of stomach

FIGURE 53–7. The nasogastric tube is placed so that its tip resides proximal to the proposed gastric transection site. After the stapler is placed across the stomach, a pin inserted into the stapler, and the stomach aligned carefully in the stapler, the stapler is closed on the stomach and staples are applied. A large Payr clamp is then placed across the stomach distal to the stapler, and a scalpel is used to transect the stomach adjacent to the stapler on the distal side.

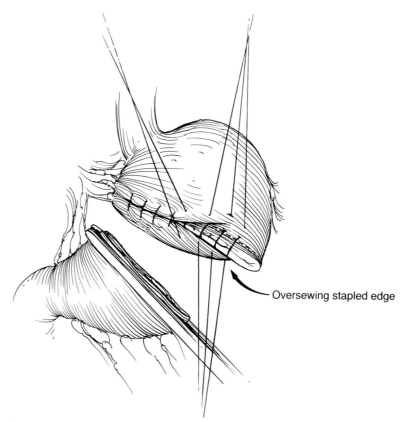

Oversewing stapled edge

FIGURE 53–8. A row of interrupted seromuscular Lembert sutures is placed to invert the row of staples in the distal stomach.

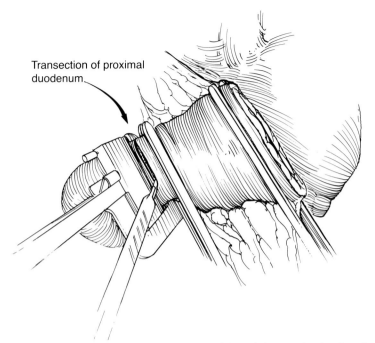

Transection of proximal
duodenum

FIGURE 53–9. The distal stomach is lifted anteriorly, and the stapler is placed across the duodenum just distal to the pylorus. A pin is inserted into the stapler, and staples are applied. Either a small Payr clamp or a large Kocher clamp is placed across the pylorus just proximal to the stapler. A scalpel is used to transect the duodenum adjacent to the proximal side of the stapler.

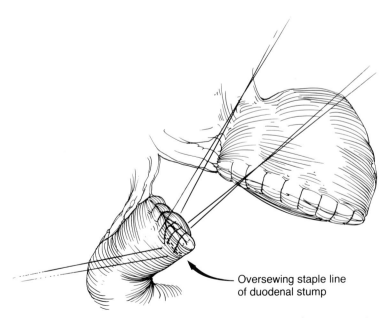

Oversewing staple line
of duodenal stump

FIGURE 53–10. The staple line is reinforced with a row of interrupted seromuscular Lembert sutures.

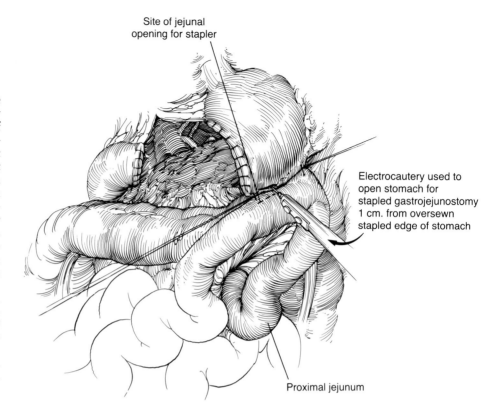

FIGURE 53–11. The transverse colon is retracted anteriorly to expose the ligament of Treitz, and the proximal jejunum is identified. A short loop of jejunum is brought anterior to the colon in an isoperistaltic fashion; with electrocoagulation, an opening is made in the greater curvature side of the stomach 1 cm. proximal to the closure of the end of the stomach in order to admit entry of one tip of a side-to-side stapler. The stapler is assembled and positioned to approximate the antemesenteric border of the jejunum to the greater curvature of the stomach. Care is taken to avoid interposing tissue between the jejunum and the stomach.

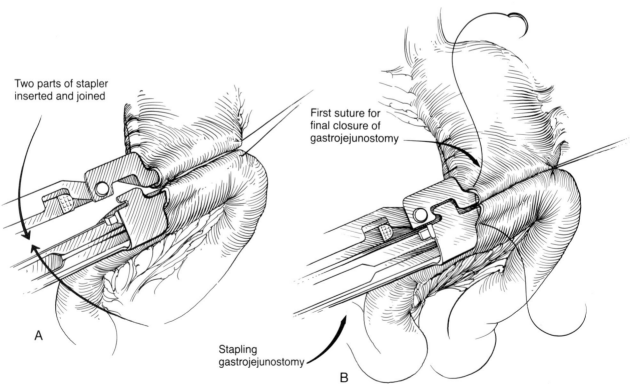

FIGURE 53–12. *A,* The stapler is clamped, and the staples are applied. *B,* Before removal of the stapler, nonabsorbable sutures are placed on either side of the stapler as corner stitches to begin closure of the defect left by the stapler. The stapler is removed.

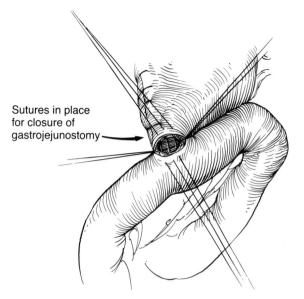

FIGURE 53–13. The previously placed corner stitches are used for retraction, and the luminal aspect of the staple line is inspected for hemostasis. Bleeding points are secured with sutures, and the stapler defect is closed with interrupted through-and-through sutures.

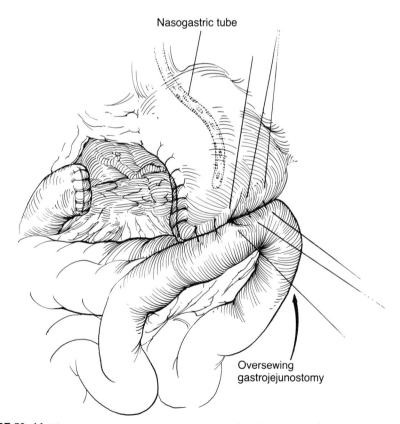

FIGURE 53–14. The gastroenterostomy is completed with a layer of interrupted seromuscular Lembert sutures. The tip of the nasogastric tube is positioned 2 cm. proximal to the anastomosis. The operative site is inspected for bleeding, all sponges and instruments are removed from the abdomen, and the incision is closed.

54

Repair of Hiatal Hernia (NISSEN)

WILLIAM C. MEYERS, MD

The Nissen fundoplication procedure for correction of esophageal reflux should be simple and quick in most patients. In fact, if much dissection is performed, at least in a primary operation, the procedure is probably being performed improperly. The main indication for Nissen fundoplication in adults is reflux esophagitis refractory to medical therapy. The best results are obtained in the absence of a pre-existing stricture, although most minor esophageal strictures are dilated at the time of operation. The Nissen fundoplication can also be performed in conjunction with other stricture-relieving procedures. The following description applies primarily to the *first-time* antireflux procedure. For example, the incision might change if performed in conjunction with a cholecystectomy; and the technique is modified when a fundoplication is performed with a highly selective vagotomy.

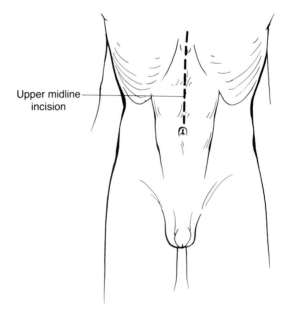

Upper midline
incision

FIGURE 54–1. The Nissen fundoplication is performed through an upper midline incision that extends superiorly, usually along the xiphoid process, and ends just above the umbilicus. Extension of the incision below the umbilicus prevents retraction of the transverse colon by the anterior abdominal wall. The lateral segment of the liver is mobilized and usually folds easily beneath a Mikulicz pad and a Deaver retractor. The thin anterior esophageal peritoneum is incised sharply. If the esophagus lies high in the chest, obscuring its visualization, the peritoneal incision is made along the crural edge; the stomach and esophagus are reduced prior to attempting encirclement of the esophagus. Most hiatal hernias are easily reduced, even when esophageal shortening is evident on the preoperative barium swallow.

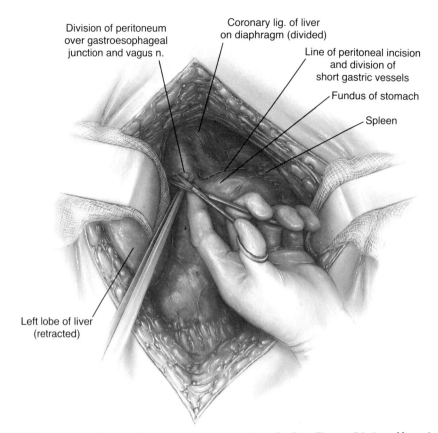

Division of peritoneum over gastroesophageal junction and vagus n.

Coronary lig. of liver on diaphragm (divided)

Line of peritoneal incision and division of short gastric vessels

Fundus of stomach

Spleen

Left lobe of liver (retracted)

FIGURE 54–2. After the preliminary maneuvers described in Figure 54–1, self-retaining retractors are inserted, usually in combination with a Deaver retractor. An upperhand or Elmed retractor elevates the sternum 5 to 6 cm. superiorly, and a Balfour retractor further supplements the exposure. When performed by an experienced surgeon, this incision and exposure are expeditious and greatly facilitate the next steps of the procedure.

FIGURES 54–3 and 54–4. The distal esophagus is bluntly but gently encircled. A plane should easily be found around the esophagus anterior to the aorta. If necessary, this plane can be found by blunt dissection higher into the mediastinum. This important maneuver can avoid blunt penetration of the esophagus or stomach in the presence of large hiatal hernias. Prior to or during this maneuver, a nasogastric tube and a Maloney dilator are placed into the stomach. One needs to palpate the tube entering the stomach in order to avoid perforation of the esophagus. Usually, a No. 18 Salem sump nasogastric tube with a No. 28 to No. 40 Maloney dilator is preferred. The purpose of placing two tubes is to hold the nasogastric tube in place after the repair is completed and the dilator is removed. The purpose of placement of these tubes is to prevent a wrap that is too tight. Two fingers are placed behind the esophagus, and an umbilical tape should be easily passed to encircle the esophagus and should be essentially bloodless. The purpose of the umbilical tape is to provide downward traction for the subsequent procedure. A 6- to 7-cm. length of distal esophagus is easily dissected bluntly, and the position of each vagal trunk is noted. The anterior (left) vagus is generally more intimately attached to the esophageal wall and, because of its position, is at risk of entrapment by the subsequent sutures.

Occasionally, several short gastric vessels are ligated and divided, as well as some thin peritoneal tissue medial and lateral to the esophagus. The dissection is directed toward delivering the esophagus inferiorly rather than dissecting along the lesser and greater curvatures of the stomach. The reason for this is that undissected perigastric tissue provides support for the subsequent wrap and prevents slippage. One cannot rely on identification of the gastroesophageal junction solely by the anatomic external branching of the vessels and nerves. The most reliable identification of the gastroesophageal junction is made endoscopically; but this is usually impractical at the time of operation, and one should veer on the superior side while placing the sutures.

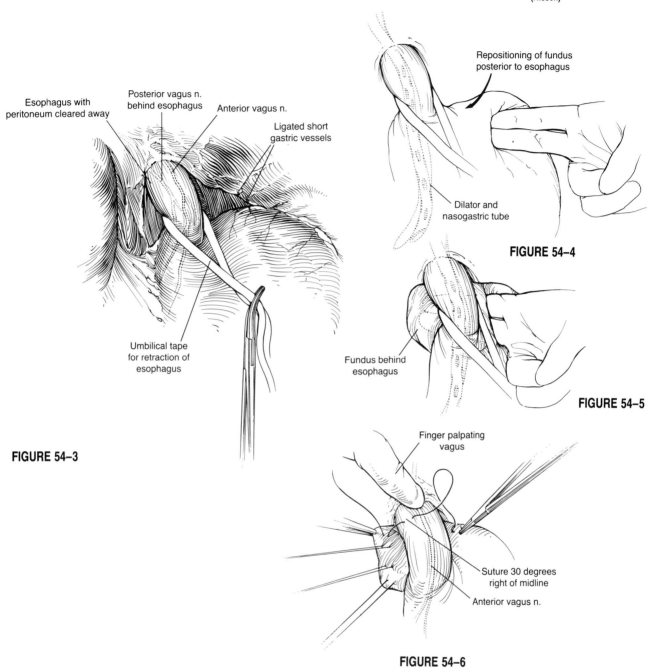

Esophagus with
peritoneum cleared away

Posterior vagus n.
behind esophagus

Anterior vagus n.

Ligated short
gastric vessels

Umbilical tape
for retraction of
esophagus

FIGURE 54-3

Repositioning of fundus
posterior to esophagus

Dilator and
nasogastric tube

FIGURE 54-4

Fundus behind
esophagus

FIGURE 54-5

Finger palpating
vagus

Suture 30 degrees
right of midline

Anterior vagus n.

FIGURE 54-6

FIGURES 54–5 and 54–6. With the distal esophagus retracted inferiorly, the gastric fundus is easily retracted posterior to the esophagus and a portion of fundus is engaged with Babcock forceps. A short wrap is performed consisting of about four sutures placed 1 cm. apart and incorporating a small site of esophageal wall. The sutures approximate the fundus to itself anteriorly and posteriorly to the esophagus. The position of the vagus nerves is noted to avoid their entrapment. The sutures should be cut *without* tension, providing a loose ("floppy") wrap. If the suture approximation appears too tight, the most inferior sutures are released and additional sutures are replaced more superiorly. Almost any nonabsorbable suture can be used, although 2–0 or 3–0 silk on swaged-on needles is preferred. Pop-off needles disengage too easily prior to completion of placement of the sutures. The Maloney dilator is removed, leaving the nasogastric tube in place.

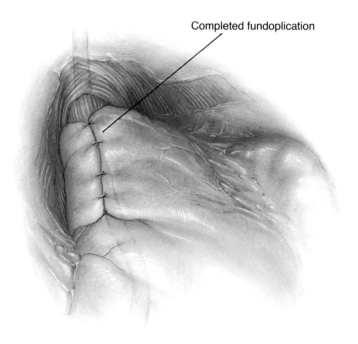

Completed fundoplication

FIGURE 54–7. The hiatal hernia defect can be reduced with additional sutures, but this is probably not an essential part of the procedure. The umbilical tape is removed; but if this is difficult, a tiny portion is left in to prevent disruption of the suture line. The field is inspected for hemostasis, the retractors and Mikulicz pads are removed, and the abdomen is closed.

55

Laparoscopic Nissen Fundoplication

THEODORE N. PAPPAS, M.D.

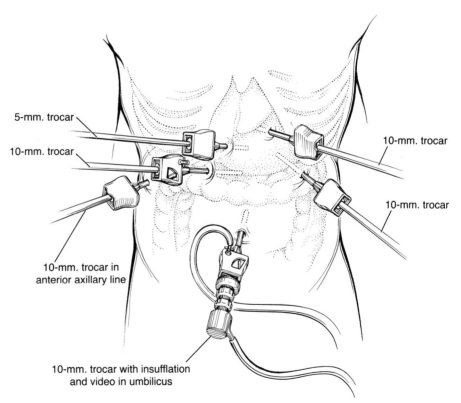

FIGURE 55–1. The appropriate placement of trocars is essential for laparoscopic Nissen fundoplication. The trocars should be placed high in the abdomen to allow adequate visualization of the hiatus. Six trocars are used, including a 10-mm. trocar at the umbilicus for the camera. A 10-mm. trocar in the left upper quadrant is necessary for placement of an Endo-Babcock clamp. A 10-mm. trocar is placed at the upper midline for an Endo-Retractor. Eventually, an Endo-Babcock is placed in the far right lateral aspect of the costal margin, and two trocars are placed in the right upper quadrant for placement of the suture. These trocars should be placed as high as possible to allow them to reach the hiatus on patients who are obese or have a broad abdomen.

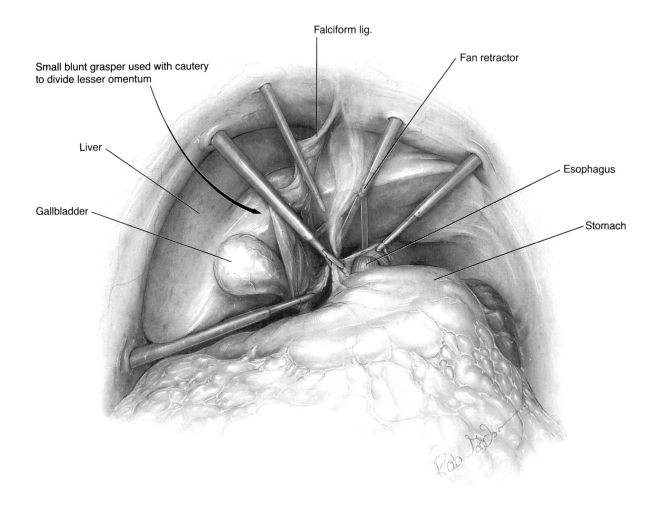

FIGURE 55–2. This illustration demonstrates the view as seen from the 10-mm. trocar at the umbilicus. The hiatus is being exposed, with the fan retractor lifting the left lobe of the liver upward. Dissection is performed by opening the gastrohepatic ligament with the cautery. Occasionally, a small accessory vessel to the left lobe of the liver is found and clipped. Once the hepatoduodenal ligament is opened, the crus of the diaphragm is mobilized from the gastroesophageal junction.

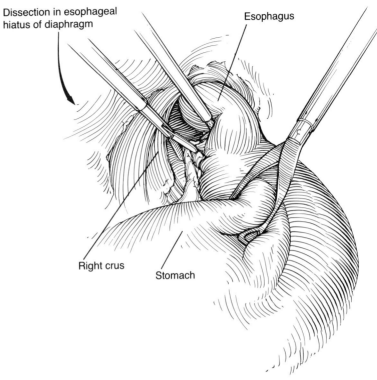

Dissection in esophageal
hiatus of diaphragm

Esophagus

Right crus

Stomach

FIGURE 55–3. Care is taken to accurately distinguish the crus from the esophagus which can be accomplished by moving a nasogastric tube in the esophagus while the gastroesophageal junction is viewed endoscopically. With the crus retracted to the patient's right and the esophagus retracted upward, the space behind the esophagus can be dissected under direct vision. Blind dissection should *not* be done.

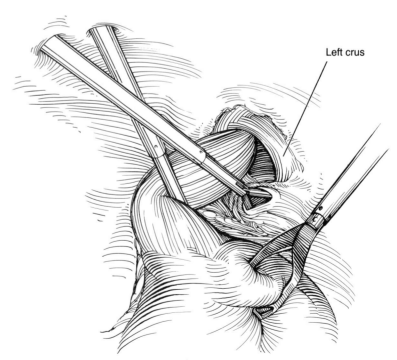

Left crus

FIGURE 55–4. The left crura are mobilized from the esophagus, and the space between this side of the esophagus and the crura is opened bluntly. Care is taken not to enter the left pleural space.

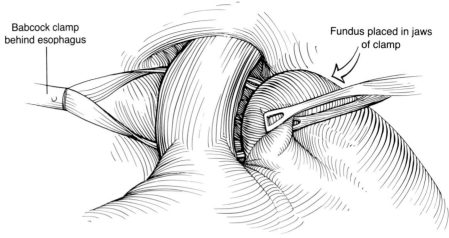

Babcock clamp
behind esophagus

Fundus placed in jaws
of clamp

FIGURE 55–5

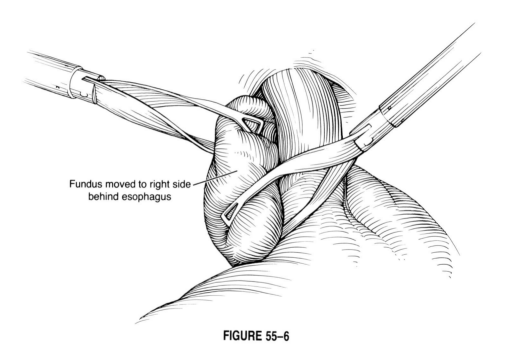

Fundus moved to right side
behind esophagus

FIGURE 55–6

FIGURES 55–5 and 55–6. An Endo-Babcock clamp is placed from the most lateral right trocar and is passed behind the gastroesophageal junction. Again, the placement of an Endo-Babcock in this area is done under direct vision. The Endo-Babcock is passed behind the gastroesophageal junction, and the fundus of the stomach is grasped and pulled behind it. At this point, the nasogastric tube is removed and a large dilator (58 or 60 French) is passed into the stomach to be certain that the wrap is not too tight.

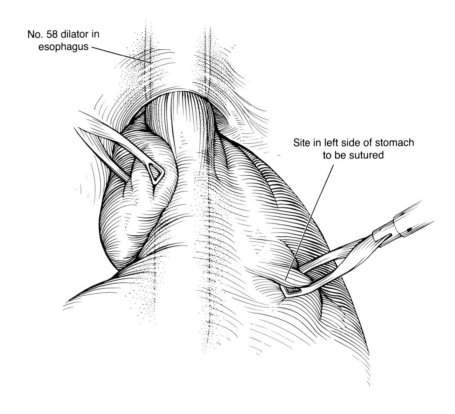

No. 58 dilator in
esophagus

Site in left side of stomach
to be sutured

FIGURE 55–7. The remainder of the fundus is brought up to the wrap in the usual manner, with certainty that the wrap is created with the same segment of stomach that was being passed around the back of the esophagus.

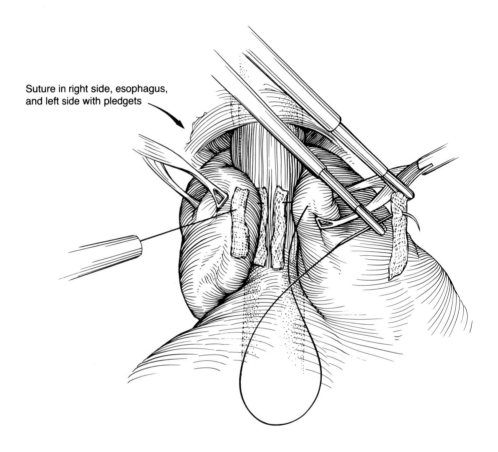

Suture in right side, esophagus, and left side with pledgets

FIGURE 55–8. Pledgets are passed into the abdomen, and a 1–0 suture is used to secure the wrap. This is done by placing four pledgets and suturing a pledget at each tissue interface. The suture is then brought back out through the trocar, and an extracorporeal knot is tied.

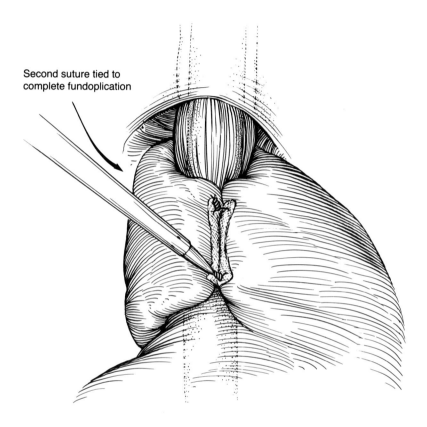

Second suture tied to
complete fundoplication

FIGURE 55–9. The second suture is placed and again tied extracorporeally on the outside. This leaves a wrap of approximately 2 cm. and, as stated above, is created over a large (58 or 60 French) bougie.

56

Total Gastrectomy

WILLIAM C. MEYERS, M.D.

Indications for total gastrectomy include primary gastric neoplasms, the Zollinger-Ellison syndrome, and *critical* surgical procedures for peptic ulcer disease. The degree of radicality of the procedure for gastric neoplasms varies considerably, according to the preference of the surgeon and the location and extent of the lesion. The procedure depicted in these illustrations was performed for a gastrinoma causing the Zollinger-Ellison syndrome. For this condition, the *entire* stomach is removed because it is the end organ for the associated peptic ulcer diasthesis. Therefore, a more radical procedure in regard to surrounding structures is not as necessary as might be indicated for an infiltrative neoplasm. For the latter, varying degrees of lymph node dissection and removal of the spleen and omentum may be appropriate.

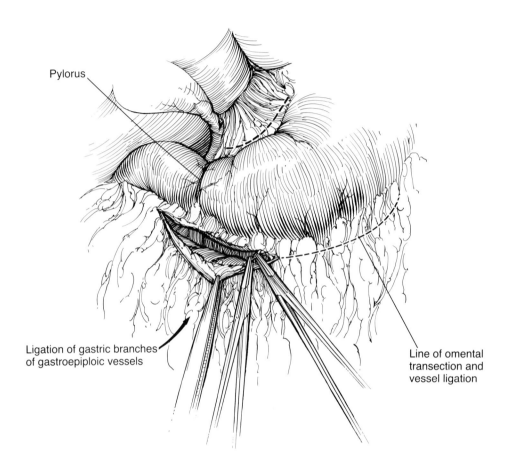

Pylorus

Ligation of gastric branches
of gastroepiploic vessels

Line of omental
transection and
vessel ligation

FIGURE 56–1. Total gastrectomy is performed through a generous upper midline incision. After thorough abdominal exploration, the stomach is closely inspected; if a tumor is present, its relationship to adjacent structures, e.g., pancreas, mesocolon, and major vessels, is determined. For gastrinoma, neoplastic involvement of the stomach is unlikely, in which case the lesser sac can usually be entered either below or above the stomach and both the greater and lesser curvatures can be mobilized. Any adhesions or peritoneal attachments to the pancreas and posterior peritoneum are divided to mobilize the entire stomach.

The stomach is devascularized, taking care to preserve the spleen. The best approach is usually to ligate the vessels of the greater curvature of gastroepiploic and inferior short gastrics first and to save the more difficult portion of the procedure, i.e., ligation of the short gastrics and diaphragmatic attachments, until later. The right and left gastric vessels are ligated and divided, usually with 2-0 silk suture ligatures. The gastric vessels are identified as two separate bundles, and the remainder of the attachments on the lesser curvature are relatively avascular.

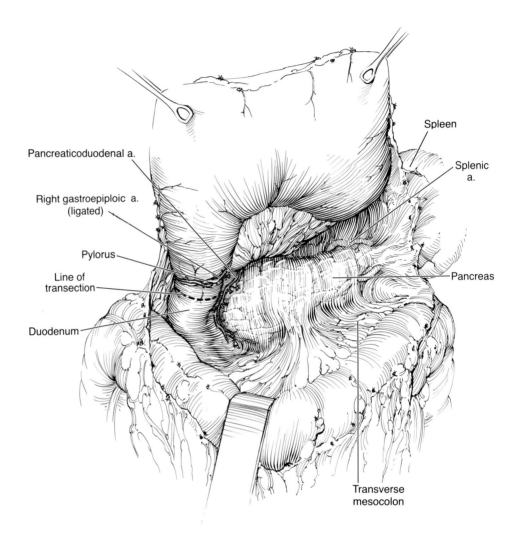

FIGURE 56–2. As the vessels are divided toward the duodenum, the right gastroepiploic artery emerges from the gastroduodenal artery in proximity to the anterosuperior pancreaticoduodenal arterial branches; this requires careful dissection. Bleeding from even a small branch in this region can obscure the anatomy and make subsequent dissection much more difficult. A small branch of the right gastric artery serving the pylorus often arises proximal to the previously ligated artery and should be ligated and divided. The dissection is extended to include at least a proximal centimeter of the duodenum. Usually, the portal triad does not require identification unless there is severe proximal duodenal peptic ulcer disease and contracture.

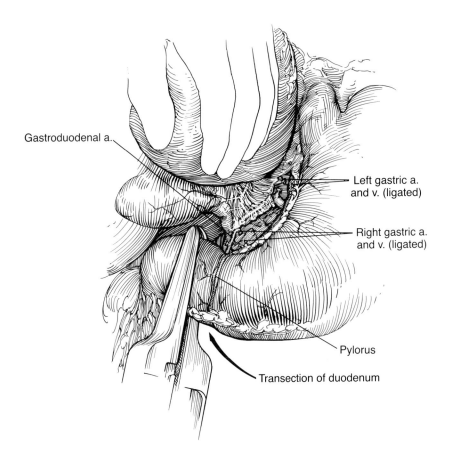

Gastroduodenal a.

Left gastric a.
and v. (ligated)

Right gastric a.
and v. (ligated)

Pylorus

Transection of duodenum

FIGURE 56–3. The duodenum is divided with the GIA stapler, making a clamp unnecessary on the proximal side. It is important to be certain that the nasogastric tube is sufficiently proximal so that it is not included in the GIA staple line. A similar maneuver is recommended when the distal esophagus is transected. Devascularization of the stomach is completed with transection of the stomach, permitting an easier dissection. Dissection of the high fundal vessels may be difficult and is facilitated by developing the angle of His, the vascular plane adjacent to the greater curvature of the gastroesophageal junction.

After completion of the devascularization, the stomach and esophagus are usually left attached until placement of the posterior row of the anastomosis has been completed. Generally, small vessels supplying the distal esophagus are divided prior to the anastomosis. It is not necessary to identify each vagal trunk because the esophageal transection provides an effective vagotomy.

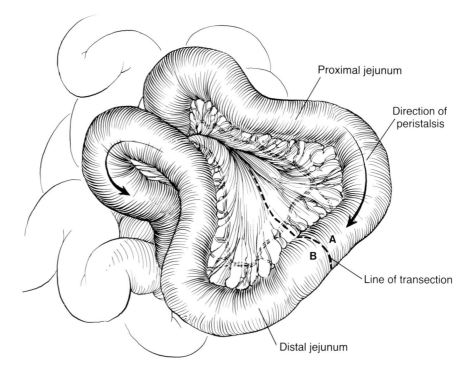

Proximal jejunum

Direction of
peristalsis

A

B

Line of transection

Distal jejunum

FIGURE 56–4. The easiest and probably best method of reconstructing esophagoenteric continuity is with a Roux-en-Y esophagojejunostomy. This method requires a minimum of 18 inches of a Roux loop in order to prevent bile reflux esophagitis. General aims in selecting the site of jejunal transection for the Roux-en-Y include an adequate length of jejunum to perform the anastomosis without tension. The transection is made as proximal as possible (toward the ligament of Treitz), and appropriate arcades on each side should be present to maintain the vascularity of both sides of the jejunum. The anastomosis can be made in either an antecolic or a retrocolic manner. The primary consideration is to select the route that causes the least tension. If either is appropriate, an antecolic anastomosis is generally preferred because of its simplicity. The ligament of Treitz is best identified by upward manual traction on the transverse colon. Operative lighting and exposure are adjusted for precise identification of the jejunal arcades. The jejunum is divided with the GIA stapler directed perpendicularly to prevent compromise of the blood supply on both sides. Additional length can usually be supplied by dividing the mesentery as long as at least one large arcade is preserved on each side. Additional relaxing incisions of other parts of the mesentery can also be helpful.

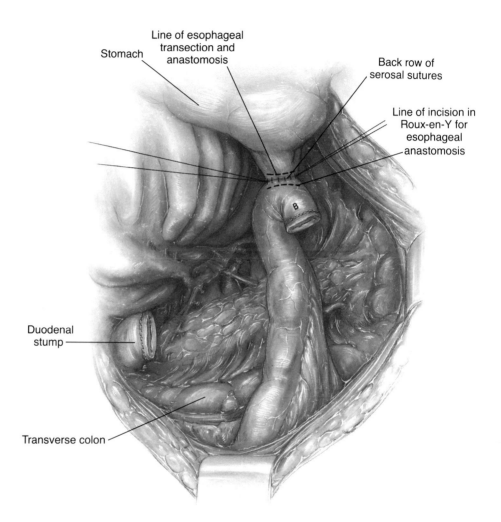

Stomach

Line of esophageal
transection and
anastomosis

Back row of
serosal sutures

Line of incision in
Roux-en-Y for
esophageal
anastomosis

Duodenal
stump

Transverse colon

FIGURE 56–5. To complete the Roux-en-Y reconstructive procedure, two anastomoses are necessary: the esophagojejunal anastomosis and an end-to-end jejunojejunal anastomosis.

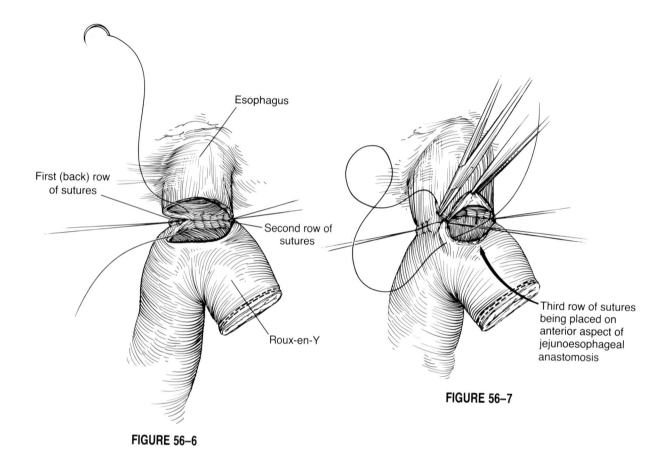

First (back) row
of sutures

Esophagus

Second row of
sutures

Roux-en-Y

FIGURE 56–6

Third row of sutures
being placed on
anterior aspect of
jejunoesophageal
anastomosis

FIGURE 56–7

FIGURES 56–6 and 56–7. The esophagojejunostomy is performed first. The preferred method of esophagojejunal anastomosis is by the hand-sewn, double-layer, interrupted, 3-0 silk suture technique. Both layers of the posterior row of sutures are placed prior to completing the transection of the esophagus. The nasogastric tube is placed through the anastomosis into the jejunal limb prior to placing the anterior row. The most important technical details of the double-layer, interrupted anastomosis are: (1) the posterior-row suture approximates serosa, muscularis, and submucosal layers but not the mucosa; (2) the end sutures are placed first; (3) the inner layers of sutures include the entire thickness of both the esophagus and the jejunum; and (4) luminal patency is best preserved by traction on the previously tied suture in a direction opposite that of the next suture.

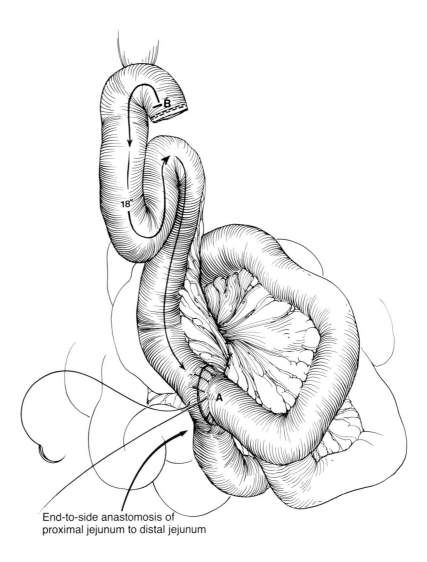

18"

B

A

End-to-side anastomosis of
proximal jejunum to distal jejunum

FIGURE 56–8. The jejunojejunostomy is performed either with a GIA–TA-55 stapler or by a hand-sewn double-layer technique.

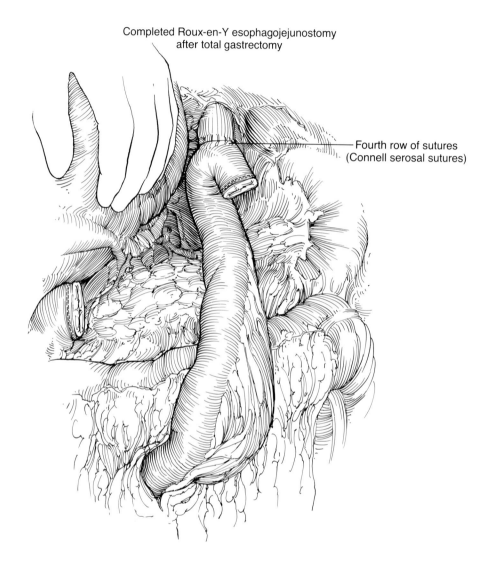

Completed Roux-en-Y esophagojejunostomy
after total gastrectomy

Fourth row of sutures
(Connell serosal sutures)

FIGURE 56–9. The hand-sewn anastomosis usually consists of interrupted sutures of 3-0 silk in the outer layer and running interlocking or Connell 3-0 chromic sutures for the inner layer. The mesenteric defect caused by the Roux-en-Y technique is closed to prevent herniation of the small bowel.

57

Total Gastrectomy (STAPLER)

HILLIARD F. SEIGLER, M.D.

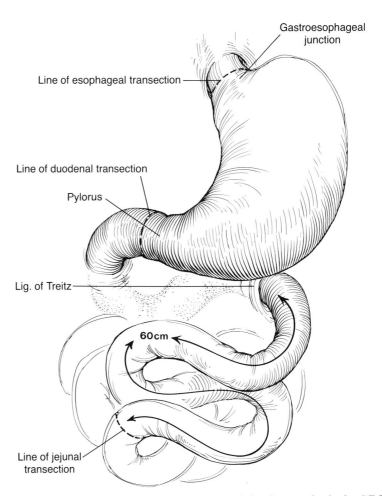

FIGURE 57–1. The stomach has been completely mobilized using both the LDS stapler and appropriate double clamping and suture ligatures for the major gastric vessels. The posterior peritoneum over the esophagus has been sharply excised, and the esophagus has been mobilized 4 inches over its terminal using blunt and sharp dissection. The first portion of the duodenum has been mobilized using a Kocher maneuver. An appropriate area of upper jejunum approximately 40 to 60 cm. from the ligament of Treitz has been selected for division of the jejunum.

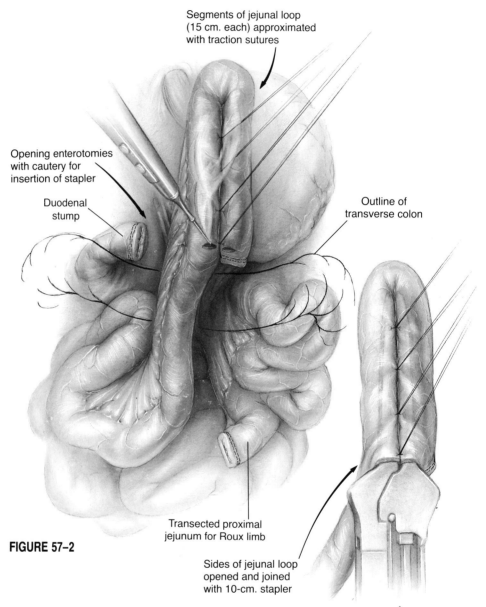

Segments of jejunal loop
(15 cm. each) approximated
with traction sutures

Opening enterotomies
with cautery for
insertion of stapler

Duodenal
stump

Outline of
transverse colon

FIGURE 57–2

Transected proximal
jejunum for Roux limb

Sides of jejunal loop
opened and joined
with 10-cm. stapler

FIGURE 57–3

FIGURE 57–2. Either the PI 30 or the PI 55 stapler is placed across the duodenum, and the instrument is fired. The proximal duodenum is clamped with a bowel Kocher clamp. This permits adequate closure of the duodenal stump. The jejunum can then be divided using the 5-cm. GIA stapler. The distal jejunum is brought up in the antecolic position, and traction sutures are placed as shown, thus fashioning a 15-cm. jejunal loop.

FIGURE 57–3. Enterotomies are then made in the antemesenteric position of the jejunal loop, and the 10-cm. GIA stapler is passed and fired, creating a jejunal pouch for gastric replacement.

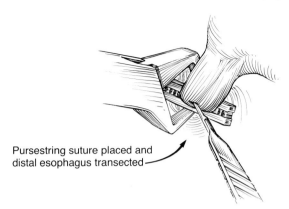

Pursestring suture placed and
distal esophagus transected

FIGURE 57–4. The pursestring device is then placed around the esophagus; the esophagus is divided, thus permitting resection of the entire stomach.

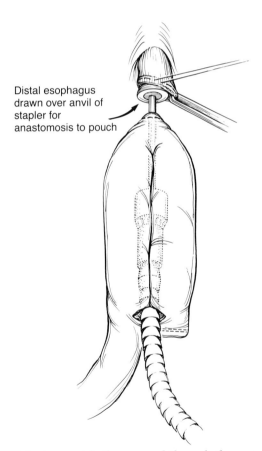

Distal esophagus
drawn over anvil of
stapler for
anastomosis to pouch

FIGURE 57–5. The EEA instrument is then passed through the open enterotomies, and the center rod is extended at the apex of the jejunal loop. Cautery is used to permit passage of the center rod without the anvil in place. A pursestring suture is then placed around the center rod to prevent tearing the jejunal wall. The anvil is secured into place, and the open end of the divided esophagus is gently passed over the anvil using Babcock clamps. The esophageal pursestring suture is gently tied around the center rod.

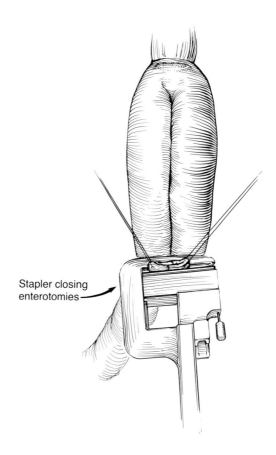

Stapler closing
enterotomies

FIGURE 57–6. The cartridge and the anvil are approximated and the EEA instrument is fired. The tissue doughnuts must be carefully inspected for the presence of complete circles of tissue. The enterotomy is closed with a PI 55 stapler.

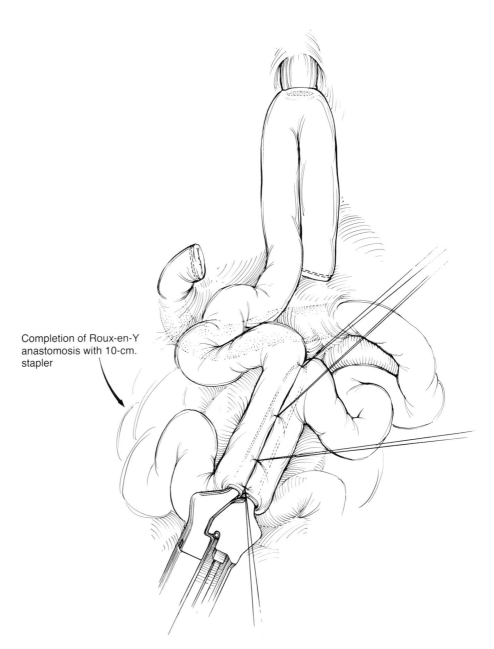

Completion of Roux-en-Y
anastomosis with 10-cm.
stapler

FIGURE 57–7. The Roux-en-Y anastomosis is completed using either a 10-cm. or a 5-cm. GIA stapler. The open enterotomies are closed with either a PI 30 or a PI 55 stapler as previously shown.

58

Pyloromyotomy for Congenital Hypertrophic Pyloric Stenosis

NICHOLAS A. SHORTER, M.D.

If a diagnosis of congenital hypertrophic pyloric stenosis is made, surgical pyloromyotomy is required. The procedure should be undertaken, however, only after the child is adequately hydrated and any electrolyte disturbances are corrected. In rare instances, this can take several days; however, with these precautions, the procedure should have almost no mortality and minimal morbidity.

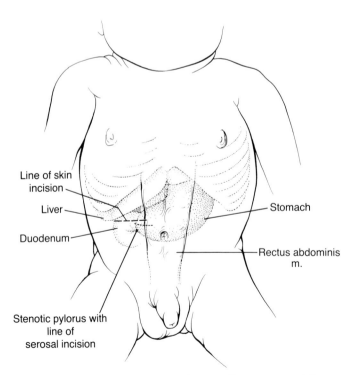

FIGURE 58–1. The abdomen is opened through a small transverse right upper quadrant incision.

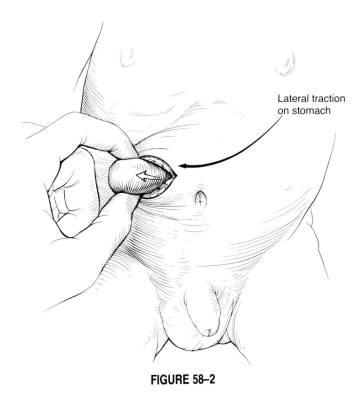

Lateral traction
on stomach

FIGURE 58–2

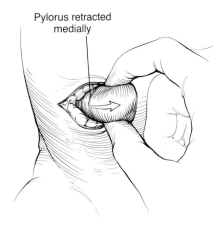

Pylorus retracted
medially

FIGURE 58–3

FIGURES 58–2 and 58–3. The stomach is grasped, and gentle traction is applied to the right followed by traction to the left, which delivers the pylorus into the wound.

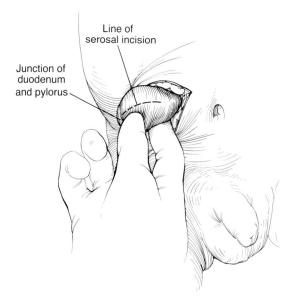

FIGURE 58–4

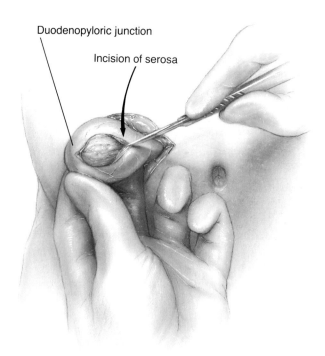

FIGURE 58–5

FIGURES 58–4 and 58–5. With the pylorus stabilized, the serosa of the pylorus is scored with a scalpel, being certain it is just proximal to the duodenopyloric junction, which can be identified by a color change from white to pink. Failure to do this may cause perforation of the very superficial duodenal mucosa. The incision should be extended a short distance onto the anterior wall of the stomach.

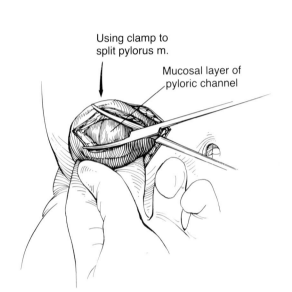

Using clamp to
split pylorus m.

Mucosal layer of
pyloric channel

FIGURE 58–6

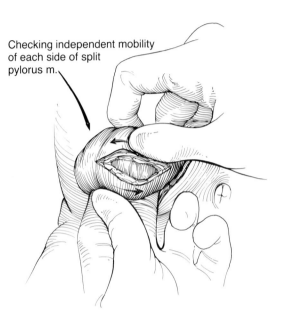

Checking independent mobility
of each side of split
pylorus m.

FIGURE 58–7

FIGURE 58–6. The pyloric muscle is then split, preferably with the blunt end of a knife handle, but a small curved clamp or one of the instruments specifically designed for this purpose is also appropriate. Bleeding is usually minimal and ceases spontaneously.

FIGURE 58–7. Completeness of the myotomy is confirmed by checking for independent movement of the two sides. One should always check for mucosal perforation by milking the duodenum backward and/or insufflating the stomach with air and squeezing it gently through the pyloric channel.

The pylorus is then replaced into the abdomen, and the incision is closed in layers with absorbable sutures. Feedings can be started within the first 24 hours postoperatively.

59

Fundoplication for Gastroesophageal Reflux in Infants and Children

ARTHUR J. ROSS, III, M.D.

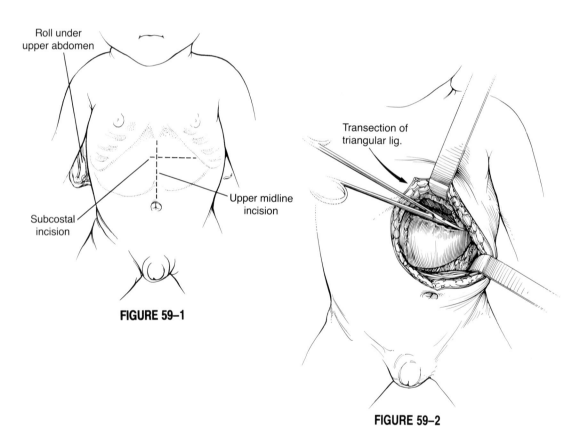

FIGURE 59–1. The child is positioned supine with a roll placed beneath the upper abdomen. Depending on the width of the costal angle and costal margin, either a midline or a subcostal incision is employed.

FIGURE 59–2. When the abdomen is entered, the viscera are packed away; extensive abdominal exploration is not routinely employed. The triangular ligament of the left lobe of the liver is taken down, and the left lobe of the liver is then retracted beneath the right lobe. The spleen is elevated on a Mikulicz pad, and the short gastric vessels along the fundus and greater curvature of the stomach are divided between clamps, doubly ligating the gastric side.

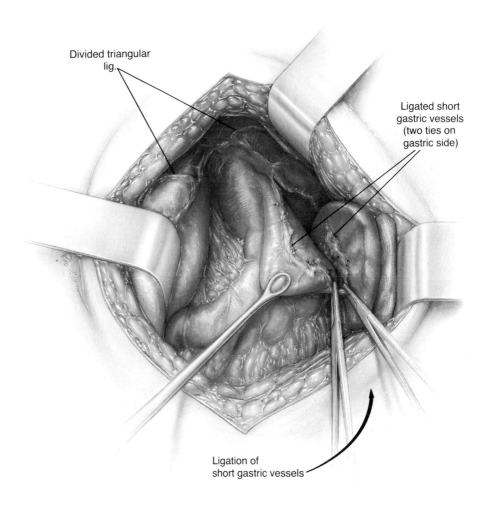

Divided triangular
lig.

Ligated short
gastric vessels
(two ties on
gastric side)

Ligation of
short gastric vessels

FIGURE 59–3. When the spleen is mobilized and freed from the fundus, it is allowed to fall back into the left upper quadrant for the remainder of the operation.

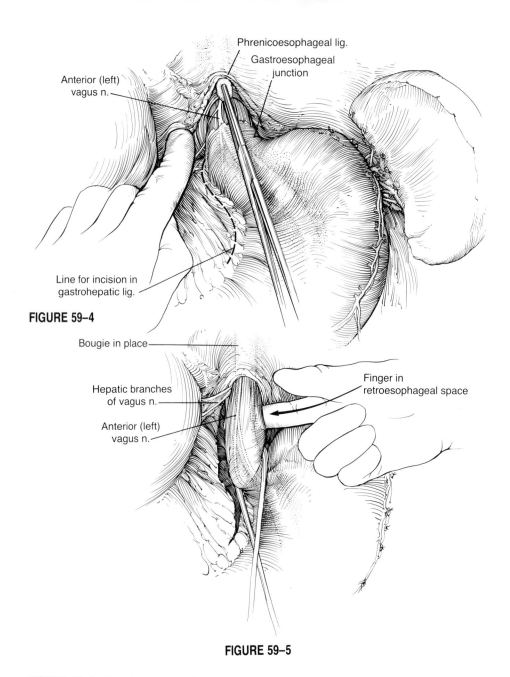

Phrenicoesophageal lig.

Gastroesophageal
junction

Anterior (left)
vagus n.

Line for incision in
gastrohepatic lig.

FIGURE 59–4

Bougie in place

Hepatic branches
of vagus n.

Anterior (left)
vagus n.

Finger in
retroesophageal space

FIGURE 59–5

FIGURE 59–4. The dissection of the gastroesophageal junction, esophagus, and retro-esophageal space is facilitated by the placement of a mercury bougie of appropriate size into the esophagus. A 24 to 28 French bougie is usually appropriate for infants, whereas larger children require a 34 to 36 French bougie; 38 to 40 French bougies are generally employed for adolescents. The placement of the bougie is especially critical in children with severe esophagitis, in whom the dissection of the esophagus and retroesophageal space can be difficult. Sharp dissection is used to open the phrenicoesophageal ligament; and, when incised, a dissector can be used to push this ligament cephalad atraumatically.

FIGURE 59–5. This type of dissection has less of a tendency to disrupt vagal tributaries. The dissection is extended over the gastroesophageal junction into the region of the gastrohepatic ligament, which is usually opened as far caudad as the left gastric artery. Attention is given to identification of the hepatic branches of the vagus, and minimal disruption of these fibers is optimal. Entry to the retroesophageal space is gained, and dissection is performed bluntly with either a finger tip or a blunt-tipped Kelly clamp. When this space is developed, a Penrose drain is passed beneath the esophagus for caudad traction, allowing exposure of the esophagus as far cephalad as the diaphragmatic crura. Both the anterior and the posterior vagus should be identified, but it is not imperative that they be separated from the esophagus and excluded from the subsequent wrap. Crural approximation is an important part of the procedure and is performed using interrupted nonabsorbable sutures.

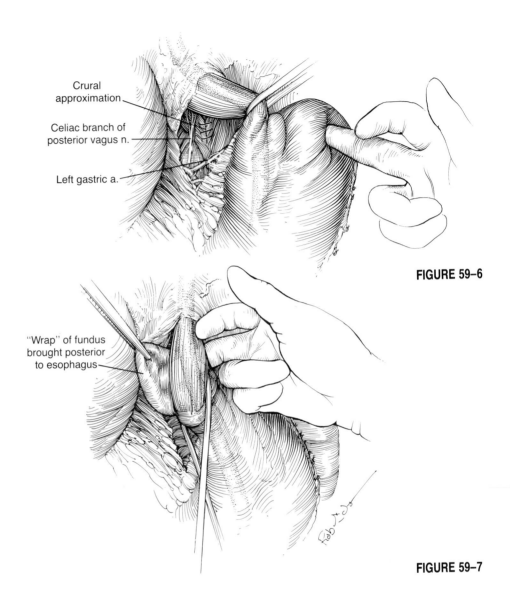

Crural
approximation

Celiac branch of
posterior vagus n.

Left gastric a.

FIGURE 59–6

"Wrap" of fundus
brought posterior
to esophagus

FIGURE 59–7

FIGURE 59–6. The goal is to pass the tip of a Kelly clamp between the opposed crura and the esophagus. The wrap is then performed. In larger patients, this can easily be done with caudal traction on the Penrose drain and by pushing the fundus posterior to the esophagus.

FIGURE 59–7. In smaller children, this technique may be somewhat cumbersome; a very good alternative is to place silk traction sutures in the region of the gastroesophageal junction. They provide sufficient caudal traction so that the Penrose drain can be removed.

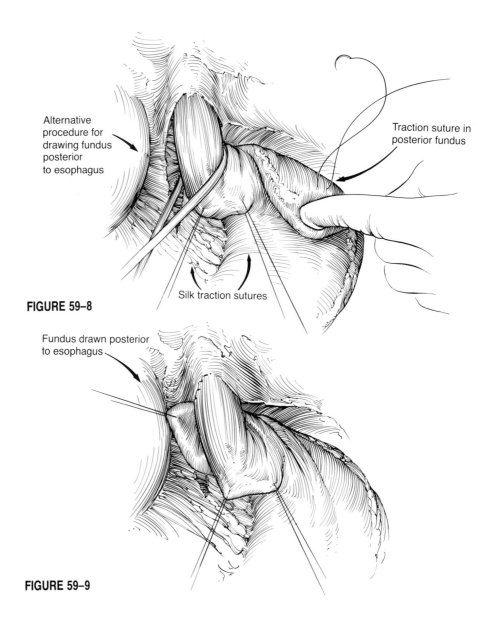

Alternative
procedure for
drawing fundus
posterior
to esophagus

Traction suture in
posterior fundus

Silk traction sutures

FIGURE 59–8

Fundus drawn posterior
to esophagus

FIGURE 59–9

FIGURE 59–8. Concurrently, another silk traction suture is placed on the posterior fundus at the site destined to become the top suture of the wrap. This suture is drawn behind the esophagus using a Kelly clamp, and it includes the fundus.

FIGURE 59–9. Cephalad traction on this suture and concurrent caudad traction on the lesser curvature–gastroesophageal junction sutures form the wrap, which, in infants and small children, should be approximately 2 cm. in length. Regardless of the technique employed, the wrap is constructed using interrupted nonabsorbable sutures, taking a bite through the esophagus in addition to both sides of the wrap.

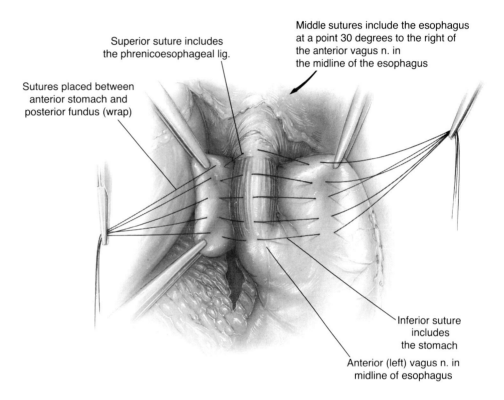

Superior suture includes
the phrenicoesophageal lig.

Middle sutures include the esophagus
at a point 30 degrees to the right of
the anterior vagus n. in
the midline of the esophagus

Sutures placed between
anterior stomach and
posterior fundus (wrap)

Inferior suture
includes
the stomach

Anterior (left) vagus n. in
midline of esophagus

FIGURE 59–10. The most cephalad suture also incorporates the phrenicoesophageal ligament. An attempt is made to construct the wrap such that the open end of the C is approximately 30 degrees off the midsagittal plane toward the patient's right side. As appropriate, the wrap is completed by having nonabsorbable sutures approximating the wrap to the diaphragm.

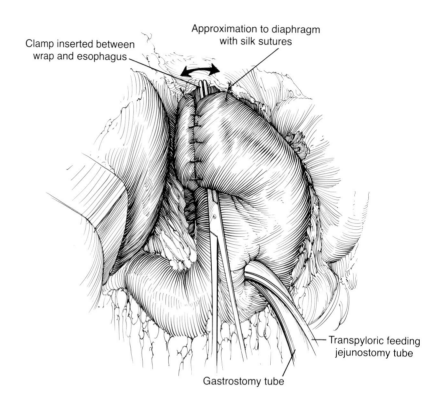

Clamp inserted between
wrap and esophagus

Approximation to diaphragm
with silk sutures

Transpyloric feeding
jejunostomy tube

Gastrostomy tube

FIGURE 59–11. The well-constructed wrap easily allows a Kelly clamp to move between it and the underlying esophagus. The use of a gastrostomy is not required in all patients; however, it is sound policy to employ a gastrostomy in children who are brain damaged and neuromuscularly impaired.

An additional option is the concurrent placement of a transpyloric jejunal feeding tube, which does not require an additional gastrotomy or skin incision.

60

Closure of Perforated Peptic Ulcer

THEODORE N. PAPPAS, M.D.

Exploration for a perforated peptic ulcer is necessary in patients (1) who have an unknown diagnosis; (2) who perforate a peptic ulcer during active ulcer therapy; (3) who would benefit from definitive ulcer operation during closure of perforated peptic ulcer; and (4) who are taking corticosteroids for systemic disease.

The patients should be adequately hydrated prior to operation. Broad-spectrum antibiotics are often used in the perioperative period.

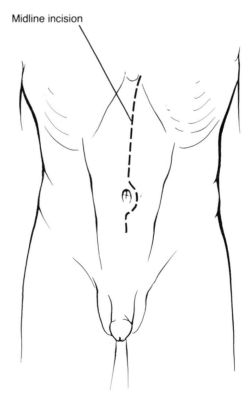

Midline incision

FIGURE 60–1. The abdomen is explored through an upper midline incision extended to the xiphoid and proximally to the left side of the xiphoid as necessary.

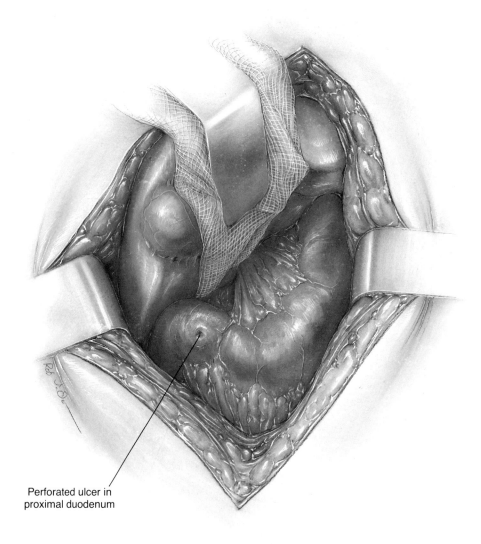

Perforated ulcer in
proximal duodenum

FIGURE 60–2. The abdomen is explored, and the cloudy peritoneal material is aspirated and sent for bacteriologic culture. On exploration of the right upper quadrant, the ulcer is usually easily visualized.

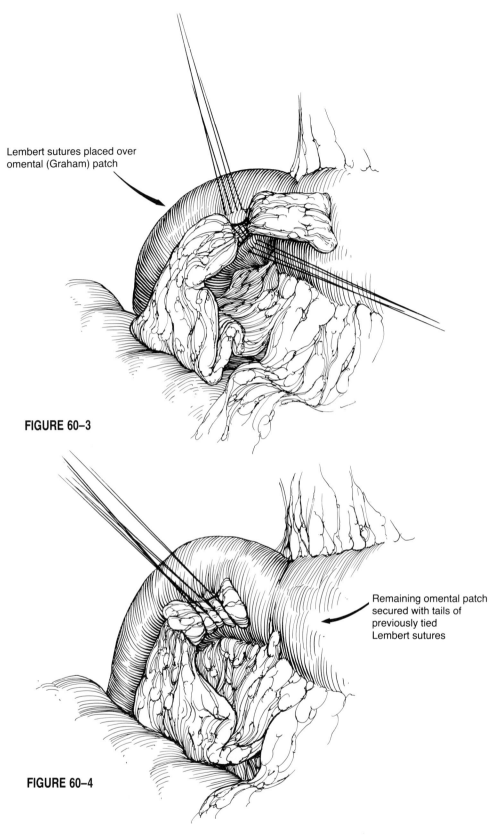

Lembert sutures placed over
omental (Graham) patch

FIGURE 60–3

Remaining omental patch
secured with tails of
previously tied
Lembert sutures

FIGURE 60–4

FIGURE 60–3. After adequate exploration of the upper abdomen, the retractor is inserted.
If simple closure of the ulcer is deemed the appropriate treatment, 3-0 silk sutures are
placed in a Lembert manner across the ulcer.

FIGURE 60–4. Once these sutures are in place, a piece of omentum is placed across the
base of the ulcer; the sutures are then tied snugly in an effort to close the hole with the
patch of omentum.

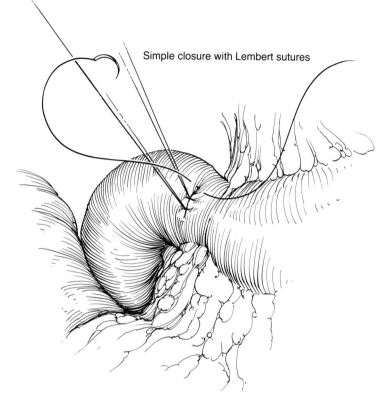

Simple closure with Lembert sutures

FIGURE 60–5

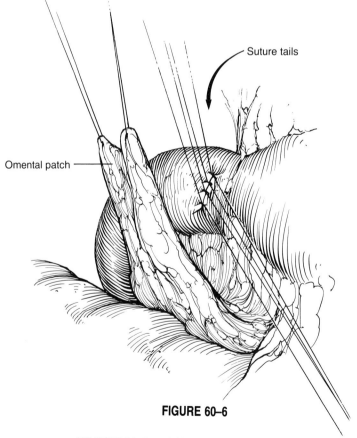

Suture tails

Omental patch

FIGURE 60–6

FIGURES 60–5 and 60–6 *See legend on opposite page*

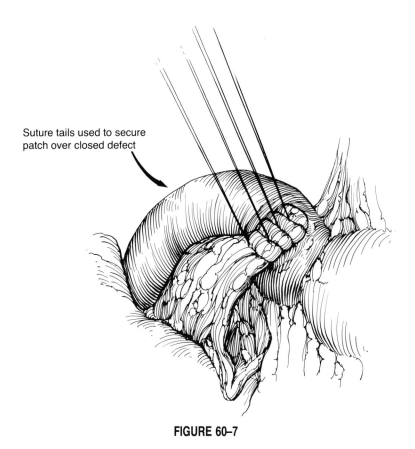

Suture tails used to secure
patch over closed defect

FIGURE 60–7

FIGURES 60–5 to 60–7. An alternative technique is to tie the sutures first and close the defect, followed by placement of the omental tag across the ends of the sutures and then tying them again over the omental tag. The first technique is often necessary if there is a maximal amount of edema around the perforated ulcer, making the simple closure somewhat difficult.

The abdomen should be generously irrigated with warm saline solution to decrease the bacterial content. The abdomen is closed.

61

Truncal Vagotomy

THEODORE N. PAPPAS, M.D.

If a decision is made to perform a *definitive* ulcer operation during exploration for perforation, a vagotomy and pyloroplasty can be done. (See Chapters 47, 48, 49, and 50.) If a vagotomy and pyloroplasty is chosen, the pyloroplasty is usually accomplished through the perforated ulcer bed.

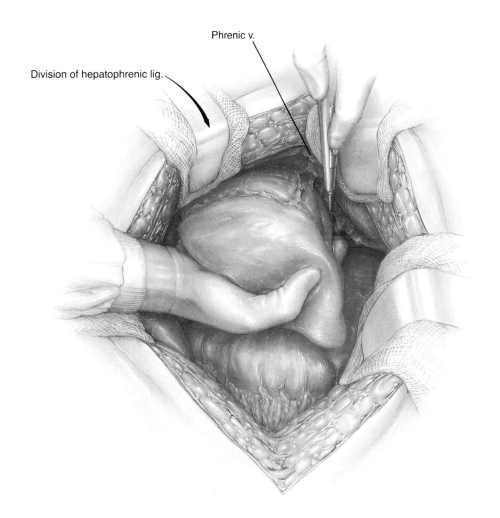

Phrenic v.

Division of hepatophrenic lig.

FIGURE 61–1. Truncal vagotomy is accomplished by placing a retractor in the upper abdomen with firm upward retraction at the hiatus. The patient is placed in reverse Trendelenburg position, and the abdominal contents are packed out of the wound, exposing the gastroesophageal junction. The left lobe of the liver is then taken down by placing the right hand behind the liver and pulling the lobe downward. This exposes the hepatophrenic ligament, which is incised with electrocautery. At this point, care is taken not to enter a large phrenic vein that is embedded in the diaphragm in this region. If this vein is entered, troublesome bleeding is usually encountered.

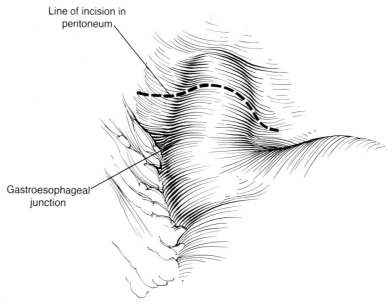

FIGURE 61–2. The left lobe of the liver is packed toward the midline, and the gastro-esophageal junction is easily visualized. The peritoneal reflection at the diaphragm is then incised to expose the esophagus.

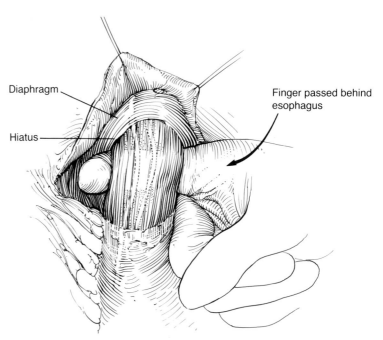

FIGURE 61–3. Once this area of peritoneum is completely incised, the index finger is placed around the esophagus to encircle it at the hiatus. Care is taken to pass the finger around the esophagus above the diaphragm. This is done to be certain that the posterior vagus is included in this encircling maneuver.

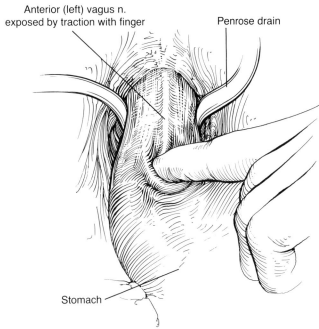

Anterior (left) vagus n.
exposed by traction with finger

Penrose drain

Stomach

FIGURE 61–4. A Penrose drain is passed behind the esophagus, and the anterior vagus is exposed by downward pressure on the gastroesophageal junction. This places tension on the anterior surface of the esophagus. The anterior vagus is a prominent structure that is usually easily seen lying in the substance of the esophagus.

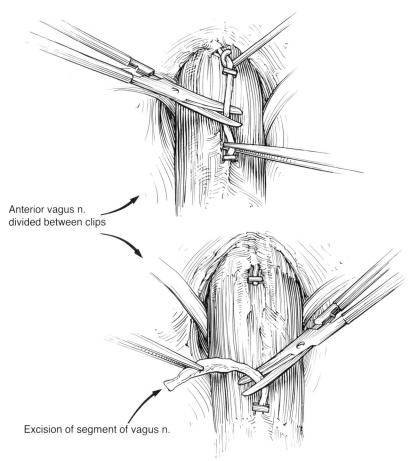

Anterior vagus n.
divided between clips

Excision of segment of vagus n.

FIGURE 61–5. The nerve hook is passed around the vagus, and it is clipped superiorly and inferiorly. A specimen of the vagus is sent to the pathologist for histologic confirmation.

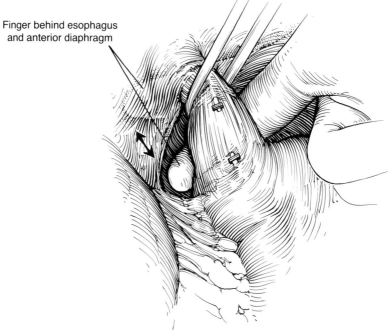

Finger behind esophagus
and anterior diaphragm

FIGURE 61–6. The posterior vagus is localized by anterior retraction of the esophagus by traction on the Penrose drain. When the index finger of the right hand is placed around the esophagus, the vagus nerve is felt on the back wall of the esophagus and is the larger posterior vagus. If the Penrose drain was placed incorrectly around the back of the esophagus and the posterior vagus was excluded, it will of course not be found with this maneuver. If difficulty is encountered, palpation superiorly on the esophagus may occasionally localize the posterior vagus before it is separated from the esophageal tissue. If it is still not encountered, care should be taken to expose tissue on the crus of the diaphragm—and in the periaortic region in the thin patient—because the posterior vagus can occasionally be found in these tissue planes.

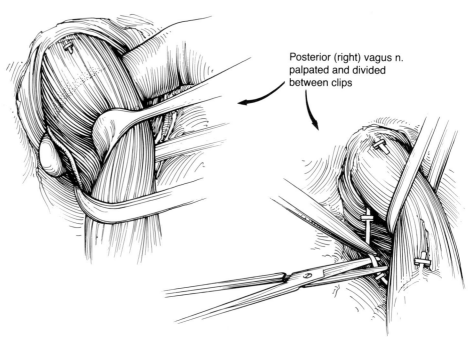

Posterior (right) vagus n.
palpated and divided
between clips

FIGURE 61–7. The posterior vagus is similarly clipped and divided and sent to the pathologist.

62

Laparoscopic Truncal Vagotomy and Gastrojejunostomy

THEODORE N. PAPPAS, M.D.

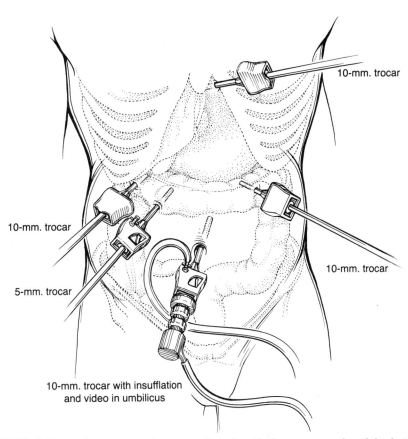

FIGURE 62–1. Truncal vagotomy is accomplished with five trocars placed high in the upper abdomen just near the costal margin to facilitate exposure to the hiatus. The abdomen is insufflated through a supraumbilical incision with a Veress needle. A 10-mm. trocar is then placed just above the umbilicus, particularly in patients with long abdomens, to be certain that the camera can reach the hiatus. Under direct vision, a second 10-mm. trocar is placed high in the upper midline adjacent to the xiphisternum and to the left of the falciform ligament. This trocar is used to place a retractor to expose the left lobe of the liver. The surgeon stands on the right side of the table and operates through two ports: a 5-mm. trocar and a 10-mm. trocar. These are placed under direct vision and represent the base of an isosceles triangle, with the apex of the triangle being the hiatus. This allows the surgeon to operate with both hands. The assistant stands on the patient's left side and operates through a 10-mm. trocar placed near the costal margin.

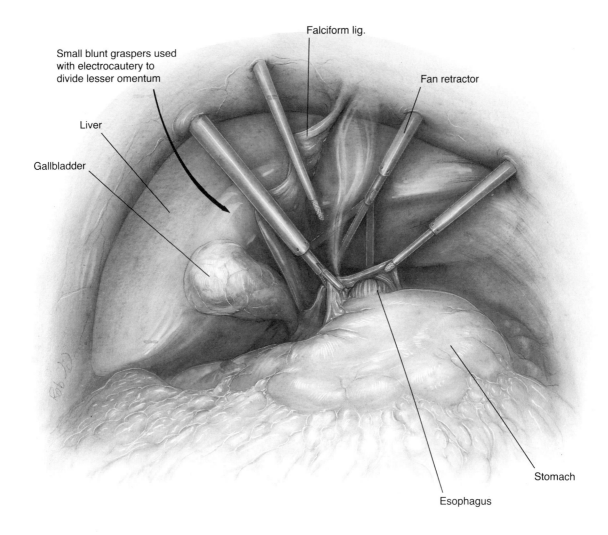

Small blunt graspers used
with electrocautery to
divide lesser omentum

Falciform lig.

Fan retractor

Liver

Gallbladder

Stomach

Esophagus

FIGURE 62–2. The internal anatomy is illustrated with the stomach in the foreground. The upper fan retractor is used to retract the left lobe of the liver and provides exposure to the gastroesophageal junction. The left upper quadrant retractor can be used to reflect the crest of the diaphragm upward or, more commonly, to draw the stomach inferiorly with an Endo-Babcock. The surgeon operates from the right side of the table, exposing the esophageal hiatus.

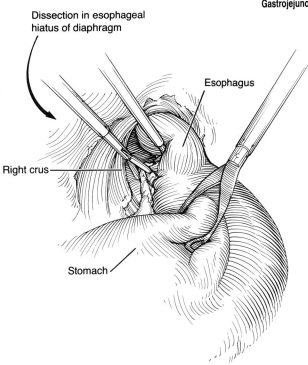

FIGURE 62-3. The hiatal dissection is illustrated. The surgeon creates a plane between the right crus of the diaphragm and the esophagus. This is done initially with sharp dissection and eventually with blunt dissection. The esophagus is then retracted to the left with a blunt dissector while the posterior dissection behind the esophagus is done under direct vision. In this way, the posterior vagus can eventually be visualized.

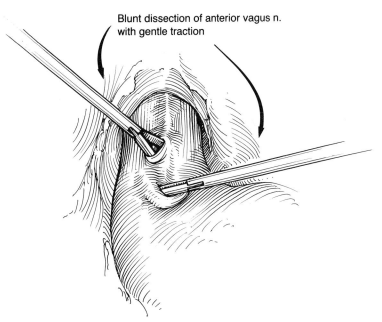

FIGURE 62-4. The anterior vagus lies within the substance of the esophageal wall. It can be visualized laparoscopically, particularly if minimal hemorrhage is created in the dissection.

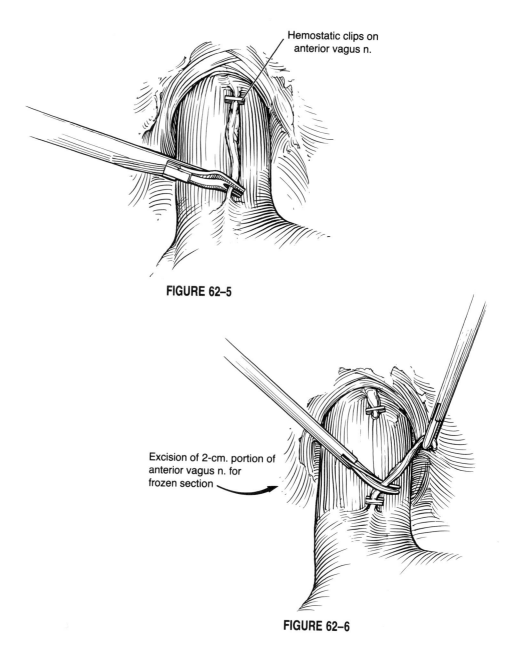

Hemostatic clips on
anterior vagus n.

FIGURE 62–5

Excision of 2-cm. portion of
anterior vagus n. for
frozen section

FIGURE 62–6

FIGURES 62–5 and 62–6. The blunt dissector is used to localize the anterior vagus, and clips are placed superiorly and inferiorly. The vagus is divided, and a section is sent to surgical pathology for confirmation.

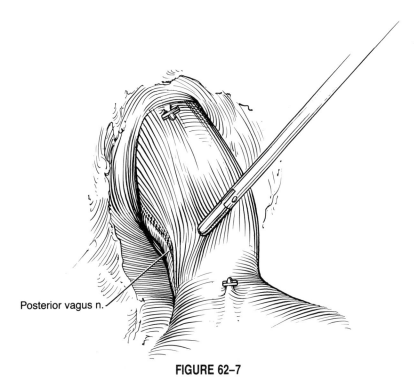

Posterior vagus n.

FIGURE 62-7

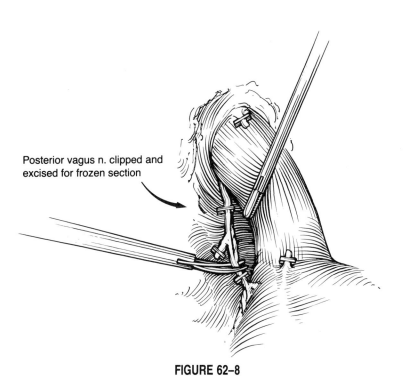

Posterior vagus n. clipped and
excised for frozen section

FIGURE 62-8

FIGURES 62-7 and 62-8. The posterior vagus nerve can be seen by retracting the esophagus to the left. The nerve should be divided high in the hiatus above the criminal nerve of Grassi. Clips are placed superiorly and inferiorly, and the specimen is sent to surgical pathology.

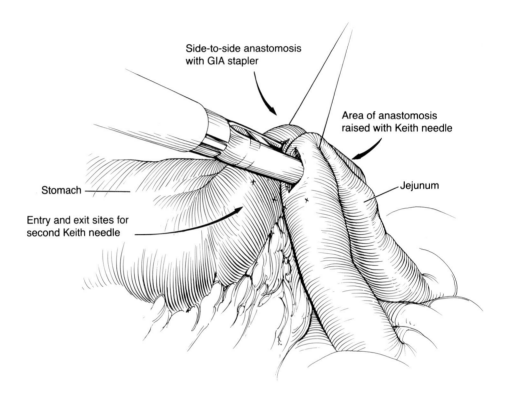

Side-to-side anastomosis
with GIA stapler

Area of anastomosis
raised with Keith needle

Stomach

Jejunum

Entry and exit sites for
second Keith needle

FIGURE 62–9. Following truncal vagotomy, one should perform the drainage procedure of choice. A laparoscopic gastrojejunostomy is depicted, and, if this procedure is attempted, a 12-mm. trocar is placed in the right upper quadrant for the Endo-GIA stapler. The procedure is begun by identifying the ligament of Treitz and selecting a segment of jejunum that can be approximated easily to the greater curvature of the stomach. A Keith needle is placed through the anterior abdominal wall, and an appropriate portion of stomach and a segment of small bowel are approximated with the needle. The Keith needle is then passed out the intra-abdominal wall, and the suture is retracted upward. This tents the small bowel and the stomach together such that enterotomies can be made in the appropriate manner. The Endo-GIA stapler is then placed, and three firings of the Endo-GIA 30 are made. This creates an adequate anastomosis.

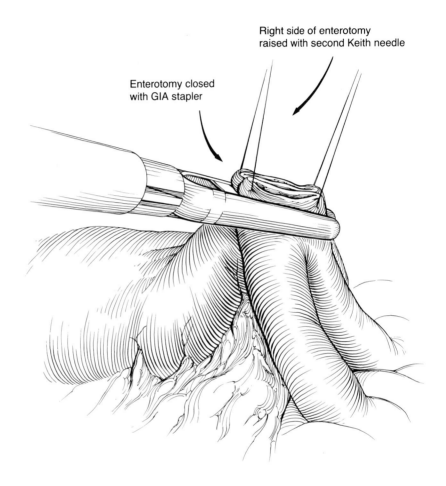

Right side of enterotomy
raised with second Keith needle

Enterotomy closed
with GIA stapler

FIGURE 62–10. A second Keith needle is placed, and the orientation of the anastomosis is changed such that an Endo-GIA stapler can be used to close the enterotomies.

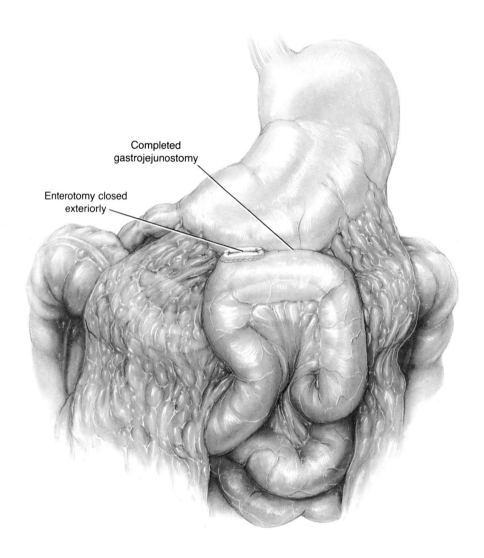

Completed
gastrojejunostomy

Enterotomy closed
exteriorly

FIGURE 62–11

63

Highly Selective Vagotomy

THEODORE N. PAPPAS, M.D.

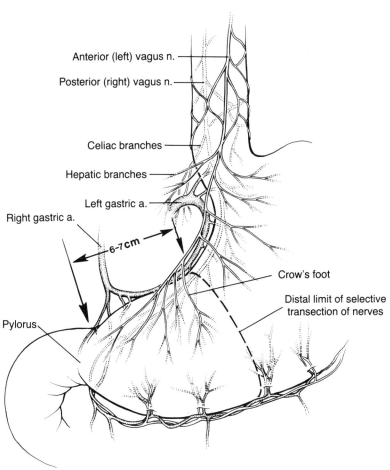

FIGURE 63–1. The most common indication for a highly selective vagotomy is intractable peptic ulcer disease. Highly selective vagotomy is accomplished by measuring 6 to 7 cm. cephalad from the pylorus. This marks the region of the antrum of the stomach. In addition, the anatomic landmarks separating the fundus from the antrum include the crow's foot of the vagus nerve, which can easily be seen on the anterior surface of the stomach.

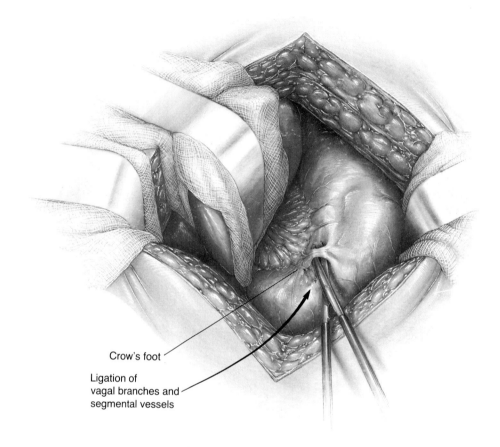

Crow's foot

Ligation of
vagal branches and
segmental vessels

FIGURE 63–2. Just cephalad to the crow's foot, the entire lesser curvature is devascularized in an effort to remove all vagal fibers in this region.

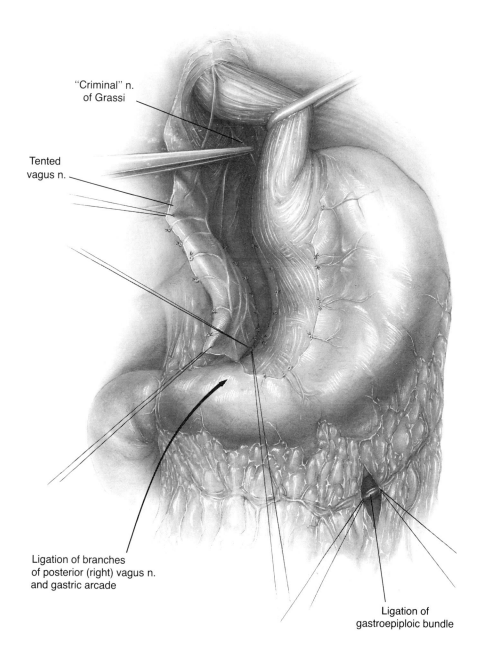

"Criminal" n.
of Grassi

Tented
vagus n.

Ligation of branches
of posterior (right) vagus n.
and gastric arcade

Ligation of
gastroepiploic bundle

FIGURE 63–3. Devascularization is done by dividing the anterior and posterior blood supply and vagal fibers with small Crile clamps. These are tied with 3–0 and 4–0 silk sutures. Care is taken to divide these vessels on the surface of the stomach in both the anterior and the posterior planes to avoid injuring the main trunk of the vagus. In this manner, the entire lesser curvature is devascularized to the gastroesophageal junction. At this point, the vagus nerve can be tented laterally.

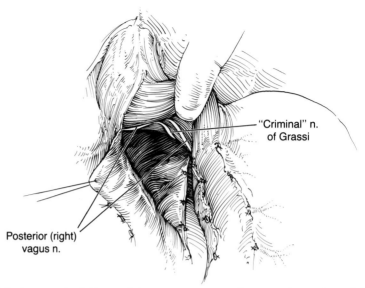

FIGURE 63–4. Any residual fibers of the vagus nerve to the posterior region of the upper stomach (the "criminal" nerve of Grassi) can be divided.

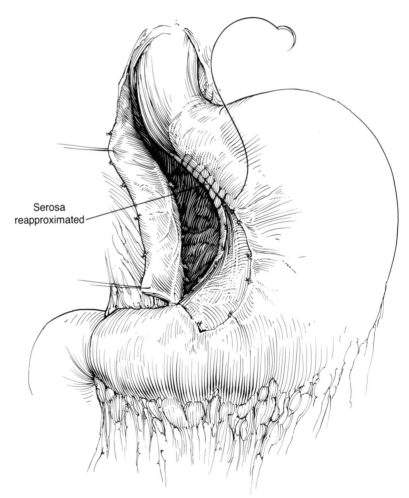

FIGURE 63–5. The serosa of the lesser curvature of the stomach is then reapproximated with interrupted 3–0 Lembert silk sutures.

64

Gastrojejunostomy

WILLIAM P. J. PEETE, M.D.

In patients with obstructive duodenal disease who have a long or redundant transverse colon, or in those with a lengthy transverse mesocolon of average thickness or less, a loop gastrojejunostomy *posterior* to the colon is often recommended.

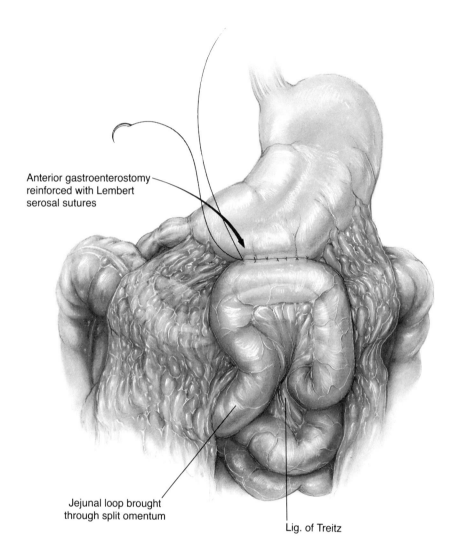

Anterior gastroenterostomy
reinforced with Lembert
serosal sutures

Jejunal loop brought
through split omentum

Lig. of Treitz

FIGURE 64–1. The gastroenterostomy may be done *anterior* to the colon when the transverse mesocolon is short or fat. If the omentum is also fat, it is helpful to remove it or divide it vertically. The ligament of Treitz is identified, and a 15- to 25-cm. loop of jejunum is drawn up and attached to the distal antrum with traction sutures so that the off loop is placed proximally adjacent to the stomach. The anastomosis may be stapled in the same manner as the side-to-side anastomosis shown in Chapter 65, or it may be hand sewn as shown in the posterior gastrojejunostomy procedure.

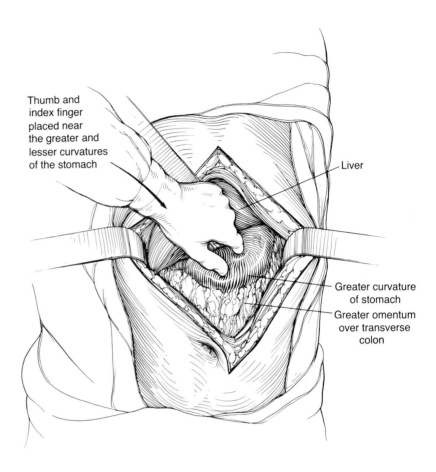

Thumb and
index finger
placed near
the greater and
lesser curvatures
of the stomach

Liver

Greater curvature
of stomach

Greater omentum
over transverse
colon

FIGURE 64–2. For an anastomosis *posterior* to the transverse colon, a midline incision is usually made from the xiphoid to the umbilicus. After inspecting the stomach and duodenum for obstruction, for which the operation is usually done, the surgeon or assistant may press with thumb and index finger on the anterior wall of the distal stomach; and the omentum and transverse colon are then held forward and upward.

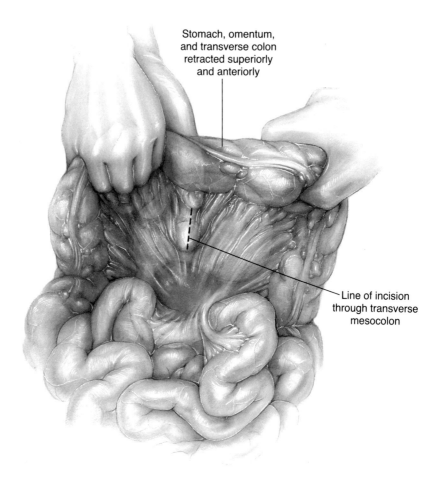

Stomach, omentum, and transverse colon retracted superiorly and anteriorly

Line of incision through transverse mesocolon

FIGURE 64–3. The thumb and index finger are located through the stomach and transverse mesocolon from the posteroinferior aspect of the transverse mesocolon to identify a point where the stomach may be drawn through the mesentery. The mesentery is incised vertically between the points identified by the thumb and index finger. Care is taken to avoid large vessels.

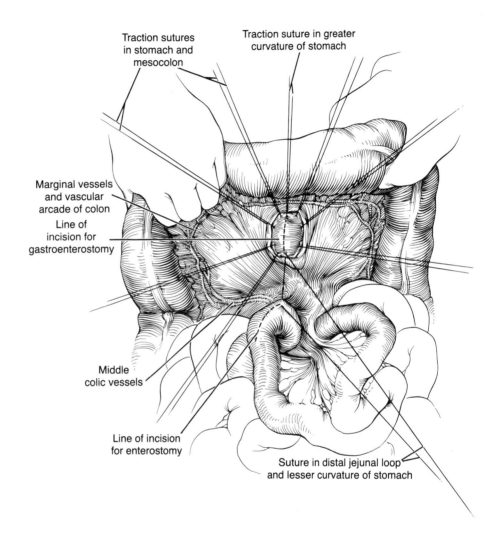

Traction sutures
in stomach and
mesocolon

Traction suture in greater
curvature of stomach

Marginal vessels
and vascular
arcade of colon

Line of
incision for
gastroenterostomy

Middle
colic vessels

Line of incision
for enterostomy

Suture in distal jejunal loop
and lesser curvature of stomach

FIGURE 64–4. Traction sutures placed near the greater and lesser curvatures serve to secure the stomach to the mesentery. Additional sutures are placed to hold the mesentery above the anastomosis and to prevent obstruction by the mesentery trapping the jejunal loop.

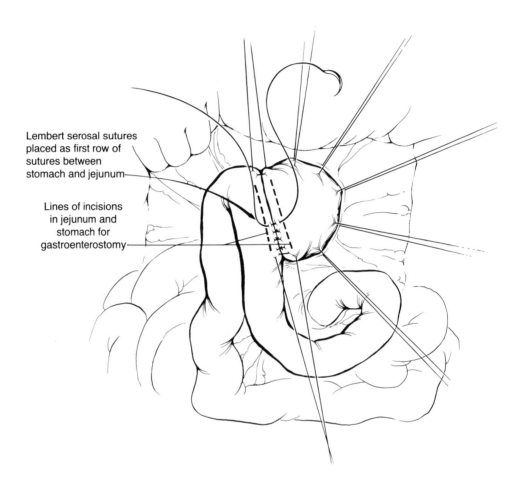

Lembert serosal sutures
placed as first row of
sutures between
stomach and jejunum

Lines of incisions
in jejunum and
stomach for
gastroenterostomy

FIGURE 64–5. The ligament of Treitz is identified, and a loop of jejunum (15- to 25-cm. long) is brought to lie comfortably adjacent to the stomach. It is fixed into position with traction sutures so that the proximal jejunum lies near the lesser curvature.

A posterior layer of seromuscular interrupted or continuous 3-0 silk sutures is placed as the first row of sutures in the anastomosis. The colon and proximal stomach may be returned to the abdomen, and the jejunum and stomach to be anastomosed are brought out of the abdomen and protected from the incision with Mikulicz pads.

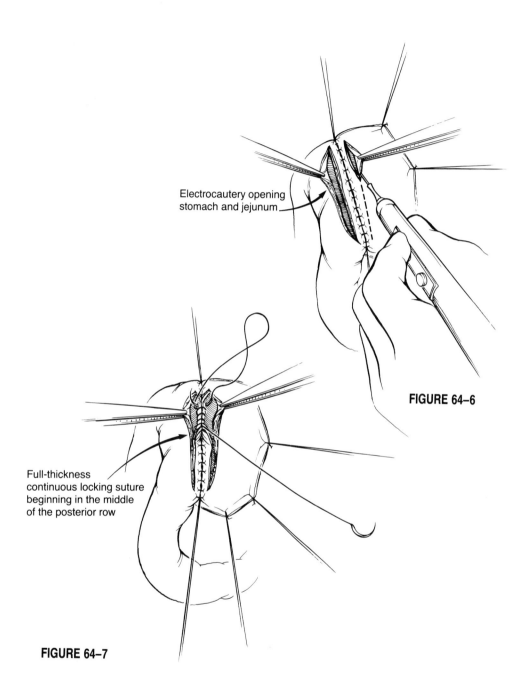

Electrocautery opening
stomach and jejunum

FIGURE 64-6

Full-thickness
continuous locking suture
beginning in the middle
of the posterior row

FIGURE 64-7

FIGURE 64-6. The stomach and jejunum are opened with vertical and longitudinal incisions, respectively. Each incision should be about 6 cm. long and made with electrocautery.

FIGURE 64-7. A full-thickness 3-0 chromic catgut suture is placed, joining and inverting the back wall of the gastroenterostomy, beginning at the ends of the incisions nearest the center of the anastomosis. This is the beginning of the second row of sutures.

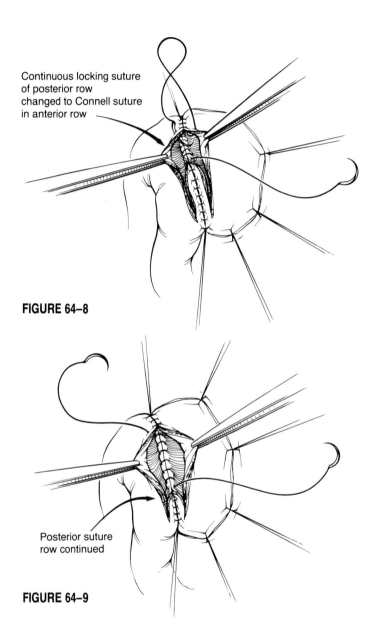

Continuous locking suture
of posterior row
changed to Connell suture
in anterior row

FIGURE 64-8

Posterior suture
row continued

FIGURE 64-9

FIGURE 64-8. The suture is taken around the corner to be continued anteriorly as a Connell suture to begin the third row.

FIGURE 64-9. The inner posterior layer of sutures is continued from the starting point near the center of the anastomosis in the opposite direction to complete the third row of sutures.

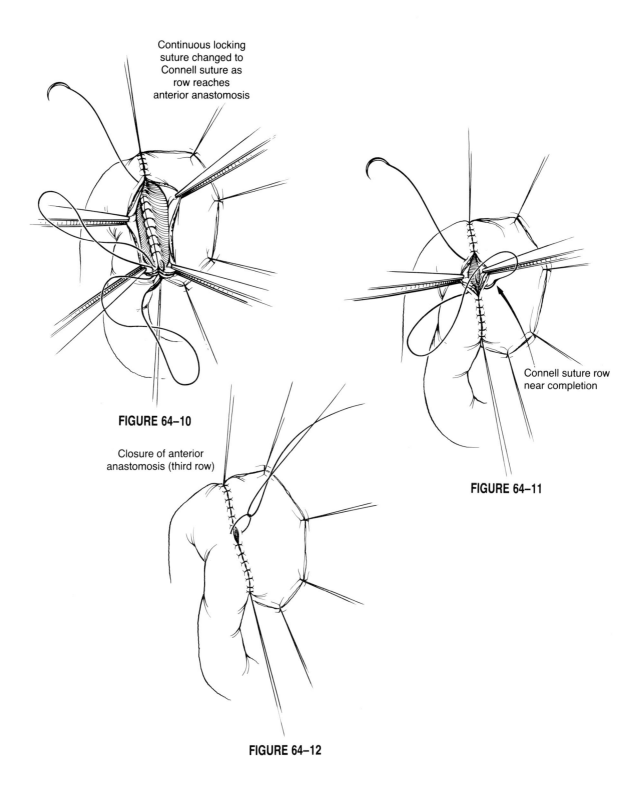

Continuous locking
suture changed to
Connell suture as
row reaches
anterior anastomosis

FIGURE 64–10

Connell suture row
near completion

FIGURE 64–11

Closure of anterior
anastomosis (third row)

FIGURE 64–12

FIGURES 64–10 and 64–11. Connell sutures are placed at the lesser curvature to begin the inner anterior full-thickness layer.

FIGURE 64–12. The gastroenterostomy is closed with inversion.

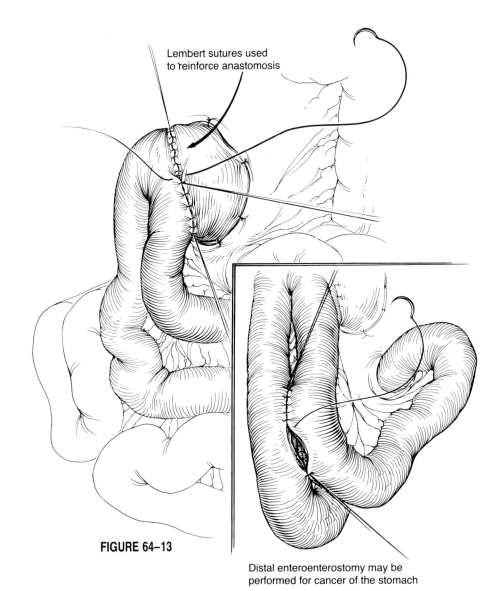

Lembert sutures used
to reinforce anastomosis

FIGURE 64–13. Lembert seromuscular sutures are used to
reinforce the anastomosis.

FIGURE 64–14. A distal enteroenterostomy may be per-
formed in patients with in-
operable stomach or duodenal
cancer to increase palliation.
The side-to-side anastomosis
may be hand sutured as
shown in the posterior gastroenterostomy, or it may be
stapled as shown in Chapter
65.

FIGURE 64–13

Distal enteroenterostomy may be
performed for cancer of the stomach

FIGURE 64–14

65

Gastrojejunostomy (STAPLER)

HILLIARD F. SEIGLER, M.D.

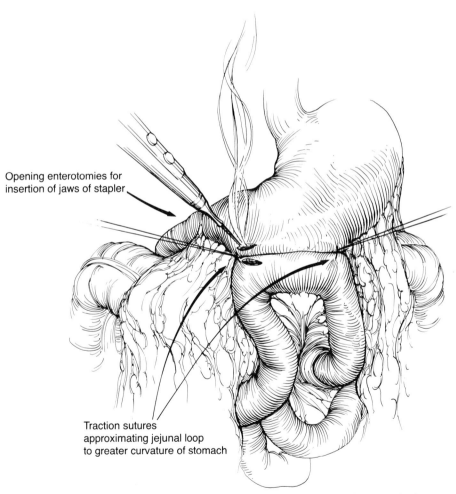

Opening enterotomies for
insertion of jaws of stapler

Traction sutures
approximating jejunal loop
to greater curvature of stomach

FIGURE 65–1. An appropriate area of upper jejunum 18 to 20 inches distal to the ligament of Treitz should be selected and carefully oriented. Traction sutures should be placed, securing the antimesenteric border of the jejunum to the inferior border of the antrum. The jejunal loop can be either retrocolic or antecolic. The antecolic position is illustrated. Small enterotomies should then be made using cautery, and careful hemostasis should be obtained.

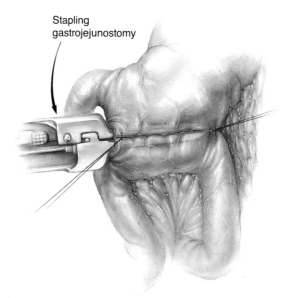

Stapling gastrojejunostomy

FIGURE 65–2. If the gastric wall is not greatly thickened or inflamed, a 4-cm. anastomotic stapler can be used. If the stomach wall is thickened secondary to chronic obstruction, the 10-cm. stapling device should be used. After the anastomotic stapling device has been fired, careful visualization of the staple row should be accomplished by direct inspection. Hemostasis can be obtained by using either low-current cautery or suture ligatures.

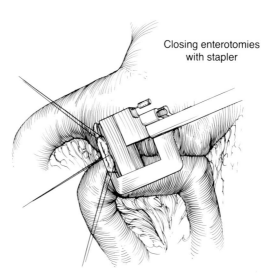

Closing enterotomies with stapler

FIGURE 65–3. The open enterotomies can be approximated using traction sutures, and full thickness of the intestinal wall should be aligned through the PI 55 stapler. Excess tissue should be excised using the scalpel, and hemostasis should be obtained using cautery.

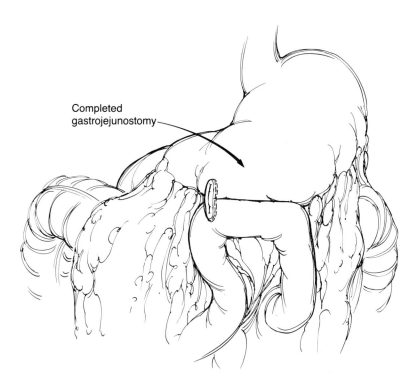

Completed
gastrojejunostomy

FIGURE 65–4. Both staple rows should be carefully inspected for continuity and hemostasis. Adequacy of the gastrojejunostomy can be demonstrated by palpation.

66

Enterotomy for Gallstone Ileus

WILLIAM C. MEYERS, M.D.

Gallstone ileus is an unusual complication of gallstone disease. The problem is obstruction of the small bowel caused by a gallstone that passed through a fistula into the gastrointestinal tract. Obstruction can occur in any part of the tract from the esophagus to the rectum, but the usual site of obstruction is the ileum because of its relatively small caliber compared with the jejunum. The problem is approached by relief of the intestinal obstruction and the underlying biliary problem. It is usually hazardous to treat both problems surgically at the same time. This condition also usually occurs in elderly patients, often with underlying medical problems. As a result of the fistulous process, there is usually dense scarring in the right upper quadrant, which is best initially avoided. When a calcified stone is noted in the lower abdomen of a patient with small bowel obstruction, the diagnosis can be a classic one for the astute clinician.

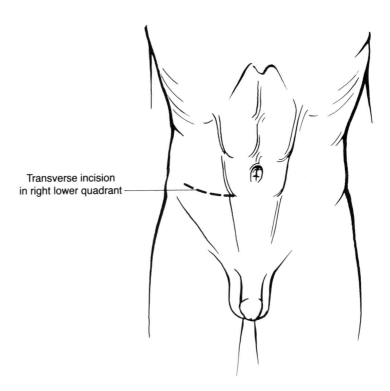

Transverse incision
in right lower quadrant

FIGURE 66–1. The incision is usually transverse, beginning in the right lower quadrant, although the location of the incision may change according to the site of the stone when this is known preoperatively.

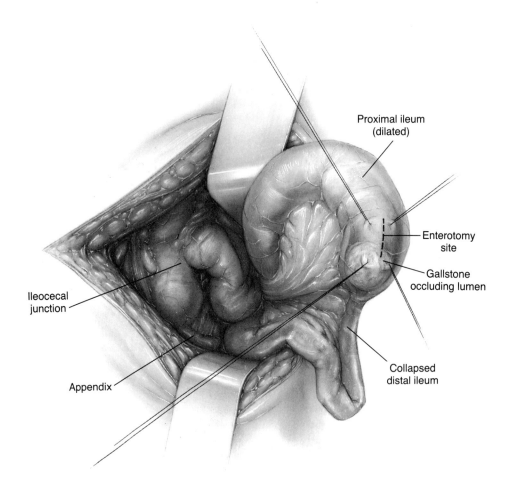

Proximal ileum
(dilated)

Enterotomy
site

Gallstone
occluding lumen

Collapsed
distal ileum

Ileocecal
junction

Appendix

FIGURE 66–2. The intestine is delivered into the operative field through the incision, and the site of obstruction is determined. The ileum distal to the obstruction is usually collapsed, whereas the proximal ileum is distended.

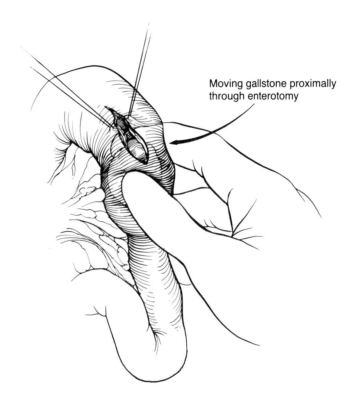

Moving gallstone proximally
through enterotomy

FIGURE 66–3. The stone may be palpated at the site of the obstruction. Traction sutures
are placed for an incision to be made several centimeters proximal to the stone, which
is delivered through the enterotomy. The intestine should be carefully examined for the
presence of other large stones, which can cause similar obstruction. Proximal stones can
be moved distally and removed through the same enterotomy. The enterotomy is closed
in the standard manner using two layers, one interrupted with 2–0 silk and the other a
Connell type with running chromic suture.

67

Roux-en-Y Gastrojejunostomy

WILLIAM C. MEYERS, M.D.

A Roux-en-Y gastrojejunostomy is usually performed after a previous ulcer procedure has been done. The usual indications are bile reflux, gastritis, or the dumping syndrome. The patient may have had a previous Billroth I or Billroth II operation or a vagotomy with drainage with either pyloroplasty or gastrojejunostomy. A conversion of a Billroth II arrangement to the Roux-en-Y gastrojejunostomy is depicted in the illustrations.

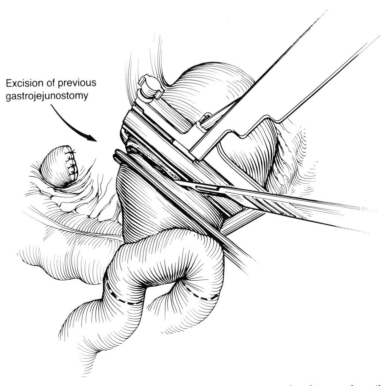

Excision of previous gastrojejunostomy

FIGURE 67–1. Usually, the area of the gastrojejunostomy can be dissected easily unless there is significant marginal ulceration. A plane is found along the mesenteric side of the bowel and stomach, with attention not to injure the mesenteric vessels.

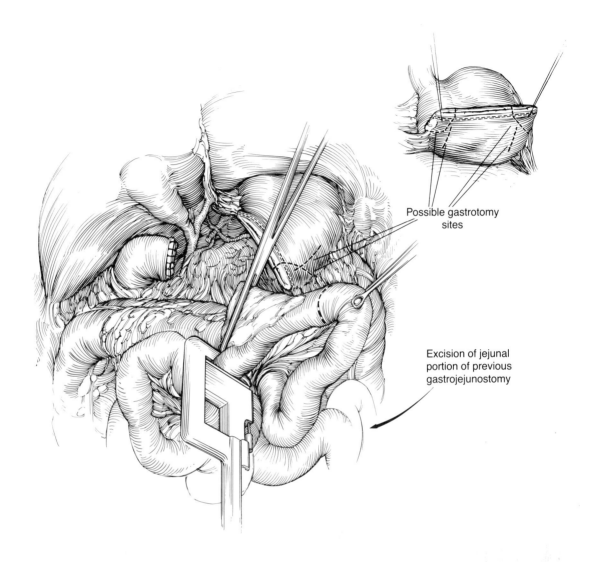

Possible gastrotomy
sites

Excision of jejunal
portion of previous
gastrojejunostomy

FIGURE 67–2. A generous portion of proximal stomach is usually removed with the gastrojejunostomy as well as several inches of jejunum.

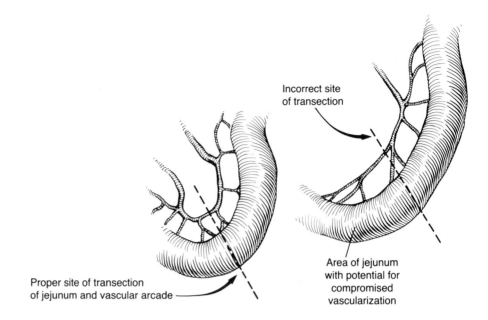

FIGURE 67–3. The site for transection of the jejunum is selected to optimize preservation of the vascular arcade.

FIGURE 67–4. After excision of the gastrojejunostomy, the distal jejunal end is brought up for anastomosis. Several sites of anastomosis are acceptable. A straight anterior anastomosis should be avoided, but even that will work well in most cases. A gastrojejunocolic fistula with posterior anastomoses was a problem prior to the era of the vagotomy, but it is not a problem today. One should be certain to create a length of at least 40 cm. (18 inches) between the gastrojejunostomy and the jejunojejunostomy to maximize prevention of bile reflux.

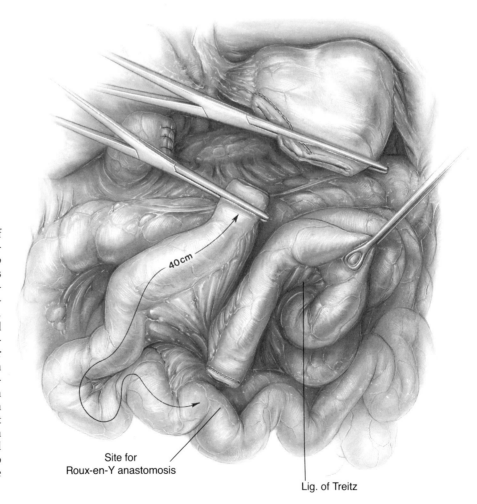

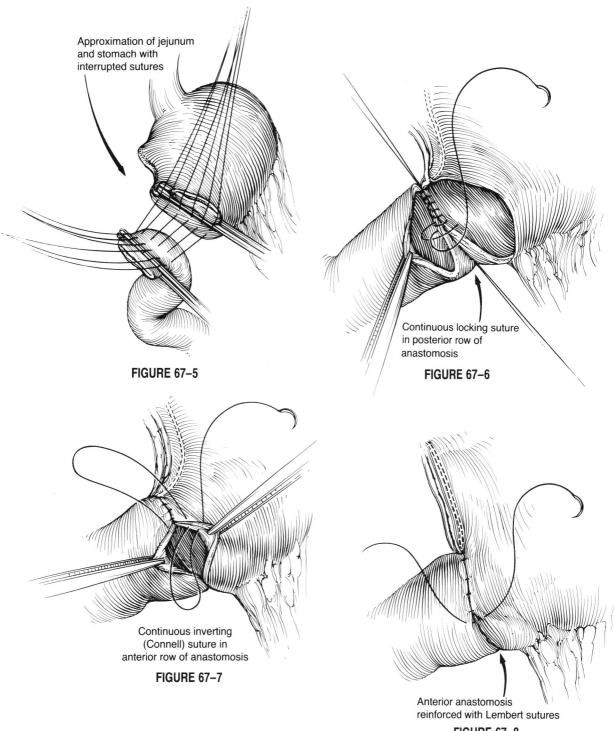

Approximation of jejunum
and stomach with
interrupted sutures

FIGURE 67–5

Continuous locking suture
in posterior row of
anastomosis

FIGURE 67–6

Continuous inverting
(Connell) suture in
anterior row of anastomosis

FIGURE 67–7

Anterior anastomosis
reinforced with Lembert sutures

FIGURE 67–8

FIGURE 67–5. Both the gastrojejunostomy and the jejunojejunostomy are performed in the standard manner either by sutures or with the stapler. It is not uncommon to use a hand-sewn anastomosis for the gastrojejunostomy and a stapling procedure for the jejunojejunostomy. Depicted is a hand-sewn anastomosis along the greater curvature of the stomach after excision of a portion of the TA-90 staple line.

FIGURE 67–6. It is important to reinforce the corner where the hand-sewn anastomosis meets the staple line with an extra silk suture.

FIGURE 67–7. Continuous Connell chromic sutures are placed for the anterior wall of the anastomosis.

FIGURE 67–8. The anastomosis is then reinforced with Lembert sutures.

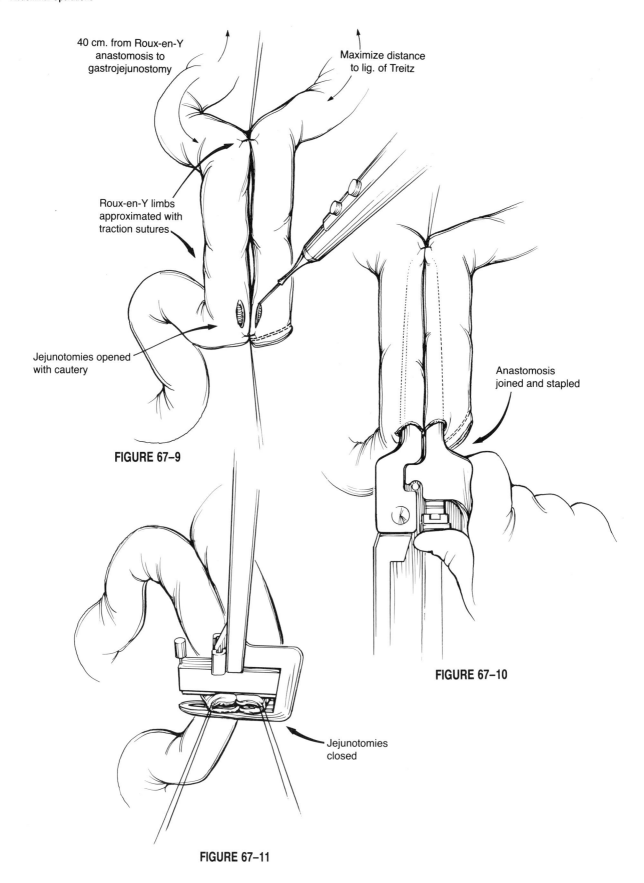

40 cm. from Roux-en-Y anastomosis to gastrojejunostomy

Maximize distance to lig. of Treitz

Roux-en-Y limbs approximated with traction sutures

Jejunotomies opened with cautery

FIGURE 67–9

Anastomosis joined and stapled

FIGURE 67–10

Jejunotomies closed

FIGURE 67–11

FIGURES 67–9 to 67–11 *See legends on opposite page*

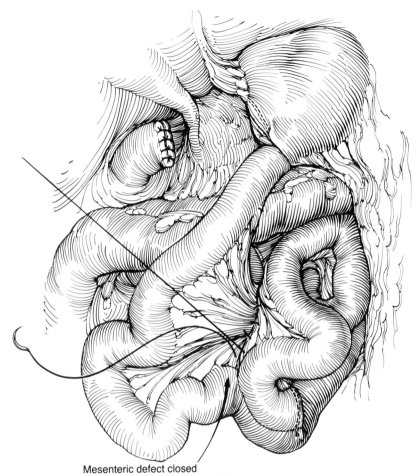

Mesenteric defect closed

FIGURE 67-12. The only mesenteric defect that needs to be closed is that between the Roux segment and the proximal jejunum.

FIGURE 67-9. The jejunojejunostomy should be performed at least 40 cm. from the gastrojejunostomy. Traction sutures are placed approximating Roux-en-Y limbs, and enterotomies are made using cautery at the point of anastomosis.

FIGURE 67-10. The GIA stapler is inserted through the jejunotomies, closed, and fired.

FIGURE 67-11. The TA-55 stapler is used to close the jejunotomies after inspection for hemostasis.

68

Roux-en-Y Gastrojejunostomy (STAPLER)

HILLIARD F. SEIGLER, M.D.

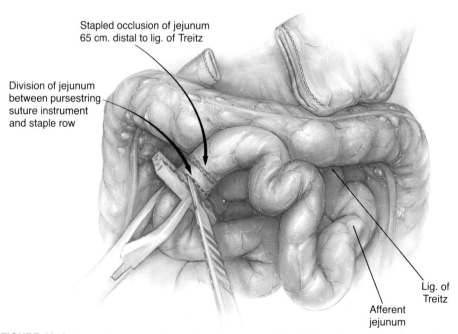

FIGURE 68–1. A partial gastrectomy has been completed. The stapled duodenal stump is secure, as is the stapled gastric pouch. An area of jejunum approximately 40 cm. from the ligament of Treitz is mobilized, a pursestring device is applied to the distal jejunum, and the proximal jejunum is stapled with either a PI 30 or PI 55 stapler, depending on bowel size.

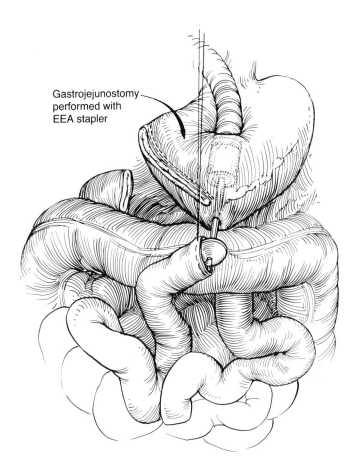

Gastrojejunostomy
performed with
EEA stapler

FIGURE 68–2. A gastrotomy is made on the anterior surface of the gastric pouch, and the EEA instrument is passed with the anvil not in place. The center rod is fully extended to the posterior and inferior portion of the gastric pouch 2 to 3 cm. away from the previously constructed staple row. With the Bovie, the center rod is passed through the posterior stomach wall; a pursestring suture is tied securely in place, thus preventing tear of the gastric wall at the location of the center rod. The anvil is then placed; with either Allis clamps or Babcock clamps, the open end of the distal jejunum is carefully slipped in and the pursestring suture is tied gently to the center rod. The EEA cartridge and anvil are approximated, and the instrument is fired. The EEA instrument is removed, and the tissue doughnuts are carefully inspected for completeness. The anastomosis can be directly visualized through the gastrotomy opening after the EEA instrument has been removed.

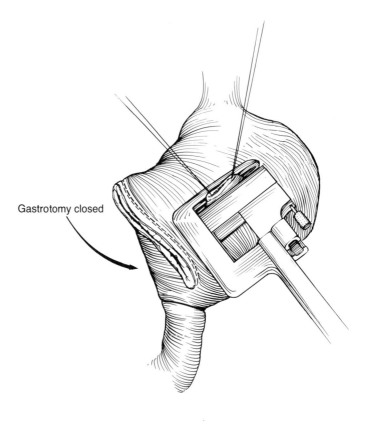

Gastrotomy closed

FIGURE 68–3. The gastrotomy is closed by using either approximating sutures or Allis clamps to place the tissue through the PI 55 stapler.

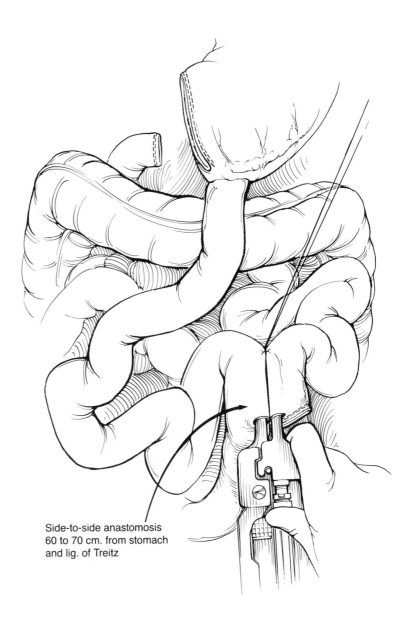

Side-to-side anastomosis
60 to 70 cm. from stomach
and lig. of Treitz

FIGURE 68–4. A side-to-side anastomosis to reconstitute the jejunum is constructed. Enterotomies are made with the Bovie in the antimesenteric position after an anchoring suture has been placed. Either a 5-cm. or 10-cm. GIA instrument can be used for construction of the anastomosis.

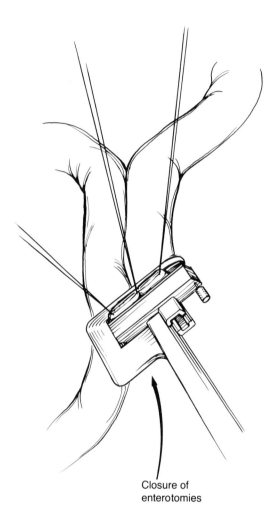

Closure of
enterotomies

FIGURE 68–5. The staple row should be carefully inspected for complete hemostasis prior to closing the enterotomies with a PI 55 stapler.

69

Meckel's Diverticulectomy

THEODORE N. PAPPAS, M.D.

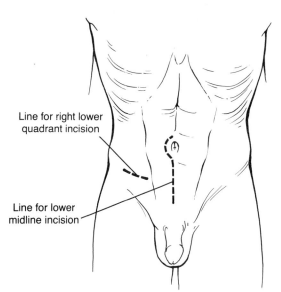

Line for right lower
quadrant incision

Line for lower
midline incision

FIGURE 69–1. In the unusual circumstance when a patient is explored after a preoperative diagnosis of Meckel's diverticulum for bleeding or diverticulitis, a periumbilical or lower midline incision can be performed. Meckel's diverticulectomy is usually performed during exploration for appendicitis through a right lower quadrant incision or removed through a midline incision during exploration for an acute abdomen. Occasionally, the diverticulum is incidentally removed during operations for other reasons. The terminal ileum and the Meckel's diverticulum are mobilized into the wound.

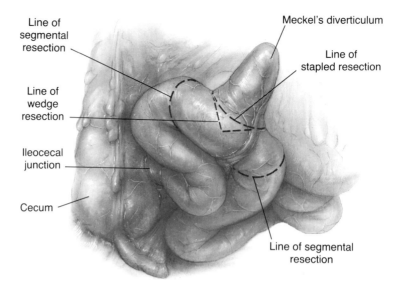

Line of
segmental
resection

Meckel's diverticulum

Line of
stapled resection

Line of
wedge
resection

Ileocecal
junction

Cecum

Line of segmental
resection

FIGURE 69–2

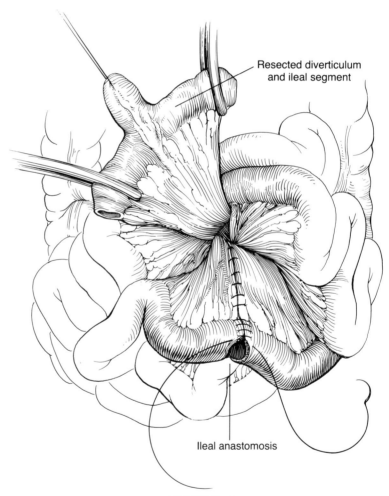

Resected diverticulum
and ileal segment

Ileal anastomosis

FIGURE 69–3

FIGURES 69–2 and 69–3. A decision is made at this time whether small intestinal continuity should remain intact and the diverticulum should be excised alone, or whether a small bowel resection should be performed (see Fig. 69–3.) It should be emphasized that a separate artery and vein in the mesentery of the Meckel's diverticulum should be ligated to prevent intramesenteric hemorrhage. Most Meckel's diverticuli can be excised by transecting the base of the diverticulum, which can be performed easily with a TA-30 stapler.

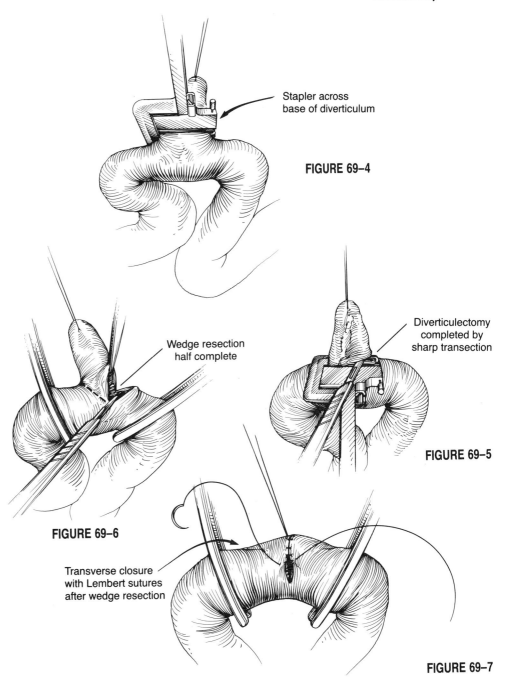

FIGURE 69-4

Stapler across
base of diverticulum

Wedge resection
half complete

Diverticulectomy
completed by
sharp transection

FIGURE 69-5

FIGURE 69-6

Transverse closure
with Lembert sutures
after wedge resection

FIGURE 69-7

FIGURE 69-4. The stapler is placed across the base of the diverticulum, being certain not to compromise the lumen of the small intestine.

FIGURE 69-5. The stapler is fired, and the specimen is removed with a No. 15 blade. The staple line does not require inversion in this situation.

FIGURE 69-6. If inflammation at the base of the Meckel's diverticulum requires a wedge resection of the small bowel, the diverticulum can be removed in this manner and the bowel reanastomosed, avoiding compromise of the bowel lumen. Active bleeding secondary to gastric mucosa in the Meckel's diverticulum should be treated with segmental resection.

FIGURE 69-7. The bowel is reanastomosed by closing the open end of the intestine transversely with a single layer of interrupted 3-0 silk Lembert sutures.

70

Appendectomy

JOHN P. GRANT, M.D.

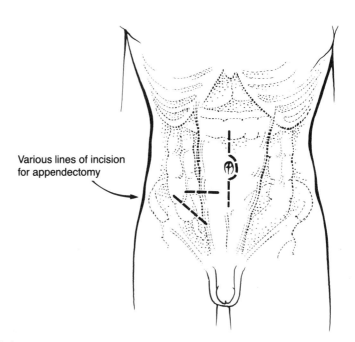

Various lines of incision for appendectomy

FIGURE 70–1. The incision can be placed in one of several locations. Some prefer the right lower quadrant with a muscle-splitting technique. Others prefer the right lower quadrant transverse incision overlying the rectus muscle with reflection of the muscle medially. Whenever the diagnosis is in question, a midline incision is certainly appropriate.

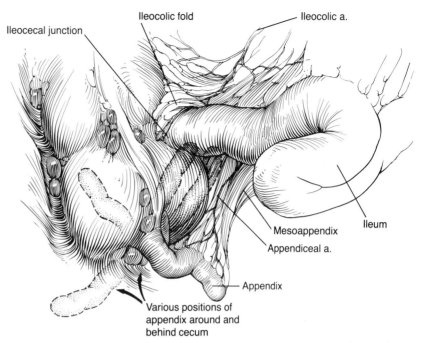

Ileocecal junction
Ileocolic fold
Ileocolic a.
Mesoappendix
Ileum
Appendiceal a.
Appendix
Various positions of
appendix around and
behind cecum

FIGURE 70–2. The appendix is located at the junction of the taeniae of the colonic wall at the tip of the cecum. It is supplied by the appendiceal artery, which must be ligated during removal of the appendix. It may be located in nearly any position, including retrocecal, extending upward toward the hepatic flexure of the colon.

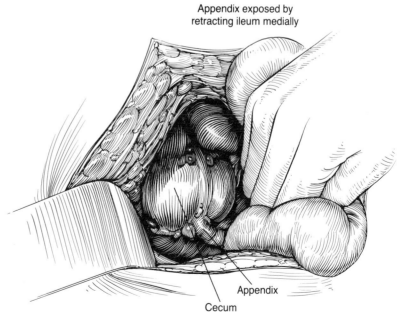

Appendix exposed by
retracting ileum medially

Appendix
Cecum

FIGURE 70–3. Upon entry into the abdomen, the small intestine is mobilized medially; the cecum is identified in the right lower quadrant. The appendix is often identified visually, but, if not, it can easily be identified by palpation, as it will be swollen and firm. Adhesions of the omentum can usually be bluntly dissected free.

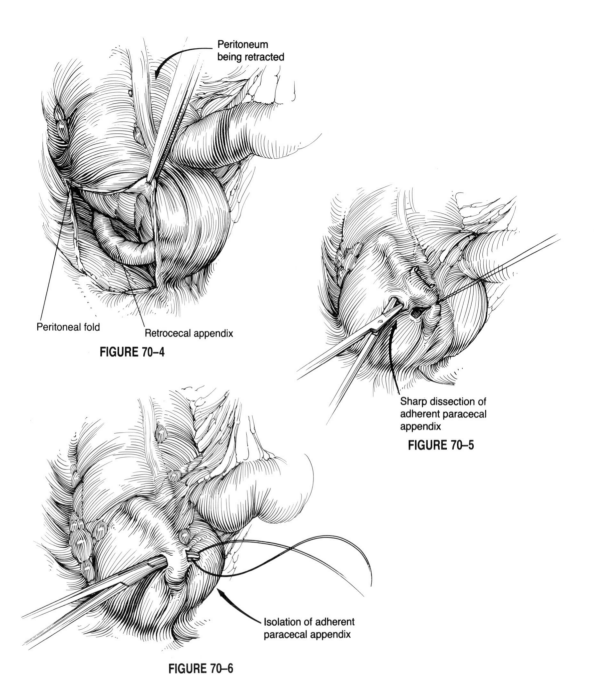

Peritoneum
being retracted

Peritoneal fold

Retrocecal appendix

FIGURE 70–4

Sharp dissection of
adherent paracecal
appendix

FIGURE 70–5

Isolation of adherent
paracecal appendix

FIGURE 70–6

FIGURE 70–4. If the appendix is retrocecal, the lateral peritoneal reflection must be incised and the cecum mobilized medially and anteriorly. The appendix can then be freed by blunt and sharp dissection.

FIGURES 70–5 and 70–6. If the appendix is paracecal, dense adhesions are bluntly dissected for exposure.

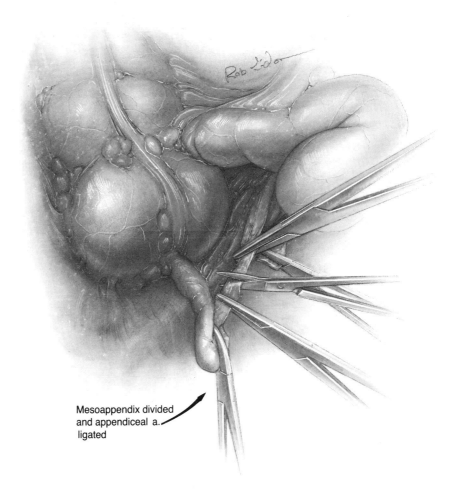

Mesoappendix divided
and appendiceal a.
ligated

FIGURE 70–7. After mobilization of the appendix, the mesoappendix is divided between clamps and carefully ligated to ensure hemostasis. The division is continued until the neck of the appendix at its junction with the cecum is completely cleared.

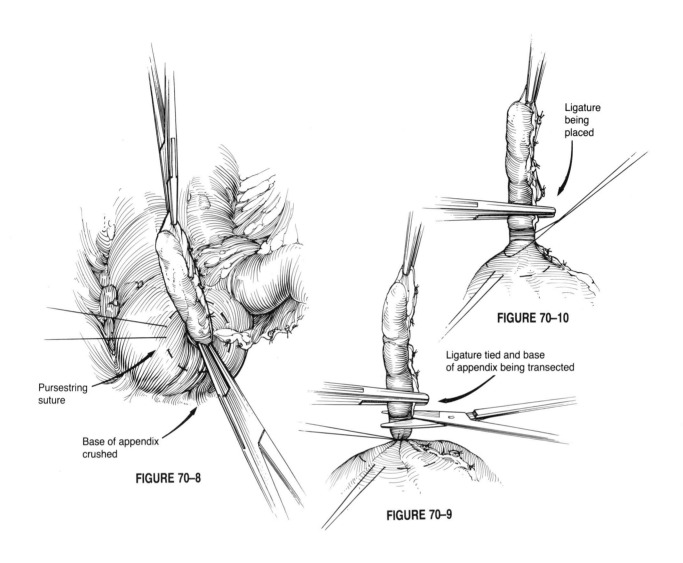

Ligature
being
placed

FIGURE 70–10

Ligature tied and base
of appendix being transected

FIGURE 70–9

Pursestring
suture

Base of appendix
crushed

FIGURE 70–8

FIGURES 70–8 to 70–10. A pursestring suture is placed at the base of the appendix approximately 1.0 cm. from the junction to allow for invagination of the stump. Two hemostats are placed at the base of the appendix to crush the tissue. The lower hemostat is removed, and a 1–0 chromic catgut ligature is placed.

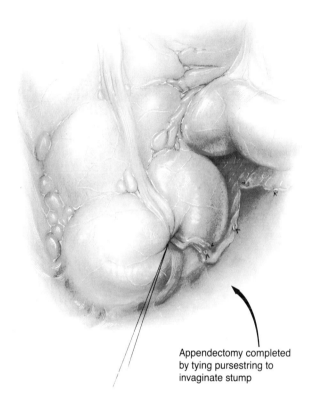

Appendectomy completed
by tying pursestring to
invaginate stump

FIGURE 70–11. The appendix is divided and the stump invaginated by securing the pursestring suture. Drains are rarely indicated. The distal ileum is examined for presence of a Meckel's diverticulum. The wound is closed in layers, leaving the skin open if an abscess is present.

71

Laparoscopic Appendectomy

THEODORE N. PAPPAS, M.D.

Laparoscopic appendectomy is an alternative to open appendectomy for use in selected patients. This technique is particularly applicable in women in whom diagnostic uncertainty exists. With a nasogastric tube and Foley catheter in place, the patient is placed in the Trendelenburg position. A small infraumbilical incision is made, and a Veress needle is placed. The abdomen is insufflated with three liters of carbon dioxide or until the insufflation pressure exceeds 10 mm. Hg.

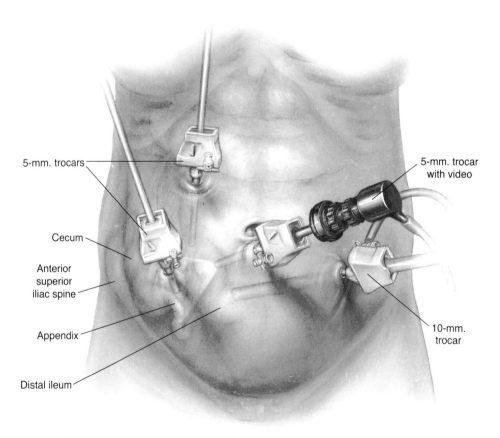

FIGURE 71–1. A 5-mm. trocar is placed in the umbilical incision, and a 5-mm. video laparoscope is placed. The other two 5-mm. trocars are placed in the right side of the abdomen. An alternate technique is to place a Hasson trocar in the umbilicus to allow removal of a thickened appendix through the umbilical incision.

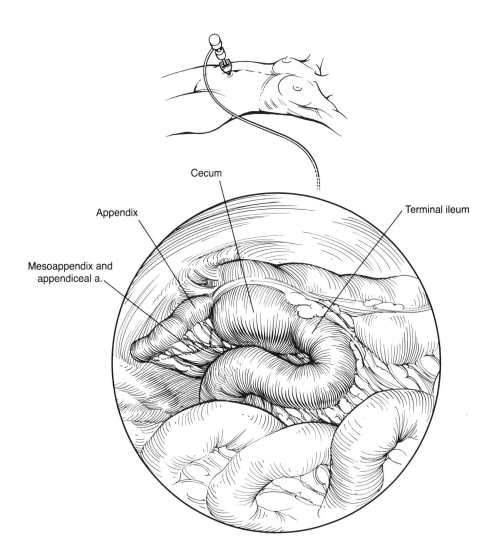

Cecum

Appendix

Terminal ileum

Mesoappendix and
appendiceal a.

FIGURE 71–2. A 10-mm. trocar is placed in the left lower quadrant in a tangential manner, thereby obviating the need for closure of the fascia at the completion of the procedure. The abdomen is visually explored, and appendicitis is confirmed. An endoloop is placed through a 5-mm. trocar, and the end of the appendix is snared for retraction. The mesoappendix is then easily visualized.

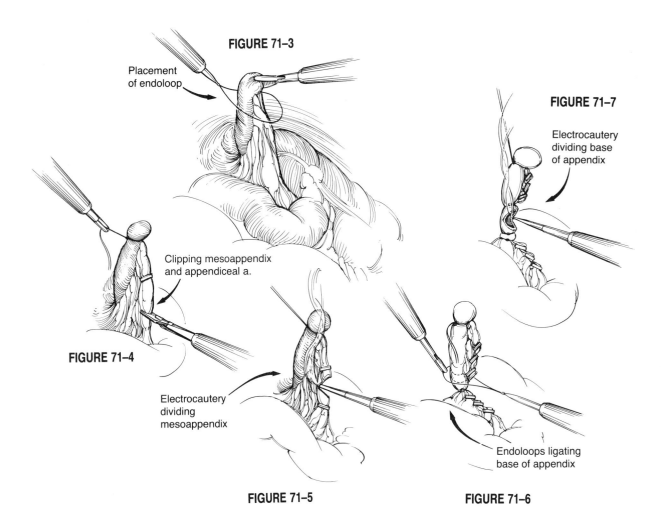

FIGURE 71–3

Placement of endoloop

FIGURE 71–7

Electrocautery dividing base of appendix

Clipping mesoappendix and appendiceal a.

FIGURE 71–4

Electrocautery dividing mesoappendix

Endoloops ligating base of appendix

FIGURE 71–5

FIGURE 71–6

FIGURES 71–3 to 71–6. The mesoappendix is dissected via the 10-mm. port. The appendiceal artery and associated fat are controlled with electrocautery and clips. When the base of the appendix is easily seen, three additional endoloops are placed sequentially on the appendix. Two are placed on the cecal side, and one is placed on the specimen side. These endoloops are secured, and the specimen is transected. An endoscopic linear stapler can be used through a 12-mm. port in the left lower quadrant to control both the appendiceal stump and appendiceal artery.

FIGURE 71–7. Electrocautery is used to cauterize the mucosa on the appendiceal stump.

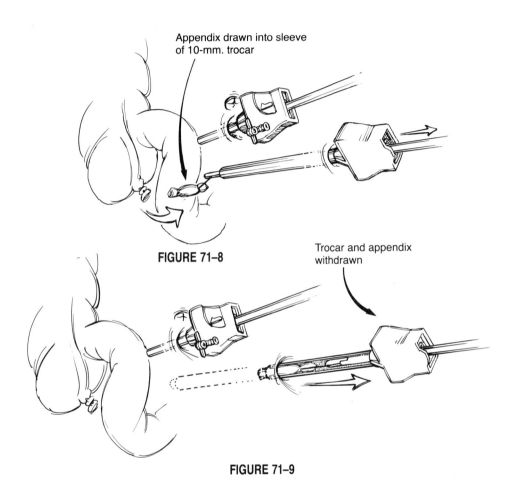

Appendix drawn into sleeve
of 10-mm. trocar

FIGURE 71–8

Trocar and appendix
withdrawn

FIGURE 71–9

FIGURES 71–8 and 71–9. The specimen is pulled into the reducing sleeve of the 10-mm. trocar and is extracted. An alternate technique is to pass the appendix into a rubber sac, which can be placed through the 10-mm. port or pulled directly out of the skin mucosa. The right lower quadrant is then generously irrigated, and the trocars removed. Steri-Strips are placed on the skin.

72

Reduction of Intussusception

NICHOLAS A. SHORTER, M.D.

The primary diagnostic and therapeutic maneuver for idiopathic intussusception is a contrast enema. When full reduction of the intussusception is unsuccessful, surgical reduction is necessary.

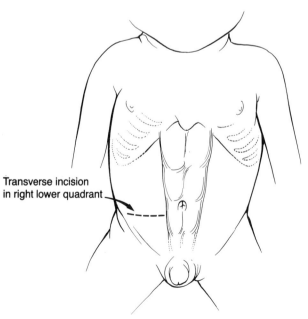

FIGURE 72–1. The abdomen is opened through an adequate right lower quadrant transverse incision.

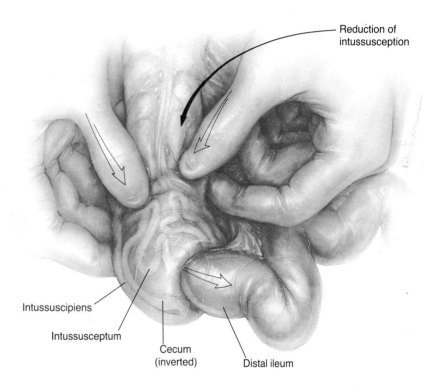

FIGURE 72–2. The intussusception is reduced by gently *pushing* it backward but not by *pulling* it, which can damage the edematous and friable bowel. Resection is indicated only for irreversible ischemia or in the rare instance when a pathologic leadpoint (polyp, tumor, Meckel's diverticulum) is identified.

Reduction alone is adequate; nothing is gained by fixing the bowel in any way, as it does not decrease the risk of recurrence. An appendectomy is usually performed.

73

Correction of Malrotation with Midgut Volvulus

ARTHUR J. ROSS III, M.D.

Malrotation is a potentially lethal anomaly that may present with intermittent vomiting or as an acute abdomen caused by midgut volvulus with intestinal ischemia. It may occasionally be diagnosed due to totally unrelated reasons. When the diagnosis has been established, surgical therapy should be planned.

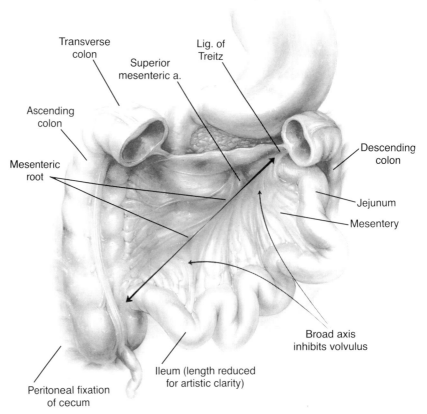

FIGURE 73–1 *See legend on opposite page*

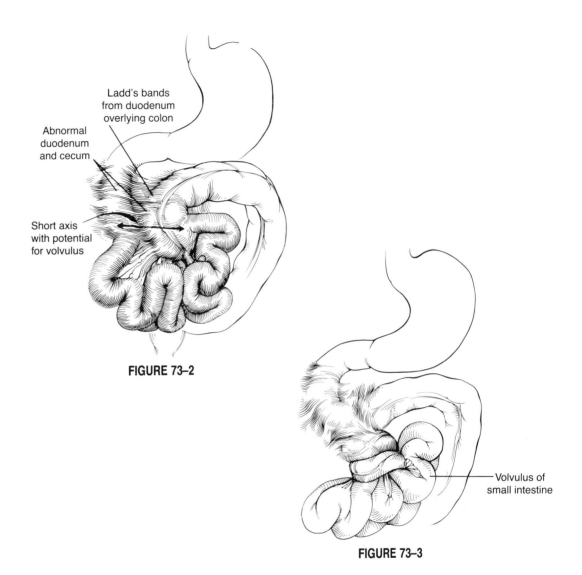

Ladd's bands
from duodenum
overlying colon

Abnormal
duodenum
and cecum

Short axis
with potential
for volvulus

FIGURE 73–2

Volvulus of
small intestine

FIGURE 73–3

FIGURES 73–1 to 73–3. Malrotation is caused by an incomplete rotation of the intestine during development. The most feared complication of this disorder of embryogenesis is volvulus, a phenomenon that rarely occurs in the presence of normal rotation of the intestine because a broad axis about the superior mesenteric artery is created by fixation of the duodenal jejunal region at the ligament of Treitz and cecum in the right lower quadrant.

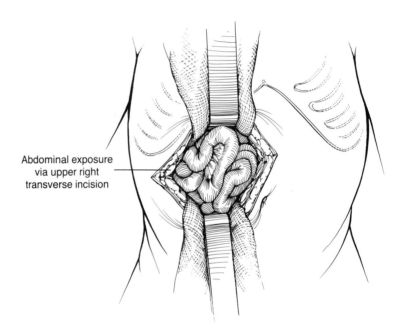

Abdominal exposure
via upper right
transverse incision

FIGURE 73–4. Nasogastric decompression is performed, along with rapid fluid resuscitation and initiation of intravenous antibiotics. One should not delay trying to correct a metabolic imbalance, which cannot be achieved until the volvulus has been managed.

The abdomen is entered through a transverse right upper quadrant incision. Rotational abnormalities can be confusing. It is helpful to deliver the entire distribution of small and large bowel very gently through the incision to define the anatomy of the anomaly. When a volvulus is present, the colon is often not seen upon entering the abdomen because it has been displaced posteriorly by the twist around the base of the mesentery. Indeed, before derotation, it will appear as though the colon is wound around the base of the mesentery. Successful reduction of the volvulus is recognized when the base is no longer encircled by the colon.

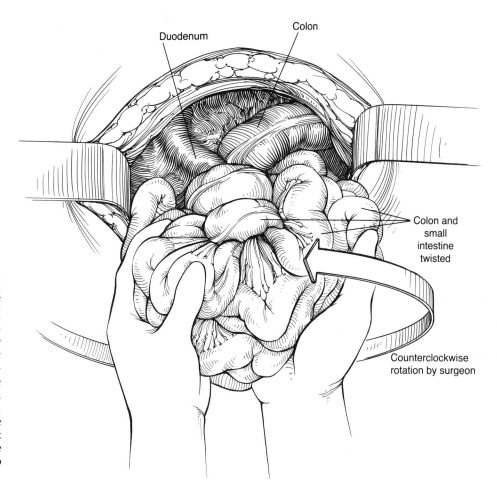

Duodenum

Colon

Colon and
small
intestine
twisted

Counterclockwise
rotation by surgeon

FIGURE 73–5. Because the volvulus is always in a clockwise direction, the entire mass of small and large bowel should be derotated in a counterclockwise direction. Under no circumstances should any bowel appearing compromised be resected until the anatomy has been defined and the volvulus reduced, because this maneuver alone usually produces a significant improvement unless the process has progressed to frank gangrene.

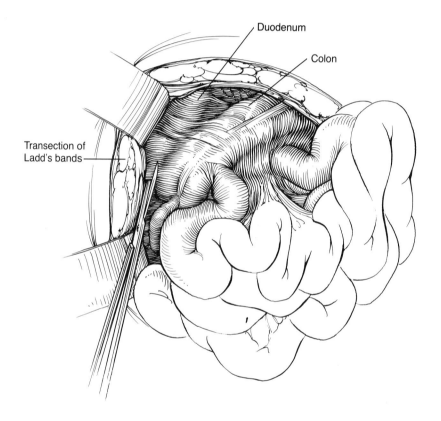

Duodenum

Colon

Transection of
Ladd's bands

FIGURE 73–6. Following derotation, the ileocecal portion of the intestine is generally drawn toward the left lower quadrant, such that Ladd's bands can be placed on appropriate tension to evaluate the degree of duodenal obstruction that they have created. As these peritoneal bands covering the duodenum are divided, the surgeon is easily able to begin the separation of the cecum and right colon from the duodenum, which allows the duodenocolic isthmus to be broadened. The superior mesenteric vessels and hepatic triad can be injured in performing this dissection; therefore, the surgeon is well advised to remain very close to the duodenal serosa to minimize the occurrence of this complication. The base of the mesentery can also be broadened when the duodenocolic isthmus has been managed, and this is accomplished by dividing the bands that attach the cecum and right colon to the base of the mesentery as well as to adjacent loops of bowel. Care should be taken not to enter into the mesentery. The final goal is to achieve sufficient broadening of the mesentery such that the right colon and cecum are mobile and lie comfortably within the region of the left gutter, whereas the duodenum and proximal jejunum lie comfortably within the right gutter.

FIGURE 73–7

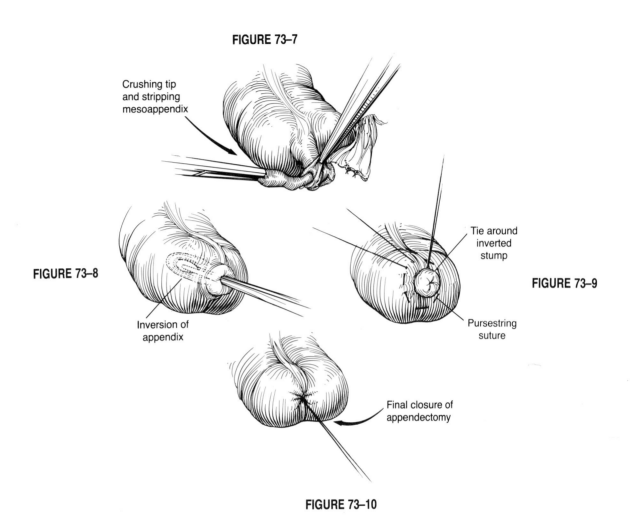

Crushing tip
and stripping
mesoappendix

FIGURE 73–8

Inversion of
appendix

Tie around
inverted
stump

FIGURE 73–9

Pursestring
suture

Final closure of
appendectomy

FIGURE 73–10

FIGURES 73–7 to 73–10. An appendectomy should be performed, and the inversion technique is preferred.

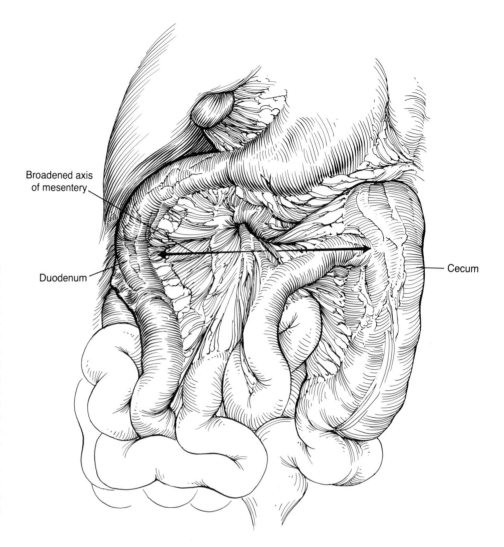

FIGURE 73–11. A nasogastric tube is passed through the pylorus and into the duodenum to exclude a duodenal web. Before closing, it is important to be certain that the intestine is replaced within the abdomen such that the duodenum and jejunum course straight downward on the right side of the abdomen and that the colon remains on the left. Fixation of the bowel in this position is neither necessary nor desirable. It is extremely rare to encounter recurrent volvulus because the bowel becomes fixed as positioned at the time of operation.

In those unfortunate cases in which either gangrenous or perforated bowel exists, that portion of the bowel must be resected. In certain instances, the judgment as to resection with primary reanastomosis versus exteriorization must be made by the surgeon as deemed appropriate. Should a substantial length of bowel be compromised, one is best advised to resect only that bowel that is definitely gangrenous and/ or perforated, with a second-look procedure scheduled about 12 to 24 hours later, when a far clearer assessment of intestinal viability can be made. This strategy is critical to avoid the creation of the short gut syndrome.

Colon

74

Right Colectomy

WILLIAM C. MEYERS, M.D.

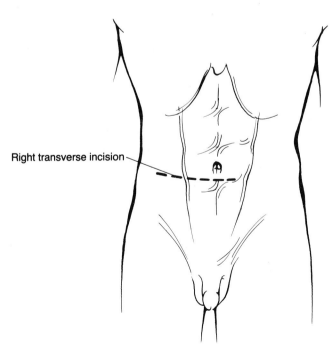

Right transverse incision

FIGURE 74-1. The easiest approach for performance of a right colectomy is through a right transverse incision just above or below the umbilicus.

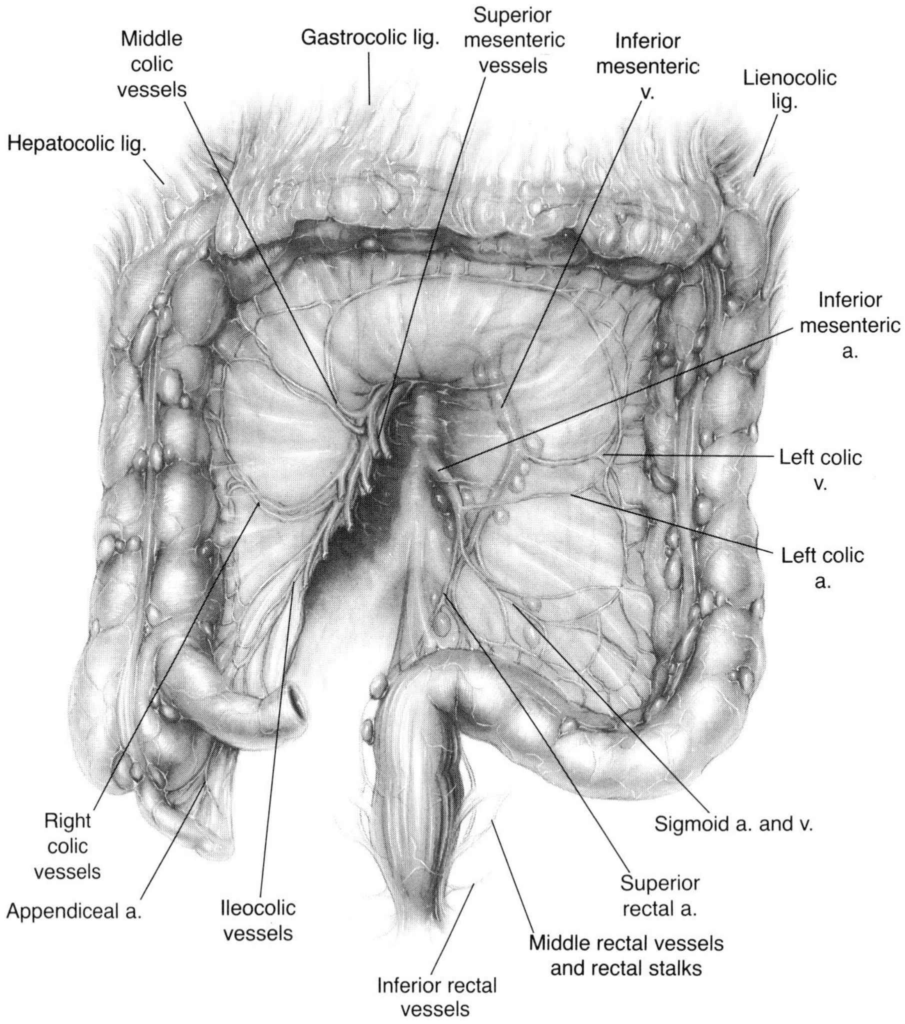

FIGURE 74–2. After general exploration for carcinoma and, in particular, examination of the liver, the first step in a right colectomy is mobilization of the right colon.

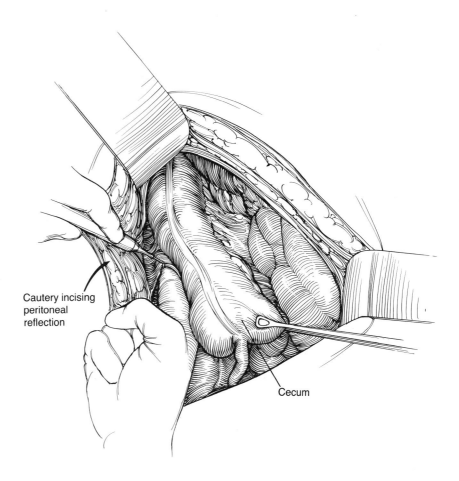

Cautery incising
peritoneal
reflection

Cecum

FIGURE 74–3. Except in the presence of cirrhosis when there is tremendous retroperitoneal hypervascularity, the best method of mobilization of the ascending colon is with
the cautery along the white line of Toldt.

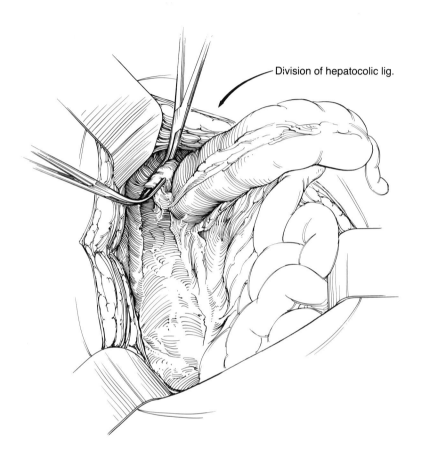

Division of hepatocolic lig.

FIGURE 74–4. A number of small vessels are usually present in the hepatocolic ligament, which is divided between Kelly clamps, and these vessels are ligated. Mobilization in this region should extend posteriorly to near the aorta.

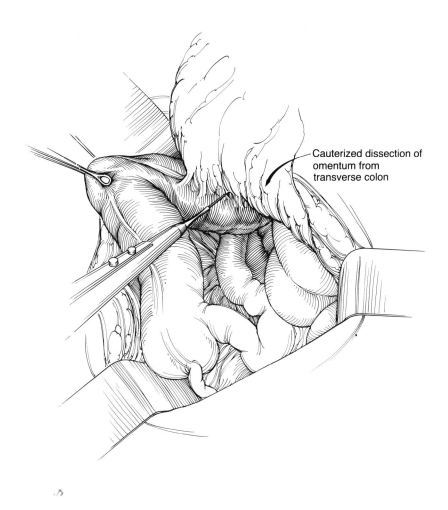

Cauterized dissection of
omentum from
transverse colon

FIGURE 74–5. The greater omentum is mobilized off the transverse colon by dissecting
along the avascular plane next to the bowel wall.

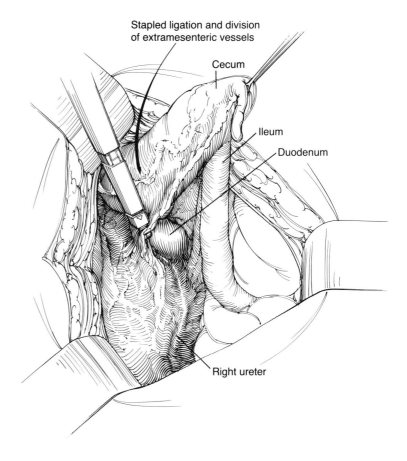

Stapled ligation and division
of extramesenteric vessels

Cecum

Ileum

Duodenum

Right ureter

FIGURE 74–6. Two structures are particularly important to identify for prevention of injury during the performance of a right colectomy: the duodenum and the right ureter located posteriorly. Injury to the duodenum increases the incidence of complications. Occasionally, a tumor may be closely adherent to the duodenum. In this situation, the best procedure is local excision of the duodenum *en bloc* with the specimen in primary two-layer repair.

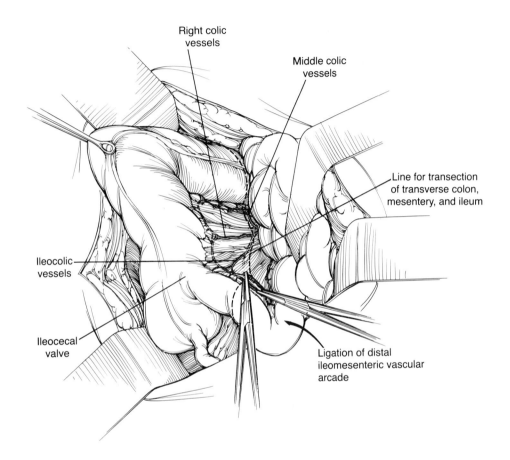

Right colic
vessels

Middle colic
vessels

Line for transection
of transverse colon,
mesentery, and ileum

Ileocolic
vessels

Ileocecal
valve

Ligation of distal
ileomesenteric vascular
arcade

FIGURE 74–7. The sites for division of the bowel are selected, and an area of relatively little vascularity approximately 2 inches proximal to the ileocecal valve is chosen, as well as a similar site just to the right of the main trunk of the middle colic vessels. Then the mesenteric vessels are divided. These include the ileocolic artery and right trunk of the middle colic vessels. The origin of the ileocolic artery is included, but branches are preserved to the left transverse colon.

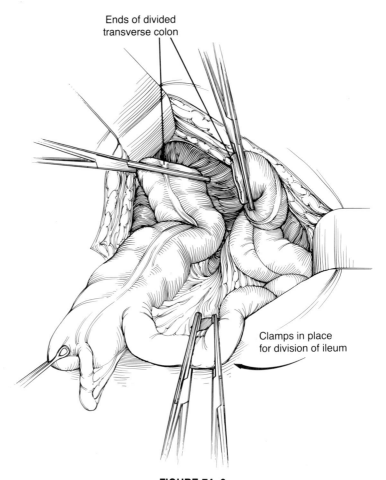

FIGURE 74-8

FIGURES 74-8 to 74-12. The anastomosis may be performed by various methods. Usually, the simplest and probably the fastest is a hand-sewn double-layer technique approximating the end of the ileum to the end of the right transverse colon. In the case of a very small caliber ileum, a stapling anastomosis may be more practical, but a direct anastomosis can usually be achieved.

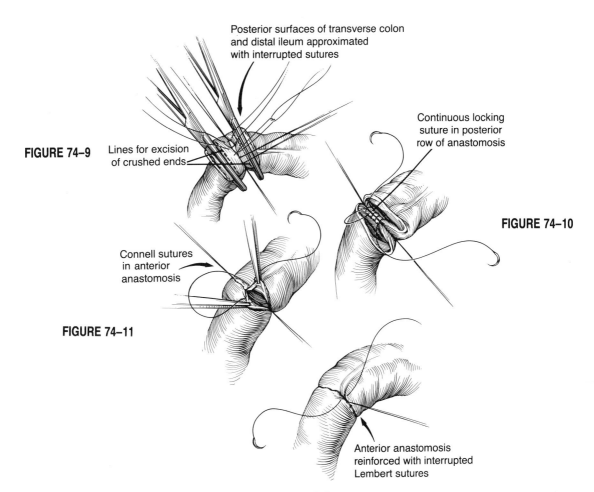

FIGURE 74–9

Posterior surfaces of transverse colon and distal ileum approximated with interrupted sutures

Lines for excision of crushed ends

Continuous locking suture in posterior row of anastomosis

FIGURE 74–10

Connell sutures in anterior anastomosis

FIGURE 74–11

Anterior anastomosis reinforced with interrupted Lembert sutures

FIGURE 74–12

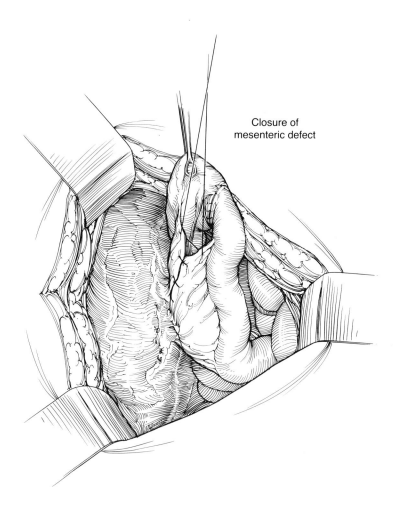

Closure of
mesenteric defect

FIGURE 74–13. Following the anastomosis, the mesenteric defect is repaired in the usual manner.

75

Right Colectomy (STAPLER)

HILLIARD F. SEIGLER, M.D.

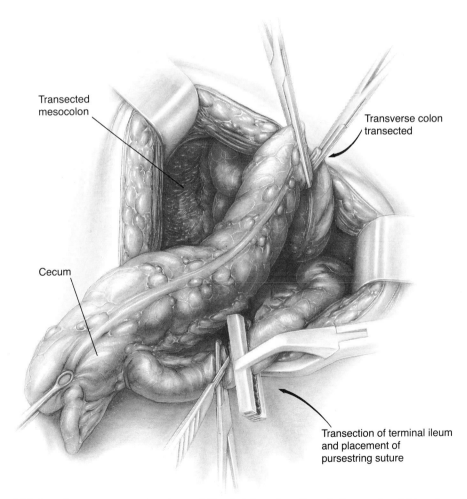

FIGURE 75–1. Demonstrated is the mobilized right colon. Bowel clamps should be placed across both the transverse colon and the distal ileum. A pursestring device can be placed across the proximal ileum.

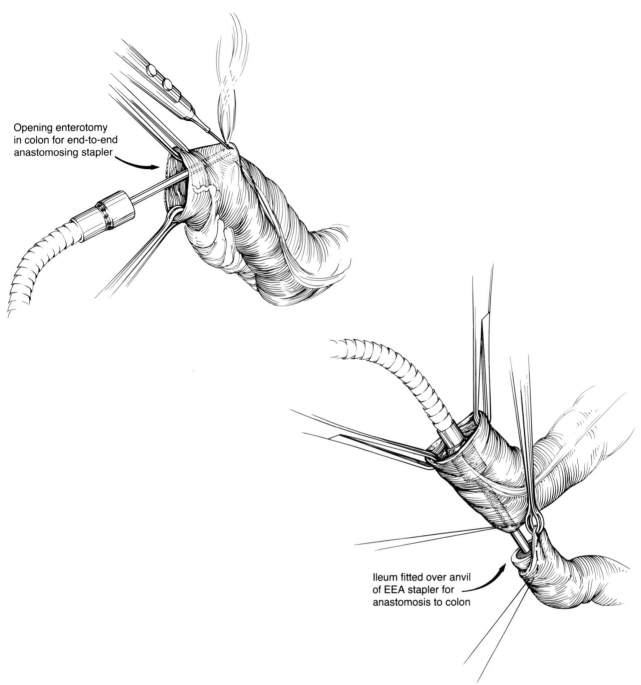

Opening enterotomy
in colon for end-to-end
anastomosing stapler

Ileum fitted over anvil
of EEA stapler for
anastomosis to colon

FIGURE 75–2. Prior to placing the anvil on the extended rod of the end-to-end stapler, the rod should be passed through the open end of the transverse colon. A small opening is made on the antimesenteric border some 3 cm. from the divided colon. A silk pursestring suture should be placed after the rod has been passed through the bowel wall.

FIGURE 75–3. The anvil is carefully secured, and the terminal ileum is passed over the anvil. The pursestring suture is then tied securely around the rod. The suture should be divided close to the rod so that the tie ends are not protruding beyond the anvil. The end-to-end stapler is approximated in a standard manner. The instrument is then fired. After the instrument has been fired, a complete turn in a counterclockwise direction is carried out, and the instrument is carefully removed through the anastomosis. Care should be taken to inspect for completeness of the two doughnuts removed from the instrument. Hemostasis should be ensured using direct visualization through the open end of the transverse colon.

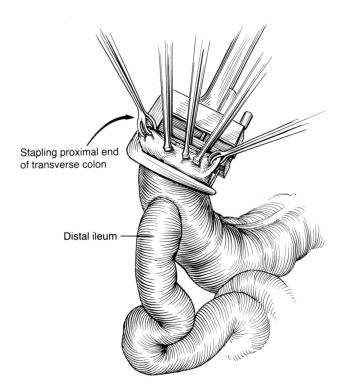

Stapling proximal end
of transverse colon

Distal ileum

FIGURE 75–4. The open end of the transverse colon should be stapled securely using either a 55-mm. or a 90-mm. PI stapler. Care should be taken to ensure that approximately 2 cm. of transverse colon is present between the stapling device and the distal ileum, thus permitting adequate blood supply to the anastomotic area. Once the excess tissue has been excised, hemostasis should be obtained with cautery.

76

Transverse Colostomy

WILLIAM C. MEYERS, M.D.

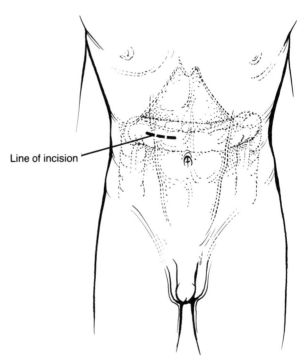

FIGURE 76–1. The standard transverse loop colostomy is made using a horizontal incision above the umbilicus.

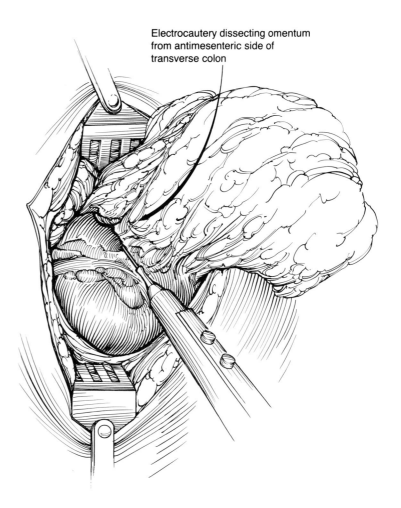

Electrocautery dissecting omentum
from antimesenteric side of
transverse colon

FIGURE 76–2. After the peritoneal cavity is entered, the transverse colon can usually be easily identified by traction on the omentum.

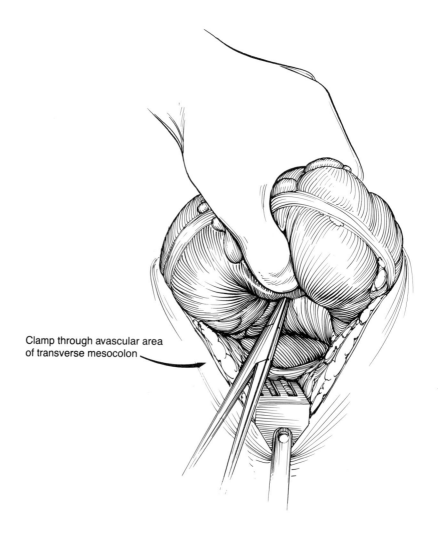

Clamp through avascular area
of transverse mesocolon

FIGURE 76–3. The taeniae coli may help to distinguish the colon from the small intestine. Because a loop colostomy is being performed rather than an end colostomy, it is not as important to identify which end is proximal. However, one should make the effort to determine orientation to avoid twisting the colon. After the omentum is cleaned from the antimesenteric side of the colon, the avascular plane is penetrated along the mesenteric side with a clamp.

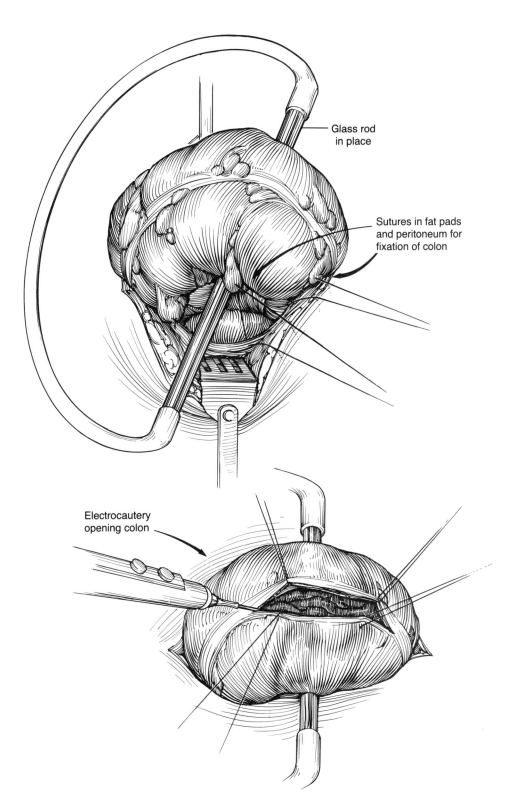

Glass rod
in place

Sutures in fat pads
and peritoneum for
fixation of colon

Electrocautery
opening colon

FIGURE 76–4. Through this opening, a rod or red rubber Robinson catheter is inserted to support the colon above the level of the skin.

FIGURE 76–5. The colon can be matured immediately or at a later time.

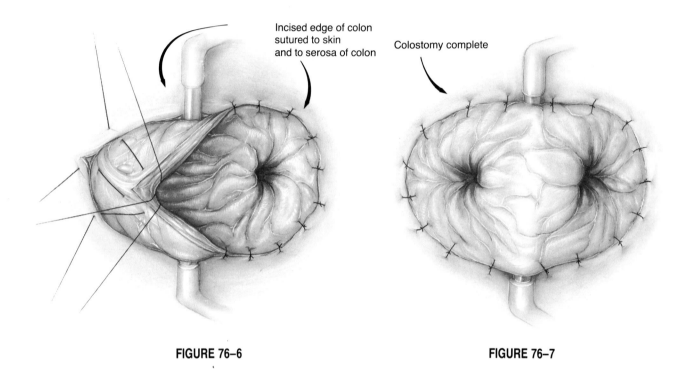

Incised edge of colon
sutured to skin
and to serosa of colon

Colostomy complete

FIGURE 76–6

FIGURE 76–7

FIGURES 76–6 and 76–7. The preferred method to mature the colostomy is to use absorbable sutures, creating a bud by including a portion of the serosa and muscularis in the suture.

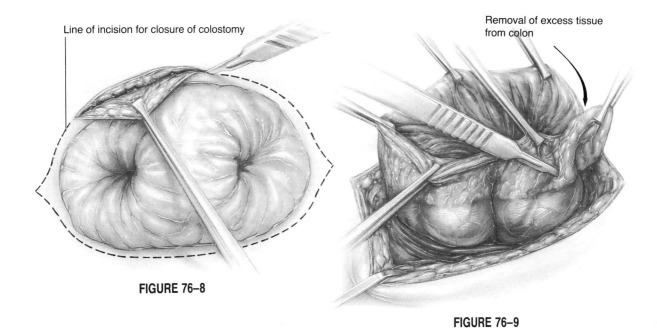

Line of incision for closure of colostomy

FIGURE 76–8

Removal of excess tissue from colon

FIGURE 76–9

FIGURE 76–8. Closure of the loop colostomy is performed using an elliptical incision around the colostomy to include a portion of skin.

FIGURE 76–9. The colon is dissected from the adjacent fascia and other tissue, and the edge of the colostomy is resected.

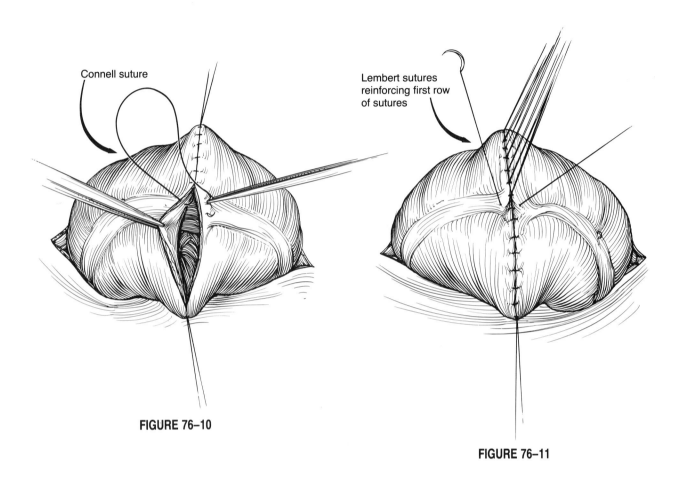

Connell suture

Lembert sutures
reinforcing first row
of sutures

FIGURE 76–10

FIGURE 76–11

FIGURES 76–10 and 76–11. A standard double-layer closure of the colostomy is performed when there is sufficient mobility to perform the anastomosis and return the colon to the abdominal cavity.

77

Laparoscopic Colostomy

H. KIM LYERLY, M.D.

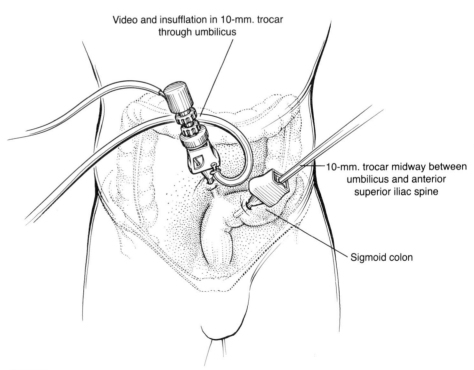

Video and insufflation in 10-mm. trocar
through umbilicus

10-mm. trocar midway between
umbilicus and anterior
superior iliac spine

Sigmoid colon

FIGURE 77–1. The patient is placed in supine position, and the abdomen is prepared and draped in a sterile manner. An orogastric tube and bladder catheter are inserted to decompress the stomach and urinary bladder. Standard insufflation through the umbilicus or in a region that can be safely insufflated is performed. Often, an open insufflation is performed with a Hasson trocar. A 10-mm. port is placed for video inspection of the intra-abdominal contents. A 10-mm. trocar is placed in the left lower quadrant, and this trocar site can be marked preoperatively at the location designated by the surgeon to be ideal for placement of the stoma. Often, a point midway between the anterior superior iliac spine and the umbilicus is satisfactory.

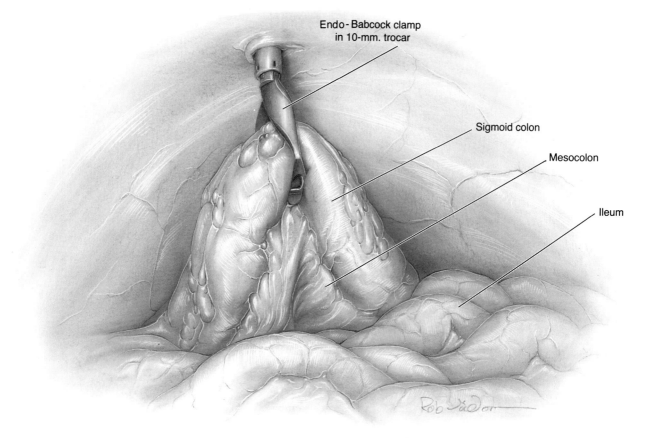

Endo - Babcock clamp
in 10-mm. trocar

Sigmoid colon

Mesocolon

Ileum

FIGURE 77–2. This view of a laparoscope pointed toward the pelvis demonstrates, to the patient's left, the sigmoid colon. Multiple loops of small bowel are noted in the inferior part of the screen. The colon is identified, and a mobile area is grasped with an Endo-Babcock. The sigmoid colon is then mobilized up to the anterior abdominal wall. Any areas of adhesions or pathologic changes that restrict mobilization are evaluated, and a freely movable portion of the sigmoid colon that can be mobilized to the anterior abdominal wall is grasped.

Once the Endo-Babcock has firmly grasped the antimesenteric border of the sigmoid colon, an elliptical skin incision is made around the trocar site. The electrocautery is then used to enlarge the opening of the 10-mm. trocar to an appropriate size for the sigmoid colostomy. Care is used to avoid entry into the peritoneal cavity in making this incision.

Stapling sigmoid colon across
distal end of loop for colostomy

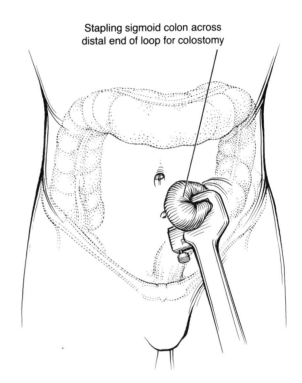

FIGURE 77–3. Once the opening for the sigmoid colostomy stoma is made, only the peritoneum lies between the operative field and the intra-abdominal contents. The 10-mm. trocar and the Endo-Babcock are then brought through the ostomy site as a loop. The loop that is brought out through the stoma site is depicted. At this point, a number of options are available. In this figure, a TA-55 stapler is used to staple the distal end of the colon. The proximal loop can then be matured in a typical manner. As an alternative, the stoma can be matured in a delayed technique. Another option for the stoma is the creation of a loop colostomy in which the distal sigmoid colon is not stapled. Finally, it is possible for the colon to be stapled and divided using a GIA stapler. The proximal stoma is matured to create a true end colostomy.

78

Left Colectomy

JOHN P. GRANT, M.D.

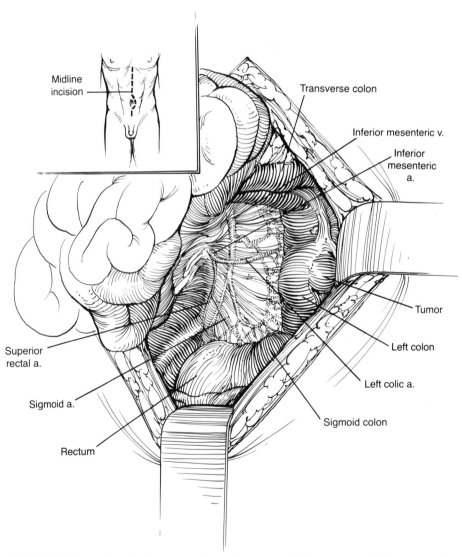

FIGURE 78–1. A midline incision is preferred, and the abdomen is carefully explored for evidence of metastatic disease or other abnormality. The small intestine is reflected to the upper left abdomen, and the sigmoid colon and descending colon are exposed.

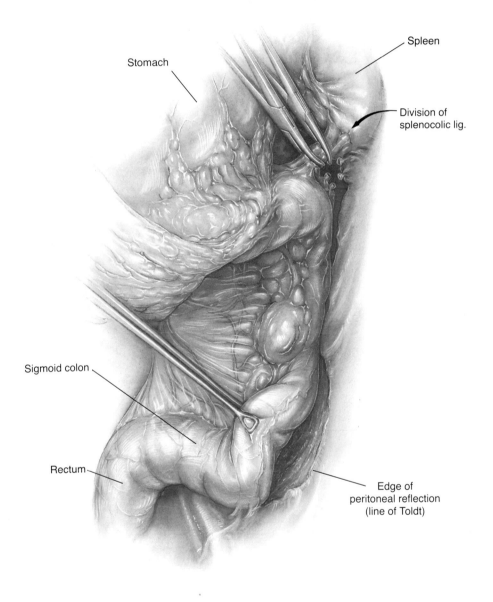

FIGURE 78–2. The lateral peritoneal reflection (line of Toldt) is incised, beginning at the sigmoid colon and continuing to the splenic flexure. The splenocolic and phrenocolic ligaments are divided between clamps and ligated.

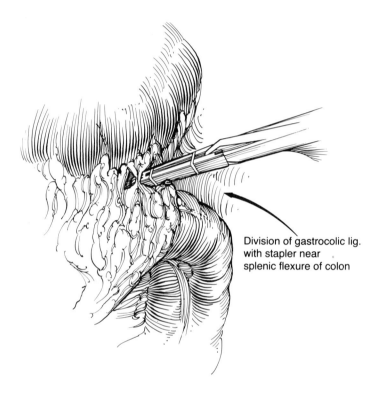

Division of gastrocolic lig.
with stapler near
splenic flexure of colon

FIGURE 78–3. The gastrocolic ligament is divided with a stapler or between clamps and ligated at a point satisfactory for adequate mobilization of the colon to perform an end-to-end anastomosis to the sigmoid colon.

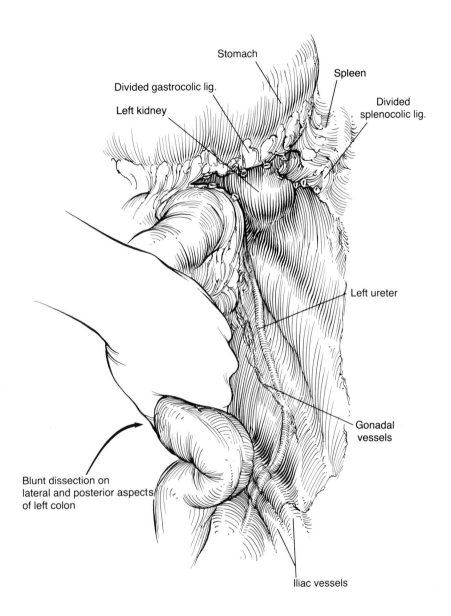

FIGURE 78–4. The left colon is reflected toward the midline by freeing the mesentery from the posterior abdomen by blunt dissection. Care is taken to identify and protect the left ureter and not to injure the left spermatic or ovarian veins.

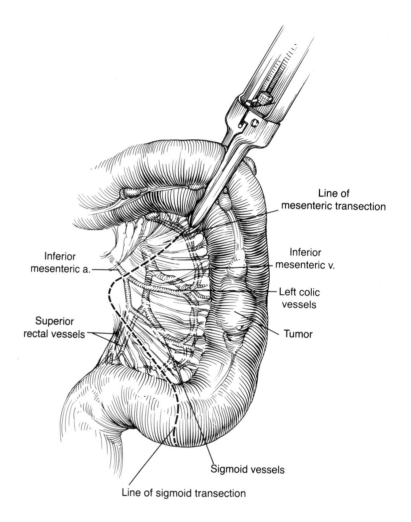

Line of
mesenteric transection

Inferior
mesenteric v.

Left colic
vessels

Tumor

Inferior
mesenteric a.

Superior
rectal vessels

Sigmoid vessels

Line of sigmoid transection

FIGURE 78–5. The mesentery is divided inferiorly and superiorly with a fan-shaped incision, which includes the left colic artery and vein, associated lymphatics, and lymph nodes. (If the lesion is benign, minimal mesentery is resected.) The abdomen is carefully packed off with Mikulicz pads to prevent soilage. The bowel is divided proximally and distally with the GIA stapler. The optimal margin on either side of the resected lesion depends on the nature of the lesion; i.e., 15 to 20 cm. for a malignant lesion and 5 to 10 cm. for a benign lesion. A colocolostomy is constructed after full mobilization of the colon to avoid tension.

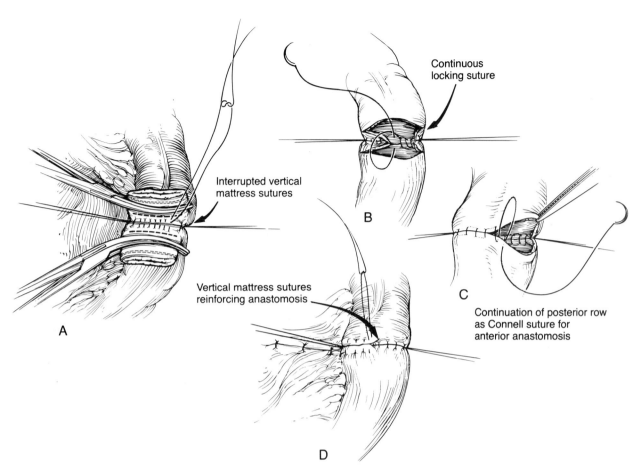

Continuous
locking suture

Interrupted vertical
mattress sutures

B

Vertical mattress sutures
reinforcing anastomosis

C

Continuation of posterior row
as Connell suture for
anterior anastomosis

A

D

FIGURE 78–6. End-to-end anastomosis: *A,* A posterior row of 4–0 silk vertical mattress seromuscular sutures is placed. *B,* The intestinal clamps are removed (or the staple line is incised), and a posterior locking suture of 3–0 chromic catgut is placed. *C,* The posterior locking suture is continued around both ends and converted to a Connell suture to accomplish serosal invagination. *D,* The anastomosis is completed by placing an anterior row of 4–0 silk vertical mattress seromuscular interrupted sutures. The mesenteric defect is closed with a 2–0 chromic catgut suture, and the bowel is returned to the abdomen, allowing the small bowel to lie in its natural position on top.

After the completion of the resection, the proximal and distal colonic segments are examined to ensure that adequate blood supply is present. Discoloration at the anastomosis should always be resected, and a new anastomosis should be made to avoid subsequent dehiscence of the anastomosis with peritonitis or abscess formation. Patency of the stoma should be confirmed by compression between the thumb and index finger.

79

Sigmoid Colectomy

JOSEPH A. MOYLAN, M.D.

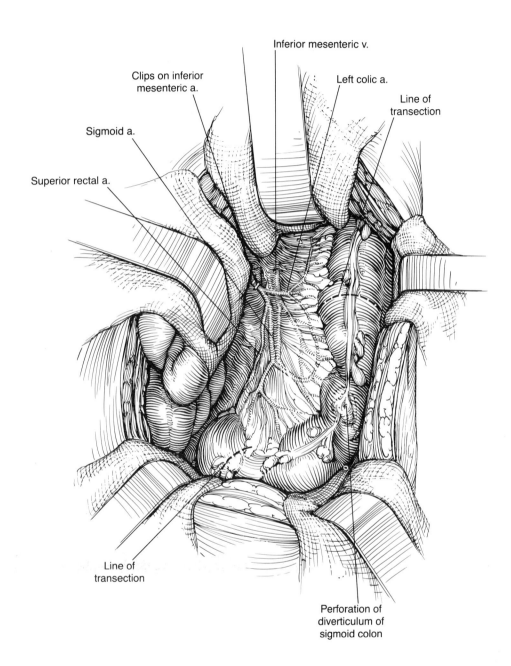

Inferior mesenteric v.

Clips on inferior
mesenteric a.

Left colic a.

Line of
transection

Sigmoid a.

Superior rectal a.

Line of
transection

Perforation of
diverticulum of
sigmoid colon

FIGURE 79–1. The abdomen is explored through a lower midline incision. After the small bowel is packed toward the upper and right side of the abdomen, sites for the division of the colon and the mesentery are identified based on the reason for the sigmoid colectomy. Adequate cancer margins are taken proximally and distally in the colon. To prevent seeding during manipulation of the colon lesion, control of the inferior mesenteric vein can be accomplished with clips. Beginning in the left lateral gutter along Toldt's line, the colon is then mobilized. The mesentery is divided to the base of the inferior mesenteric artery and vein, securing the vessels with 2–0 silk sutures.

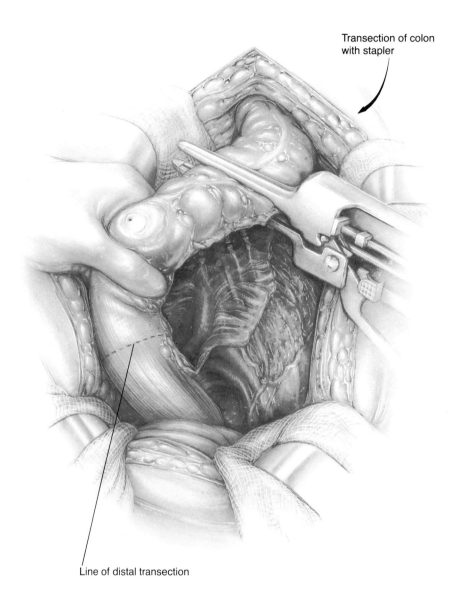

Transection of colon with stapler

Line of distal transection

FIGURE 79–2. When the mesentery has been completely divided, the colon is divided proximally and distally using the GIA stapler to prevent spillage.

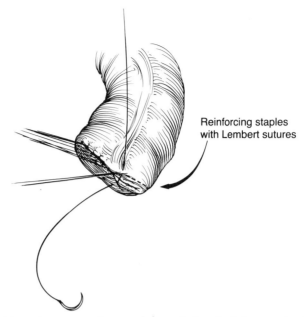

Reinforcing staples
with Lembert sutures

FIGURE 79–3. Although not mandatory, the stapled end of the proximal colon may be inverted to prevent bleeding and leakage.

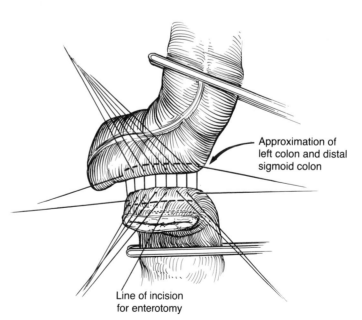

Approximation of
left colon and distal
sigmoid colon

Line of incision
for enterotomy

FIGURE 79–4. Although an end-to-end anastomosis may be appropriate, a side-to-side anastomosis is performed to ensure the largest possible opening between the proximal and the distal colon. Noncrushing clamps are placed on the proximal and distal segments. A series of serosal sutures are placed between the side of the proximal segment and the end of the distal colon, and the distal suture is excised. A linear enterotomy is made in the proximal colon.

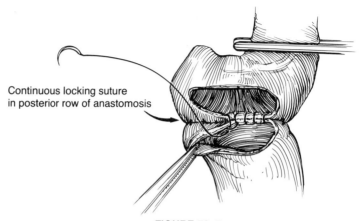

Continuous locking suture
in posterior row of anastomosis

FIGURE 79–5

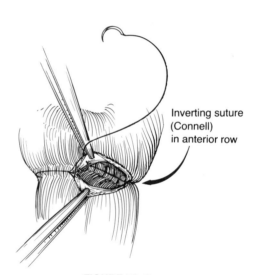

Inverting suture
(Connell)
in anterior row

FIGURE 79–6

FIGURES 79–5 and 79–6. A standard two-layer closure is performed. The inner layer is a continuous suture of an absorbable material, such as chromic catgut, Dexon, or Vicryl, with an outer layer of 4–0 interrupted silk sutures.

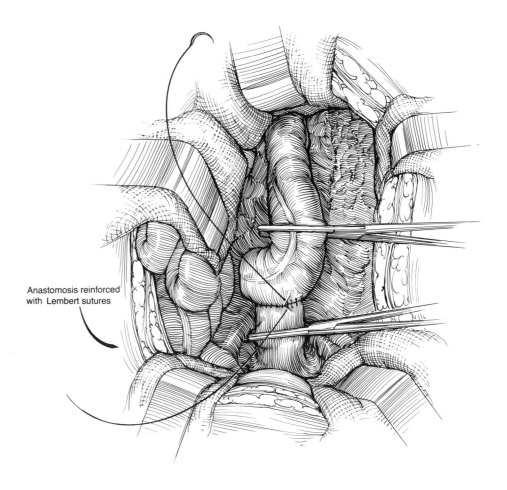

Anastomosis reinforced
with Lembert sutures

FIGURE 79–7. After the two-layer anastomosis is completed, the clamps are removed and the mesentery is closed posteriorly to prevent internal herniation and obstruction.

An alternative to the end-to-side anastomosis is the end-to-end anastomosis, which is illustrated in Figure 78–6.

80

Miles Abdominoperineal Resection

WILLIAM C. MEYERS, M.D.

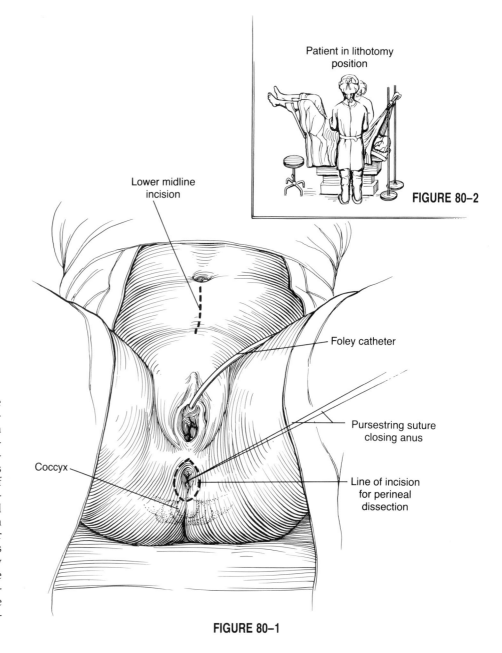

Patient in lithotomy position

FIGURE 80–2

Lower midline incision

Foley catheter

Pursestring suture closing anus

Coccyx

Line of incision for perineal dissection

FIGURES 80–1 and 80–2. The classic Miles abdominoperineal resection is performed in two parts, an abdominal dissection followed by the perineal portion. Most surgeons now perform at least part of the two stages simultaneously. The patient is placed in the lithotomy position using standard stirrups or spreader bars. The anus is sutured tight, and a Foley catheter is inserted above the thigh. A lower midline incision is made, which can be extended above the umbilicus.

FIGURE 80–1

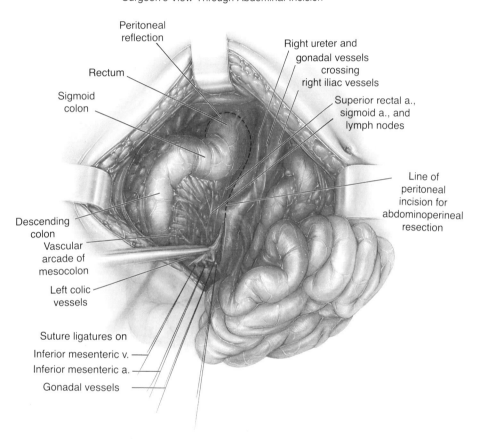

Surgeon's View Through Abdominal Incision

Peritoneal reflection

Rectum

Sigmoid colon

Descending colon

Vascular arcade of mesocolon

Left colic vessels

Suture ligatures on
Inferior mesenteric v.
Inferior mesenteric a.
Gonadal vessels

Right ureter and gonadal vessels crossing right iliac vessels

Superior rectal a., sigmoid a., and lymph nodes

Line of peritoneal incision for abdominoperineal resection

FIGURE 80–3. After careful abdominal exploration, the sigmoid colon is mobilized and the peritoneum is incised to resect all lymphatic tissue to the origin of the inferior mesenteric artery. The incision is extended anteriorly to separate the rectum from the uterus in the female, or the bladder in the male.

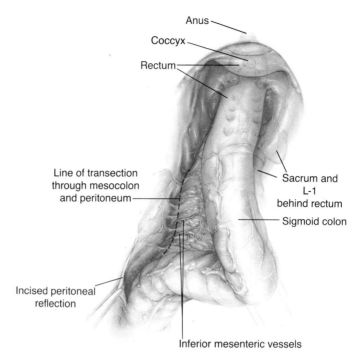

FIGURE 80-4. The mesentery of the sigmoid colon and rectum is ligated and divided to provide a plane straight down to the sacral hollow.

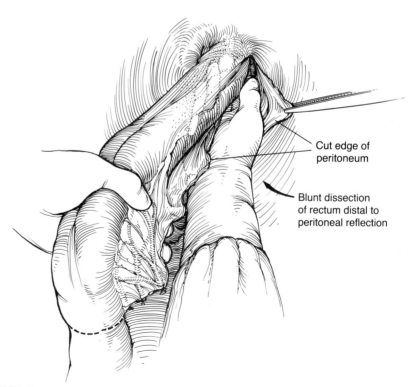

FIGURE 80-5. The plane is developed digitally, and a hand is inserted behind the rectum for blunt dissection to a point below the level of the tip of the coccyx. Care is taken to identify both ureters and to avoid injury to them throughout the procedure. A relatively bloodless posterior plane is developed, usually while a distinct "sucking" noise is heard.

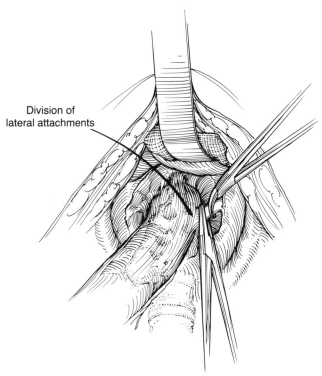

FIGURE 80–6. The primary vessels feeding the rectum are located in the lateral attachments, which are grasped with clamps, divided, and ligated. Long, large right-angle clamps are particularly useful for this maneuver.

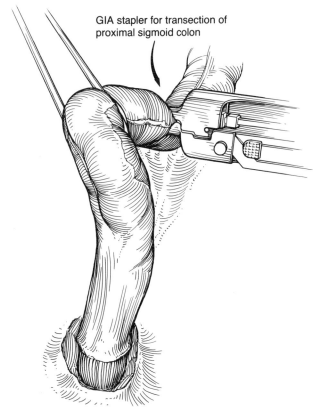

FIGURE 80–7. Prior to removal of the rectum and sigmoid colon, the GIA stapler is used to transect the colon at a convenient location and to preserve sufficient length for the colostomy.

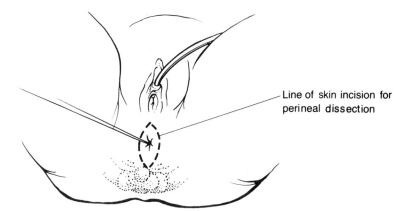

FIGURE 80–8. At or before this point, the second stage of the operation is begun. Separate instruments and a Mayo tray are placed on the surgeon's lap; the perineal dissection is initiated by an elliptical incision around the anus.

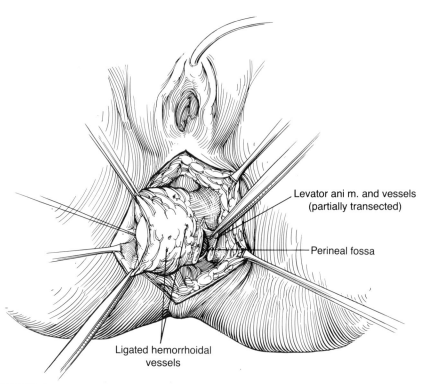

FIGURE 80–9. The coccyx is identified, and a generous amount of soft tissue is included in the dissection down to the levator ani muscles. These are incised with the cautery, the small hemorrhoidal vessels being ligated and divided.

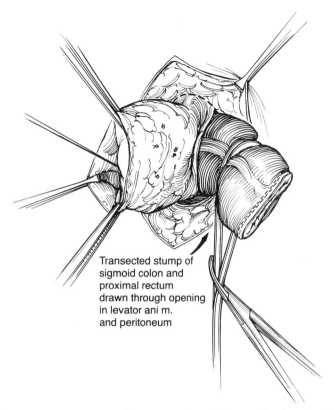

Transected stump of
sigmoid colon and
proximal rectum
drawn through opening
in levator ani m.
and peritoneum

FIGURE 80–10. The levator ani muscle is opened, and the proximal end of the specimen is retrieved and completely removed after dividing the remaining attachments. The anterior part of the perineal dissection can be reserved until later because this can be the most difficult part of the operation. In the male, Denonvilliers' fascia usually protects the prostate from the dissection. In the female, the tumor is more likely to invade anteriorly; a portion of the vagina can be included in the specimen if necessary.

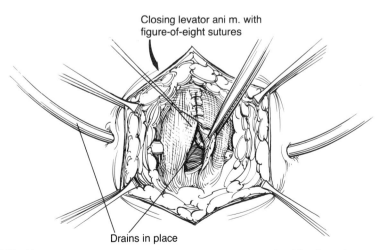

Closing levator ani m. with
figure-of-eight sutures

Drains in place

FIGURE 80–11. The levator ani muscles are reapproximated with chromic sutures after placement of two round Jackson-Pratt drains into the sacral hollow.

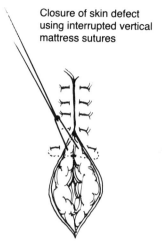

Closure of skin defect
using interrupted vertical
mattress sutures

FIGURE 80–12. The skin is closed with interrupted nylon sutures.

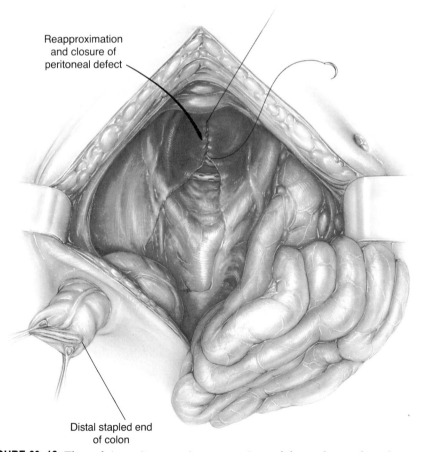

Reapproximation
and closure of
peritoneal defect

Distal stapled end
of colon

FIGURE 80–13. The pelvic peritoneum is reapproximated from above after placement of the colostomy in a predesignated location. The colostomy is matured after completion of the abdominal closure, as shown in Chapter 83, Figures 83–11 and 83–12.

81

Kock Pouch

R. RANDAL BOLLINGER, M.D., Ph.D.

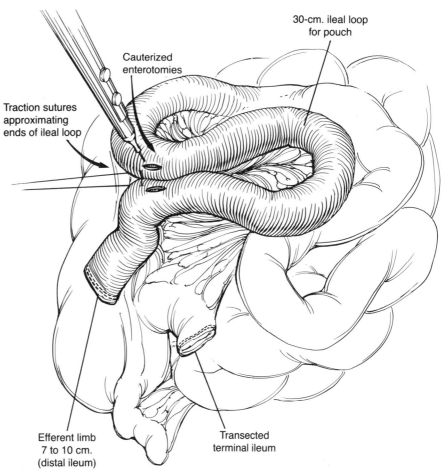

FIGURE 81-1. Exploratory laparotomy is undertaken through a midline incision. The diseased colon is removed after division of the terminal ileum with the GIA stapler. If the colon has been removed previously, the Brooke ileostomy is mobilized; any adhesions of the distal ileum or ileal mesentery are lysed. The most distal 7 to 10 cm. of ileum is preserved for the outflow tract. The length is determined by the thickness of the patient's abdominal wall and the need to create a tangential outflow tract through the rectus muscle and subcutaneous fat. The next 10 cm. is reserved for the nipple valve, which will be created by intussusception. The next 30 cm. is used for the Kock pouch. A traction suture is placed at the antimesenteric border to join the two 15-cm. segments of ileum that compose the pouch loop. All peritoneum and mesenteric fat is removed from both sides of the mesentery that supplies the 10-cm. segment reserved for the nipple valve. Care is taken to preserve the arterial supply to and venous drainage from the nipple segment. Enterotomies are made at the antimesenteric border of the afferent and efferent limbs of the Kock pouch loop.

439

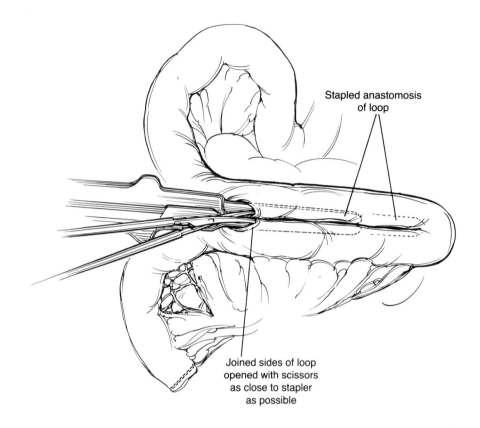

Stapled anastomosis
of loop

Joined sides of loop
opened with scissors
as close to stapler
as possible

FIGURE 81–2. The GIA stapler *without* a knife blade is used to join the pouch limbs. Scissors applied close to the stapler are used to divide the ileum superficial to the new staple line.

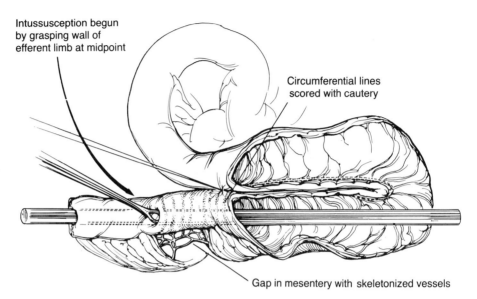

Intussusception begun
by grasping wall of
efferent limb at midpoint

Circumferential lines
scored with cautery

Gap in mesentery with skeletonized vessels

FIGURE 81-3

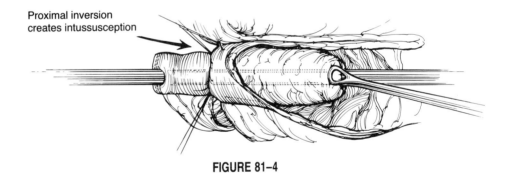

Proximal inversion
creates intussusception

FIGURE 81-4

FIGURE 81-3. The serosa of the nipple valve section is scored at 1-cm. intervals with the electrocautery to promote scarring after intussusception. Three seromuscular sutures of 3–0 silk are placed in each lateral wall to further facilitate intussusception. A 7- or 8-mm. Hegar dilator is placed through the lumen of the ileum into the open pouch to serve as a guide during the intussusception. The midpoint of the nipple segment is intussuscepted as the 3–0 silk sutures are tied sequentially.

FIGURE 81-4. A Babcock clamp placed on the leading edge of the nipple from within the pouch may facilitate inversion of the bowel to create a 5-cm. intussusception.

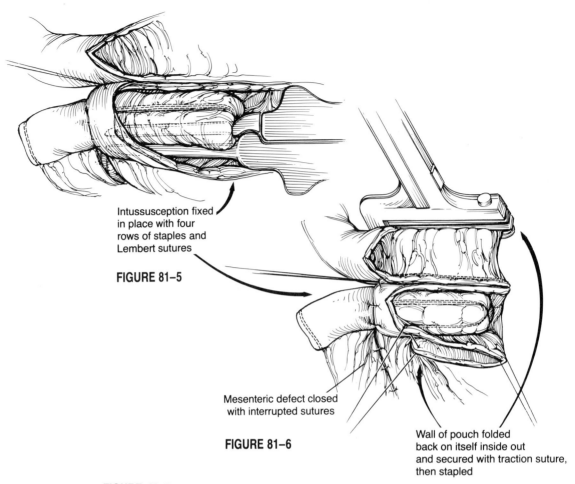

Intussusception fixed
in place with four
rows of staples and
Lembert sutures

FIGURE 81–5

Mesenteric defect closed
with interrupted sutures

FIGURE 81–6

Wall of pouch folded
back on itself inside out
and secured with traction suture,
then stapled

FIGURE 81–5. The intussusception is fixed in place with four rows of staples, again placed without a cutting blade.

FIGURE 81–6. Additional Lembert sutures are placed at the junction of the nipple valve and the outflow tract to secure the intussusception. The wall of the pouch is folded back upon itself and secured with a traction suture, then stapled with the 90-mm. stapling device.

FIGURES 81–7 and 81–8. The pouch, which is inside out, is then inverted into the normal closed position.

FIGURE 81–9. The remaining defect is closed with a running 3–0 absorbable inverting Connell suture. A second running seromuscular suture of the same absorbable material is placed for reinforcement. The pouch may be tested for leaks, and the nipple valve for continence, by instilling saline through a 30 French Robinson catheter at this point.

FIGURE 81–10. When proven intact, the pouch is sutured to the underside of the abdominal wall at the ileostomy site just above the symphysis pubis. The posterior 3–0 silk sutures are placed before drawing the outflow tract through the abdominal wall.

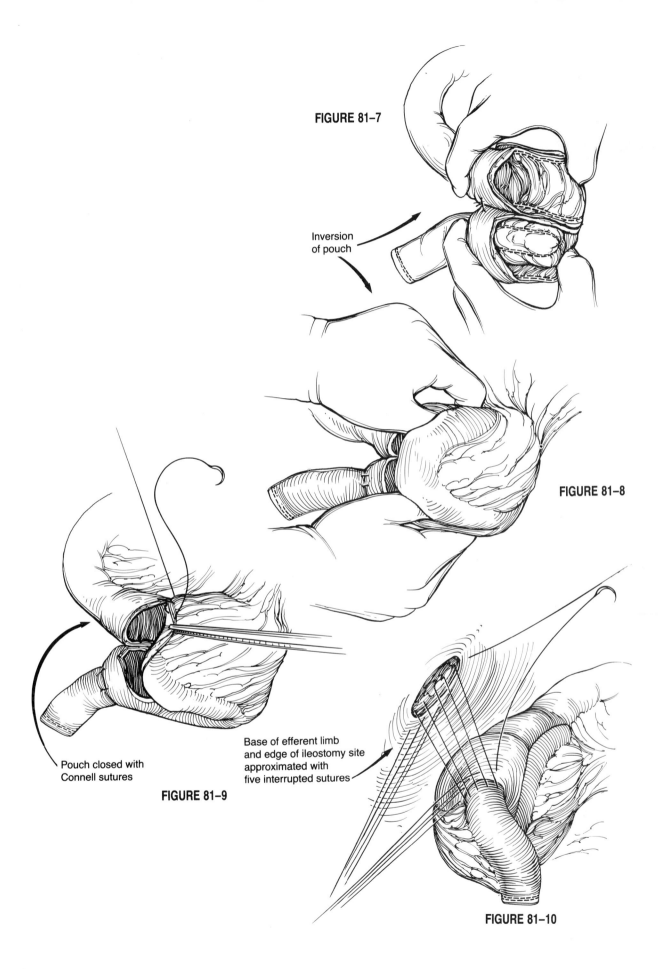

FIGURE 81-7

Inversion
of pouch

FIGURE 81-8

Pouch closed with
Connell sutures

FIGURE 81-9

Base of efferent limb
and edge of ileostomy site
approximated with
five interrupted sutures

FIGURE 81-10

443

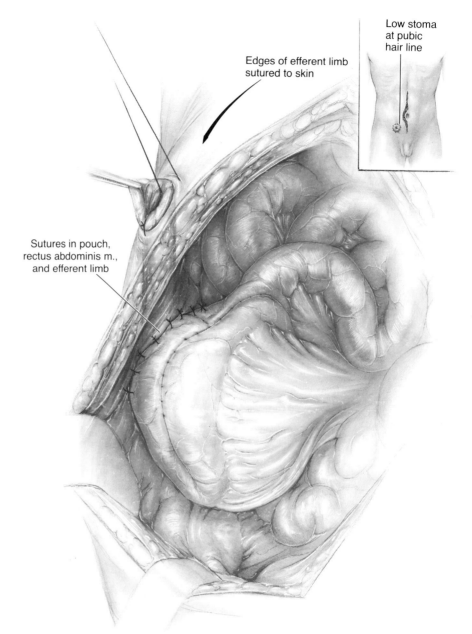

Low stoma
at pubic
hair line

Edges of efferent limb
sutured to skin

Sutures in pouch,
rectus abdominis m.,
and efferent limb

FIGURES 81–7 to 81–11. A tangential course is created from laterally at the pubic hair line to medially beneath the rectus muscle. A 2-cm. button of skin is excised, but no subcutaneous fat is removed. A cruciate opening is made in the rectus fascia. The anterior row of 3–0 silk sutures fixing the pouch to the underside of the abdominal wall is then placed and tied down. Additional seromuscular sutures are placed between the pouch and the lateral abdominal wall, extending into the pelvis to prevent pouch rotation. The mesenteric defect is closed laterally. The outflow tract is trimmed to produce a minimal 2- to 5-mm. mucosal protrusion above skin level. This will subsequently retract to skin level, which creates no problem for the patient because no external appliance is needed.

The abdomen is irrigated copiously, then closed using interrupted nonabsorbable sutures for the muscle and fascia, followed by staples for the skin. A 30 French Robinson catheter with enlarged distal holes is left inserted through the nipple valve into the pouch and is fixed to the abdominal wall to maintain the pouch in a decompressed condition for the first week of healing. The catheter is sutured to the abdominal wall with a nonabsorbable nylon suture. The tube is irrigated every 3 hours and is drained continuously into a urinary collection bag. An occlusive dressing placed over the midline wound will prevent contamination from the nearby stoma.

82

Ileoanal Anastomosis

R. RANDAL BOLLINGER, M.D., Ph.D.

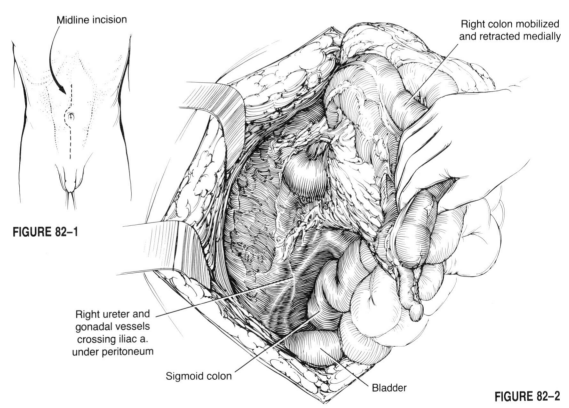

Midline incision

FIGURE 82–1

Right colon mobilized
and retracted medially

Right ureter and
gonadal vessels
crossing iliac a.
under peritoneum

Sigmoid colon

Bladder

FIGURE 82–2

FIGURE 82–1. The patient is placed in the lithotomy or supine position with the legs elevated in Allen stirrups or on spreader bars, providing simultaneous access to both the abdomen and the perineum. Through a midline incision, the abdomen is opened and explored. The liver and mesocolon of patients with inflammatory bowel disease are assessed carefully for signs of metastatic adenocarcinoma.

FIGURE 82–2. The cecum and ascending colon are mobilized, with care taken to preserve the right ureter inferiorly and duodenum superiorly. The omentum is separated from the transverse colon for later placement in the pelvis. The transverse, descending, and sigmoid colons are mobilized, and their mesentery is divided between clamps with ligatures of 2–0 silk.

445

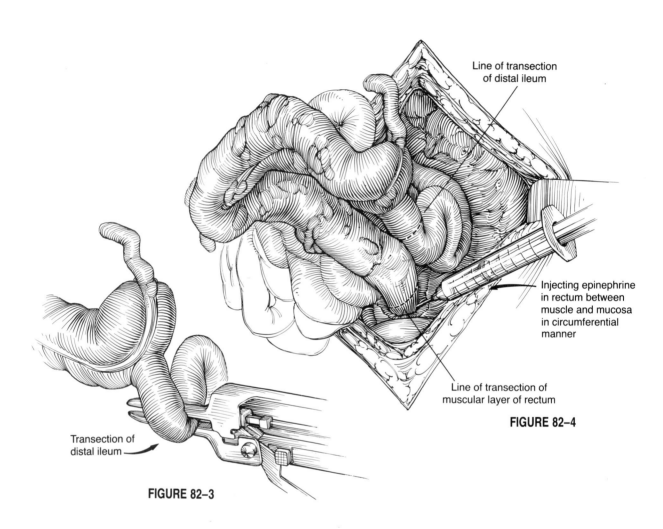

Line of transection
of distal ileum

Injecting epinephrine
in rectum between
muscle and mucosa
in circumferential
manner

Line of transection of
muscular layer of rectum

FIGURE 82–4

Transection of
distal ileum

FIGURE 82–3

FIGURES 82–3 and 82–4. The distal colon is mobilized to within 5 cm. of the peritoneal reflection. The ileum is then stapled and transected near the ileocecal valve using a GIA stapler. Epinephrine (1:100,000 in saline) is injected circumferentially into the rectum between the muscle and the muscularis mucosa in a manner to separate the layers of the bowel wall.

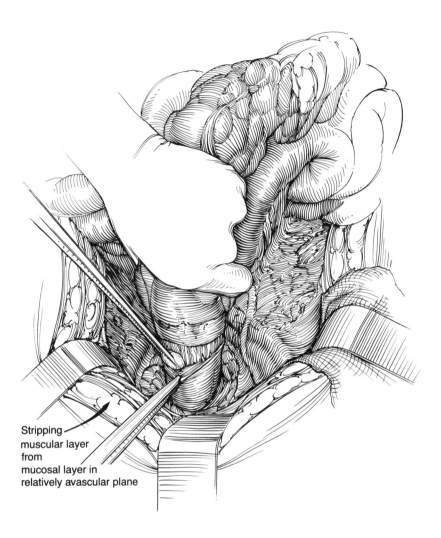

Stripping
muscular layer
from
mucosal layer in
relatively avascular plane

FIGURE 82–5. An incision is made circumferentially through the rectal serosa and muscular layers.

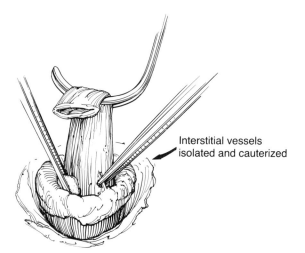

FIGURE 82–6. With traction on the mucosal tube, the muscular layers are bluntly dissected as bridging vessels are cauterized and divided. Once several centimeters of mucosa have been freed, the mucosal tube is doubly clamped and divided, and the abdominal colon is removed from the operative field. The dissection is continued inferiorly to below the levator ani muscles.

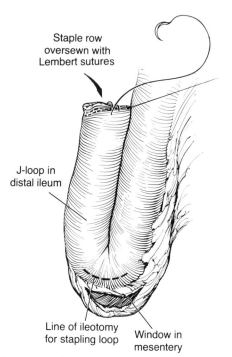

FIGURE 82–7. A J-pouch is created using the most distal 20 cm. of ileum folded back upon itself. The end staple line in the ileum is oversewn with 3–0 silk Lembert sutures. The mesentery at the tip of the pouch is cleared over a distance of 2 cm., and an enterotomy is made there for placement of the 10-cm. intestinal anastomosing stapler.

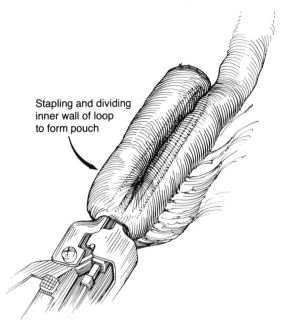

Stapling and dividing
inner wall of loop
to form pouch

FIGURE 82–8. The stapler is fired, thus dividing the bowel wall to create a 10-cm. pouch.

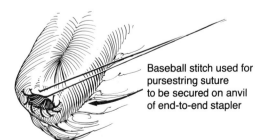

Baseball stitch used for
pursestring suture
to be secured on anvil
of end-to-end stapler

FIGURE 82–9. A 3–0 Prolene pursestring suture is placed around the enterotomy for use later to secure the pouch on the anvil of the stapler.

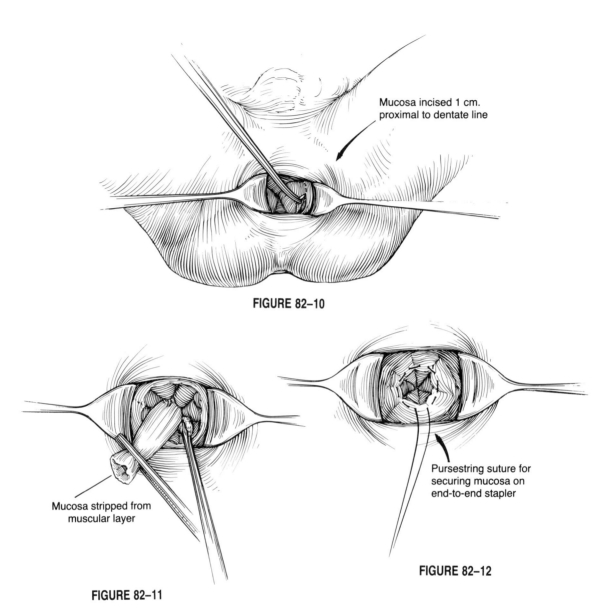

FIGURE 82–10

Mucosa incised 1 cm.
proximal to dentate line

FIGURE 82–11

Mucosa stripped from
muscular layer

FIGURE 82–12

Pursestring suture for
securing mucosa on
end-to-end stapler

FIGURE 82–10. A similar dissection is then begun from below. After pharmacologic blockade to achieve total sphincter muscle relaxation, the rectum is dilated digitally, then held open with Gelpi retractors. The mucosa is incised 1 cm. proximal to the dentate line after injecting 1:100,000 epinephrine in saline to separate the muscularis mucosa from the underlying muscle.

FIGURE 82–11. The mucosa is stripped from the muscular layer. The dissection is facilitated by inverting the mucosal remnant from above and using it to provide traction to expose the remaining mucosal attachments.

FIGURE 82–12. Once the entire mucosal tube has been removed, a pursestring of 3–0 Prolene is placed into the small mucosal remnant, which will be excised at the level of the dentate line when the EEA stapler is fired.

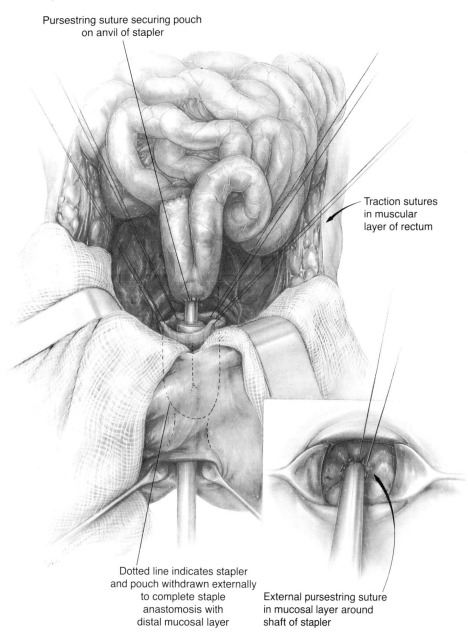

Pursestring suture securing pouch
on anvil of stapler

Traction sutures
in muscular
layer of rectum

Dotted line indicates stapler
and pouch withdrawn externally
to complete staple
anastomosis with
distal mucosal layer

External pursestring suture
in mucosal layer around
shaft of stapler

FIGURE 82–13

FIGURE 82–14

FIGURE 82–13. Traction sutures are placed in each quadrant of the rectal muscular tube.

FIGURE 82–14. A 25-mm. curved EEA stapler is inserted through the anus into the abdominal cavity. The pouch opening is placed over the anvil, and the pursestring suture is tied down. With traction on the stay sutures, the J-pouch is drawn back through the muscular tube to the dentate line, where the stapler is again opened and the distal pursestring tied down over the stapler head around the shaft of the stapling device. When the EEA stapler is fired, the remaining colonic mucosa is excised from the rectum, leaving the ileum stapled to the dentate line. A 30 French red rubber Robinson catheter may by placed into the rectum and secured to the skin of the thigh to promote drainage during the first 5 days following the operation.

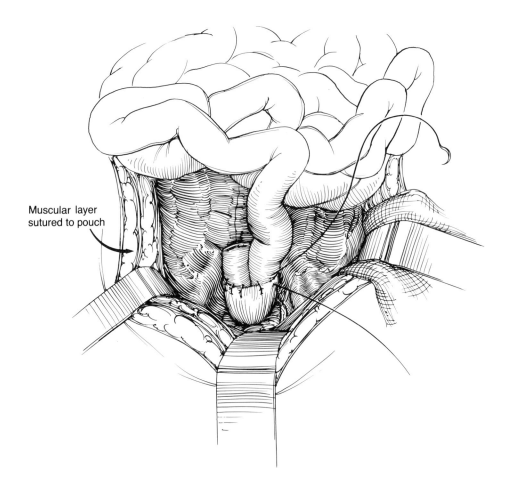

Muscular layer
sutured to pouch

FIGURE 82–15. The muscular tube is sewn with interrupted 3–0 silk seromuscular sutures to the J-pouch. The mesenteric defect of the ileum is closed with a running chromic suture.

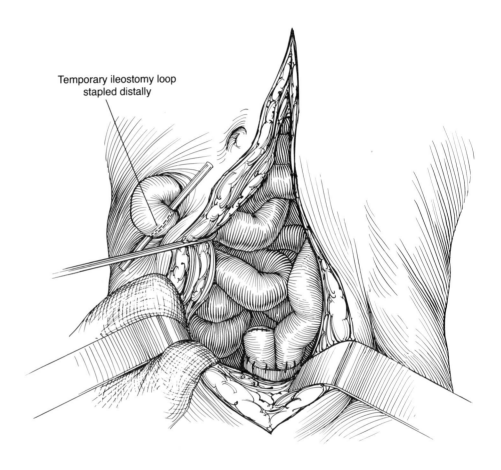

Temporary ileostomy loop
stapled distally

FIGURE 82–16. A segment of ileum proximal to the anastomosis, which reaches to the right lower quadrant abdominal wall, is identified and brought out as a temporary loop ileostomy. A Robinson catheter bridge is placed beneath the loop for the first 5 days. A staple line is placed across the distal portion of the loop to make the ileostomy totally diverting. The abdomen is then irrigated copiously with saline and antibiotic solution. Closure is accomplished with interrupted 1 nylon sutures for the rectus muscle and fascia followed by staples for the skin. An occlusive dressing is placed over the wound, after which the ileostomy is matured with six 3–0 absorbable sutures to evert and fix the mucosa. The ileostomy is taken down in 6 weeks, after healing of the rectum is complete. The second operation is usually done through the ileostomy by mobilizing the afferent and efferent limbs of ileum, excising the staple line and old ostomy, then performing a two-layered end-to-end anastomosis.

83

Subtotal Left Colectomy

ONYE E. AKWARI, M.D.

Partial left colectomy, with or without accompanying partial proximal proctectomy, is indicated for benign and malignant diseases of the large bowel distal to the splenic flexure. Carcinoma and diverticular disease are the most common indications. Excision of primary tumors mandates care to obtain adequate margins and inclusion of the associated mesentery, vessels, and lymphatics into which the tumor has spread or may have spread. However, it is generally agreed that dissection beyond the regional drainage of the involved segment is unnecessary. The timing of resection and whether or not a primary anastomosis can be safely made are matters of surgical judgment. As a general rule, left colonic anastomoses should be made electively in patients in whom satisfactory mechanical and antibiotic colonic preparation has been achieved. Patients with clinically suspected acute left colonic diverticulitis may be given a trial of medical management, with resolution of the infection in two thirds of patients. Operations may be undertaken after the acute inflammatory changes have resolved.

Lymphatic drainage parallels the regional arterial circulation. *In resections for carcinoma*, the major vessels must be resected near their origin. Therefore, carcinomas of the splenic flexure or proximal left colon require resection of the left transverse colon and the descending colon to the ascending sigmoid branch of the inferior mesenteric vessels. The left colic vessels are taken at their origin from the inferior mesenteric vessels.

Sigmoid carcinomas may require extended resection of the inferior mesenteric artery at its origin; but, usually, inclusion of the vascular trunk of the sigmoid vessels and the superior hemorrhoidal vessels permits excellent clearance, with restoration of bowel continuity at the level of the sacral promontory. It may be necessary to take down the splenic flexure in order to ensure a tension-free anastomosis in these cases.

Lesions in the upper rectum and midrectum can be approached with ligation of middle and inferior hemorrhoidal vessels as the rectum is mobilized by blunt dissection above the presacral fascia from the presacral hollow. A distal margin of 5 cm. of normal bowel beyond the tumor is generally recommended. However, experience has shown that a 2-cm. margin, and sometimes even less, is adequate. If the histologic margin is free of tumor, preservation of anal function is valued highly. No compromise, however, is acceptable in the lateral pelvic dissection and in the inclusion of the entire associated mesorectum. These precautions minimize local recurrence and local persistence of tumor in unharvested nodes in the zone of lateral spread.

Resection for diverticular and other benign diseases includes conservative removal of the involved bowel segment, although mesenteric resection may be undertaken to include a localized paracolonic phlegmon.

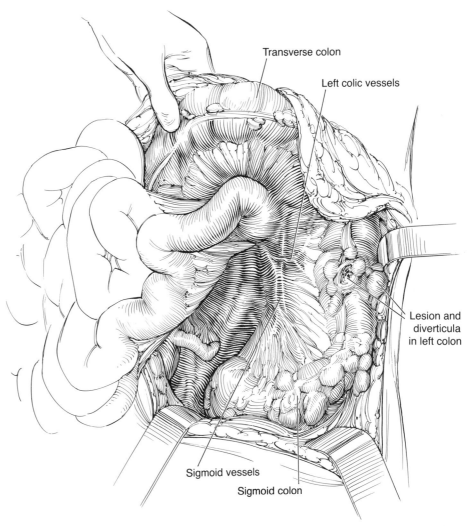

FIGURE 83–1. The lesion is approached, and the mesenteric anatomy is defined.

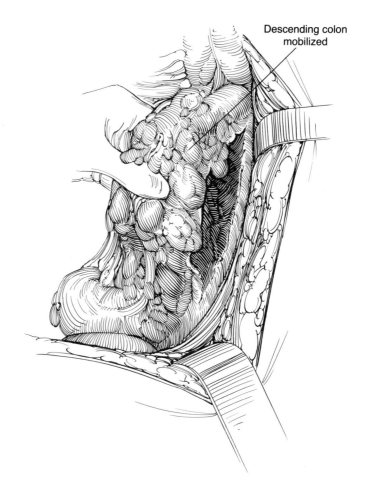

Descending colon
mobilized

FIGURE 83–2. The colon is mobilized out of the left gutter as care is exercised to protect and preserve the left ureter and its associated vessels in the retroperitoneum. The mobilization is continued distally into the pelvis. When proximal proctectomy is required for distal left colonic lesions, the peritoneum is lysed adjacent to the rectosigmoid so that the rectosigmoid is mobilized out of the proximal presacral space. With the left colonic mesentery fully elevated and the small bowel safely retracted to the right, the inferior mesenteric vessels come into full view and can be traced distally so that the superior hemorrhoidal and sigmoid vessels can be controlled between clamps and their cut ends ligated with ties of 2–0 silk.

The proximal extent of the disease and, therefore, the planned level of proximal colonic transection determines whether or not the splenic flexure of the colon must be taken down. If judged to be necessary, the splenic flexure is readily approached by superior extension of the left colonic mobilization along the left gutter, exercising great care not to apply forceful inferior traction on the splenocolic omentum. Too forceful a traction readily results in a splenic capsular tear, which may lead to annoying bleeding.

A bidirectional approach to the splenic flexure is achieved by entering the lesser omental bursa in the region of the left transverse colon and taking down the splenocolic omentum to join up with the proximal left colonic area of mobilization in the upper left gutter. Once the splenorenocolic attachment has been lysed, the splenic flexure is fully mobile.

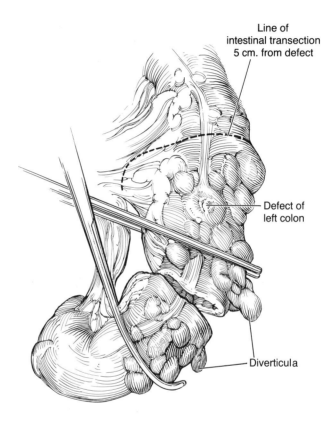

Line of
intestinal transection
5 cm. from defect

Defect of
left colon

Diverticula

FIGURE 83–3. The areas of the proposed colonic transection are now prepared, and the bowel is transected between noncrushing clamps. Control of the associated mesenteric vessels and minimal manipulation of the diseased segment should be exercised prior to bowel transection and removal of the diseased portion.

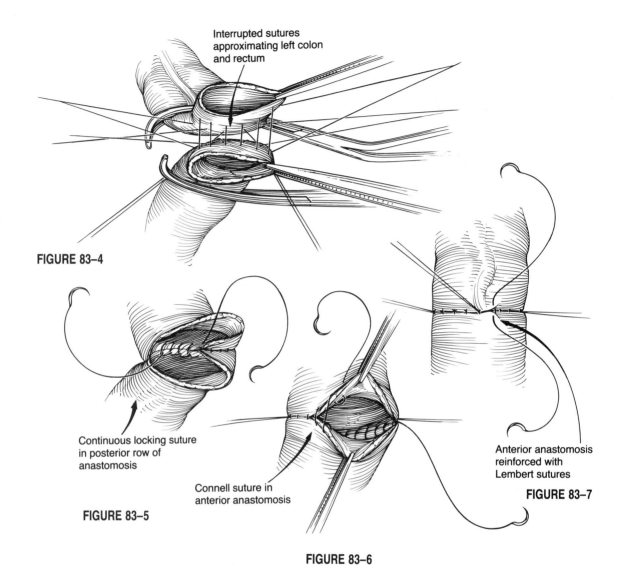

Interrupted sutures
approximating left colon
and rectum

FIGURE 83–4

Continuous locking suture
in posterior row of
anastomosis

FIGURE 83–5

Connell suture in
anterior anastomosis

FIGURE 83–6

Anterior anastomosis
reinforced with
Lembert sutures

FIGURE 83–7

FIGURES 83–4 to 83–7. An end-to-end colocolostomy in two layers is favored using an inner running suture of absorbable material and an outer interrupted row of 3–0 black silk. The inner running suture is done in a locking fashion, aiding hemostasis in the cut ends of the bowel.

Partially obstructing colonic lesions create a disparity of size that must be taken into consideration during the placement of sutures, so obstruction *per se* is not a contraindication to primary anastomosis. Primary resection and anastomosis can also be achieved in the presence of small localized pericolonic abscesses, especially when the abscess cavity can be included in the resected specimen. More difficult abscesses may permit a primary resection and anastomosis, but a covering colostomy should be performed. The covering colostomy is not an absolute protection against anastomotic leakage but does obviate the need for reoperation should leakage and/or para-anastomotic abscess develop. Percutaneous drainage of such a collection is feasible in most cases. It is the author's practice to drain left colonic anastomoses using a closed sterile suction system. Stapling instruments may be used for colonic resection and the creation of anastomosis after partial colectomy.

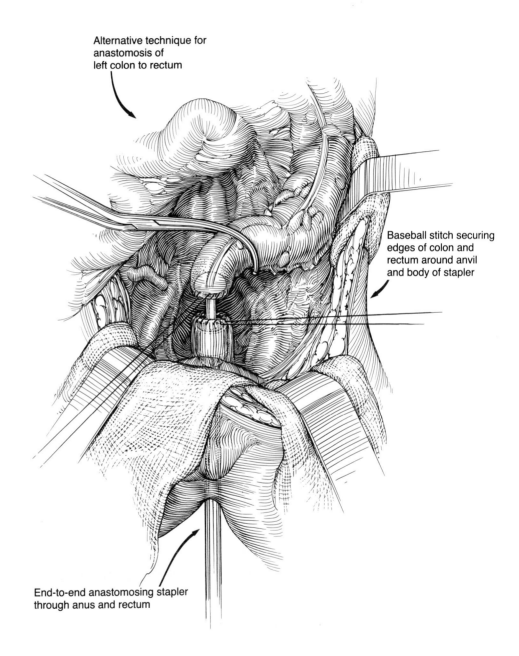

Alternative technique for
anastomosis of
left colon to rectum

Baseball stitch securing
edges of colon and
rectum around anvil
and body of stapler

End-to-end anastomosing stapler
through anus and rectum

FIGURE 83–8. After the specimen has been removed, an EEA or other intraluminal end-to-end stapling device is introduced through the anus and passed through very carefully placed pursestring sutures at the cut ends of the bowel. These running rows of 2–0 nonabsorbable smooth sutures are placed through all layers of the bowel. Once the staple head has been manipulated into the proximal segment of bowel, the sutures are tied down and the stapler is closed and fired. It is imperative that the staple line be completely free of surrounding fatty tissues and that the staples be fired with a firm squeeze so that the stapler knife cuts cleanly. The instrument is then gently rotated back and forth, with a hand supporting the suture line until the stapler slides out.

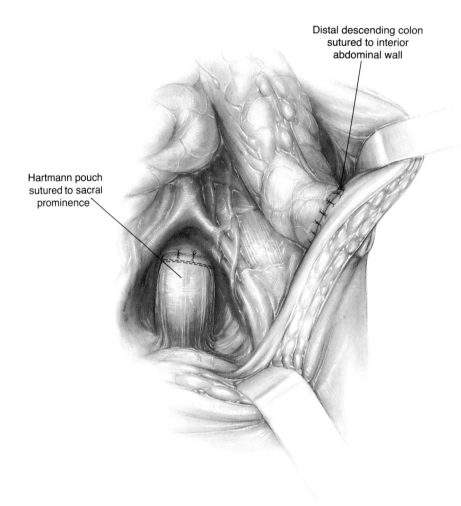

Distal descending colon
sutured to interior
abdominal wall

Hartmann pouch
sutured to sacral
prominence

FIGURE 83-9. The Hartmann operation is preferred in the presence of complicated diverticular or malignant disease such as perforated diverticulitis, massive life-threatening hemorrhage when emergency colectomy is undertaken, an internal fistula associated with sepsis, and resection of extensive pelvic cancers with a high probability of recurrence, especially in poor-risk patients and in the rare patient with an acute freely perforating carcinoma.

Management of distal colonic carcinoma using a Hartmann resection in the poor-risk patient follows the principles of resection of carcinomas occurring in this location, with dissection similar to that performed for any low anterior resection. Thus, adequate resection of the associated mesentery of the colon as well as the mesorectum is mandatory, with care exercised to achieve adequate lateral pelvic dissection. The rectum is then transected using a stapling device or is oversewn. The stump is extraperitonealized.

In distal sigmoid perforations, a reperitonealization of the distal stump is not possible. The stump is left attached by sutures of nonabsorbable material to the sacral promontory or, if the distal stump is long enough, to the anterior abdominal wall on the left side. Little, if any, need can be cited for construction of mucous fistulas, especially because this maneuver may mean leaving some diseased bowel behind.

Definitive resection of the diseased colonic segment at the initial operation is essential so that when subsequent procedures for restitution of intestinal continuity are undertaken the procedure can be performed directly without any further consideration given to issues concerning the adequacy of the previous resection.

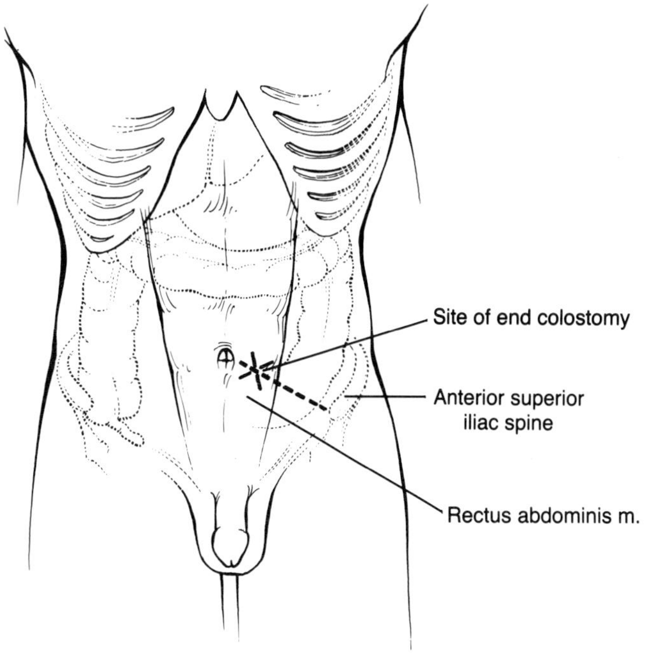

Site of end colostomy

Anterior superior
iliac spine

Rectus abdominis m.

FIGURE 83–10. After the Hartmann operation, the proximal cut end of the descending colon is exteriorized through the abdominal wall in the left lower quadrant, at a site that is marked prior to operation, as an end colostomy. Care is taken to exteriorize the stoma through the separated fibers of the lower belly of the left rectus muscle. Exteriorization of the colostomy in this manner is associated with a lower incidence of paracolostomy herniations, which are more frequent in patients in whom the stoma is exteriorized lateral to the rectus muscle.

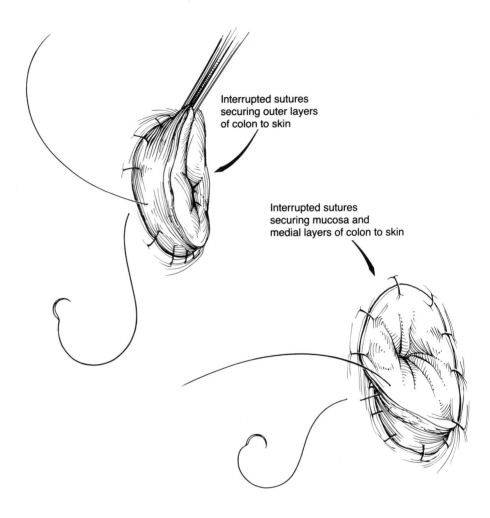

Interrupted sutures
securing outer layers
of colon to skin

Interrupted sutures
securing mucosa and
medial layers of colon to skin

FIGURES 83–11 and 83–12. The colostomy is matured primarily using interrupted sutures of absorbable material, incorporating all layers of the colon in the Brooke technique.

84

Low Anterior Resection

HILLIARD F. SEIGLER, M.D.

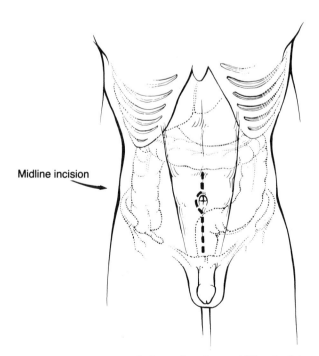

FIGURE 84–1. The abdomen is entered through a low midline incision. Low anterior resection of the rectosigmoid does not usually require mobilization of the splenic flexure.

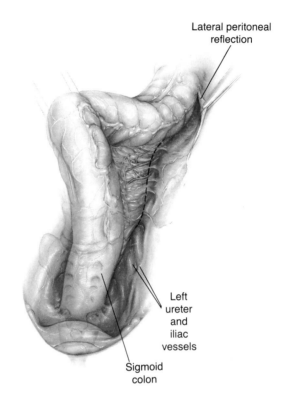

Lateral peritoneal
reflection

Left
ureter
and
iliac
vessels

Sigmoid
colon

FIGURE 84–2. The rectosigmoid is mobilized by initially dividing the lateral peritoneal
reflection. The gonadal vessels and left ureter are visualized using blunt dissection. The
peritoneum is sharply divided over the cul-de-sac of Douglas.

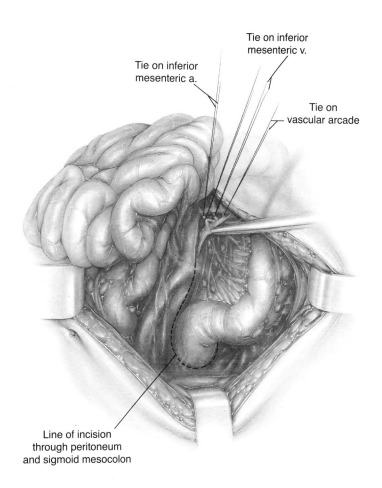

Tie on inferior
mesenteric v.

Tie on inferior
mesenteric a.

Tie on
vascular arcade

Line of incision
through peritoneum
and sigmoid mesocolon

FIGURE 84–3. The mesentery of the rectosigmoid is mobilized, and the inferior mesenteric artery and vein are isolated using blunt and sharp dissection. They are triply clamped, divided, and both free and suture-ligated. Hemostasis of the large vessel trunks is best obtained by 2–0 silk ligatures. After the major vessels are divided, the pelvic portion of the mesenteric dissection can be completed with adequate hemostasis. The lymphatic tissue in the pelvis is removed from the common iliac vessels after both the left and the right ureters have been visually identified and carefully left intact.

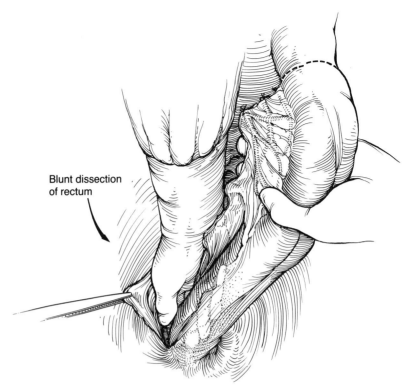

FIGURE 84–4. Blunt dissection of the upper rectum is completed using both digital maneuvers and sponge dissection. This permits retraction of the bladder anteriorly and increases the retractability of the rectum.

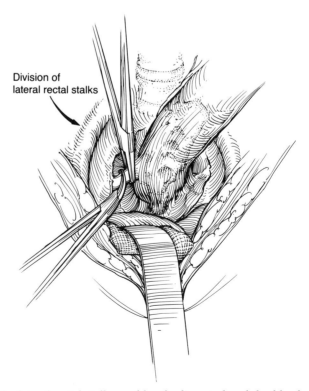

FIGURE 84–5. The lateral rectal stalks are bluntly dissected and doubly clamped, divided, and ligated with 2–0 silk sutures.

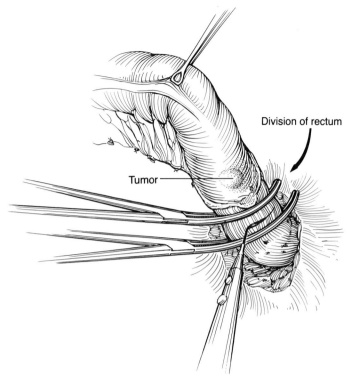

Division of rectum

Tumor

FIGURE 84–6. Bowel clamps are placed across the selected site of division of the rectum, and the bowel is divided with either a scalpel or a Bovie. The selected site should be 3 to 5 cm. below the tumor mass to ensure an adequate distal margin.

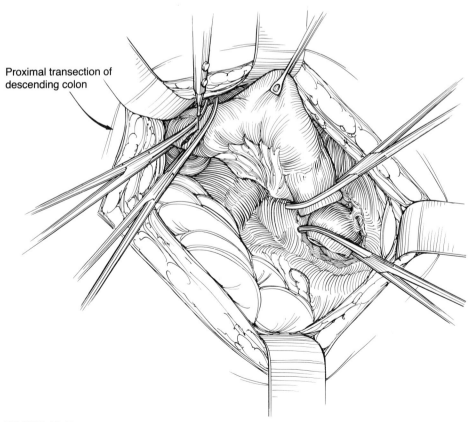

Proximal transection of descending colon

FIGURE 84–7. The bowel is clamped proximally using a bowel Kocher clamp at the inferior site and an intestinal clamp proximally.

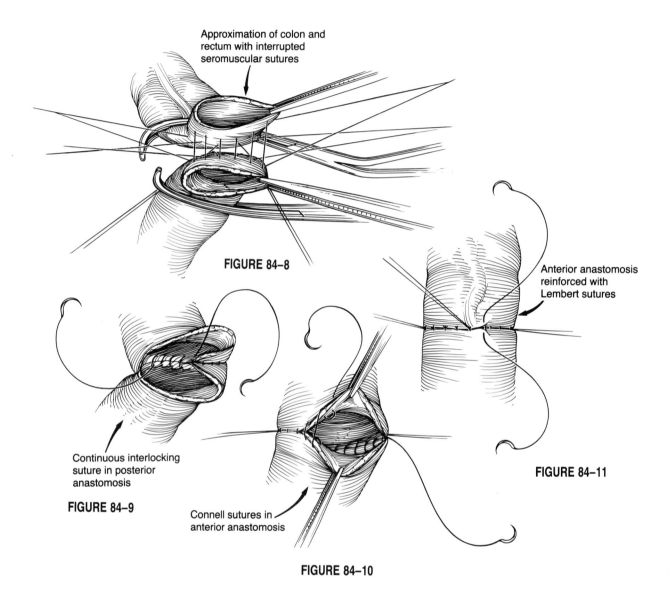

Approximation of colon and rectum with interrupted seromuscular sutures

FIGURE 84–8

Anterior anastomosis reinforced with Lembert sutures

FIGURE 84–11

Continuous interlocking suture in posterior anastomosis

FIGURE 84–9

Connell sutures in anterior anastomosis

FIGURE 84–10

FIGURES 84–8 and 84–9. The anastomosis is constructed using a posterior row of interrupted 3–0 black silk sutures in the seromuscular layer posteriorly followed by a continuous interlocking suture of chromic catgut.

FIGURES 84–10 and 84–11. Utilization of a Connell technique permits inversion of the mucosa and readies the bowel for serosa-to-serosa approximation using an outer layer of 3–0 black silk Lembert sutures. Following completion of the end-to-end anastomosis, care should be taken to ensure lack of tension.

Peritoneal and mesocolonic defects
closed with continuous sutures

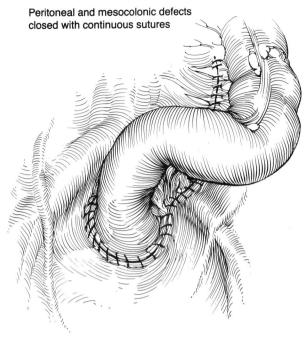

FIGURE 84–12. Reconstruction of the peritoneal floor is accomplished using either continuous catgut or interrupted silk sutures, taking care to place the anastomosis below the peritoneal closure.

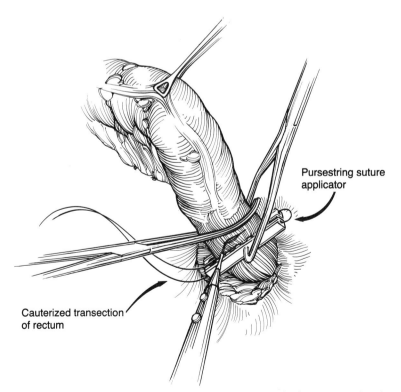

Pursestring suture
applicator

Cauterized transection
of rectum

FIGURE 84–13. If a stapled anastomosis is to be employed, the pursestring instrument can be applied to the point selected for division of the upper rectum. An angle bowel Kocher clamp is placed proximally, and the bowel is divided.

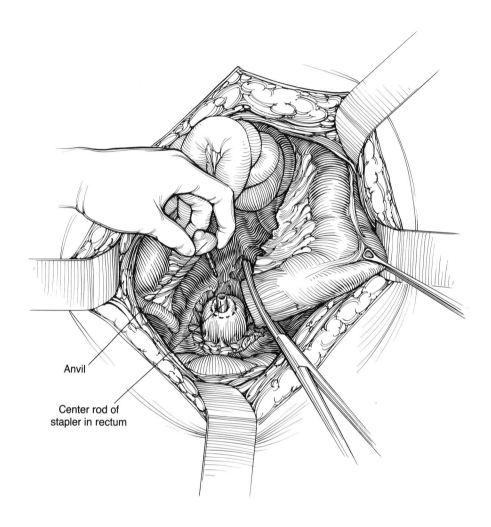

Anvil

Center rod of
stapler in rectum

FIGURE 84–14. The premium EEA instrument is used to perform the anastomosis. The instrument is introduced through the anus and is advanced to the level of the pursestring instrument. The pursestring instrument is fired and then removed. The center rod is advanced, and the anvil is applied to the center rod.

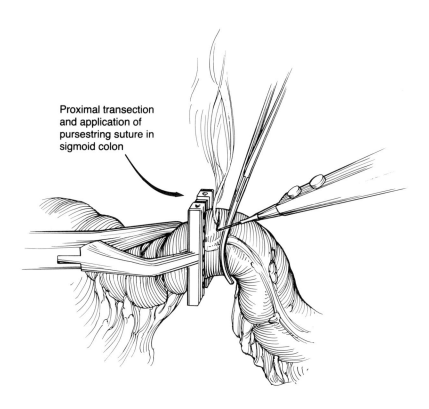

Proximal transection and application of pursestring suture in sigmoid colon

FIGURE 84–15. A second pursestring instrument is placed at the level of division of the sigmoid colon. The pursestring instrument is again fired and removed.

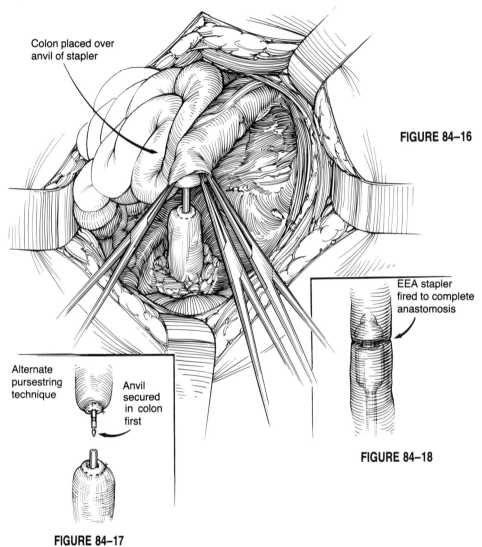

Colon placed over
anvil of stapler

FIGURE 84-16

EEA stapler
fired to complete
anastomosis

FIGURE 84-18

Alternate
pursestring
technique

Anvil
secured
in colon
first

FIGURE 84-17

FIGURE 84-16. With either three Allis clamps or three Babcock clamps, the open end of the sigmoid is placed over the anvil, and the pursestring is gently tied over the anvil to the extended center rod.

FIGURE 84-17. The anvil is approximated to the circular cartridge, and the instrument is fired.

FIGURE 84-18. The tissue doughnut should then be carefully inspected for completeness.

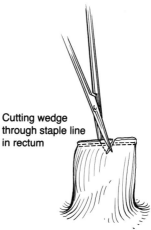

Cutting wedge
through staple line
in rectum

FIGURE 84–19. In an alternative technique, the premium EEA instrument is again used to perform the anastomosis. With scissors, a wedge is cut into the rectum through the staple line at the midpoint of the closure.

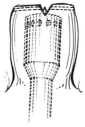

Stapler in rectum
with trocar retracted

FIGURE 84–20. The instrument is introduced transanally without the anvil and with the center rod completely recessed with the trocar tip in place.

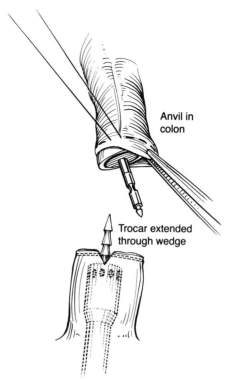

FIGURE 84–21. Once the circular staple cartridge can be felt against the stapled-off proximal rectum, the center rod can be advanced with the trocar coming through the wedged section in the center of the staple row. The divided sigmoid has the pursestring instrument in place and is fired, and the anvil is placed into the opened end of the sigmoid.

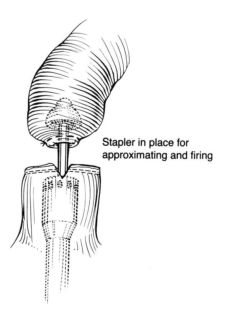

FIGURE 84–22. The pursestring is tied around the center rod, the anvil shaft is inserted into the instrument shaft, and the circular cartridge is approximated in the usual way to the anvil. The instrument is then fired. The anastomotic staple line can be inspected for hemostasis using a sigmoidoscope.

85

Laparoscopically Assisted Ileocolectomy

THEODORE N. PAPPAS, M.D.

The case depicted in Figures 85–1 to 85–12 is a laparoscopically assisted limited right colectomy. The patient's clinical presentation necessitated only a cecal resection.

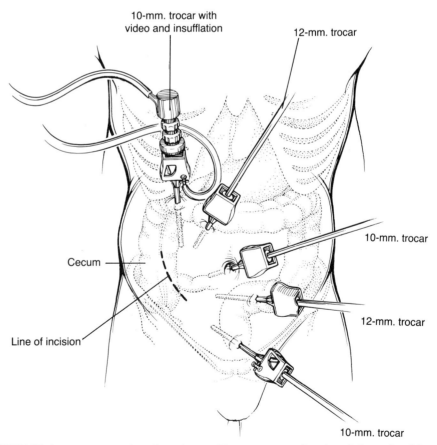

FIGURE 85–1. Trocars are placed as shown. The camera can be placed through a 10-mm. trocar in the umbilicus or through a 10-mm. trocar in the right upper quadrant. Additionally, 10- and 12-mm. trocars are placed in the right upper quadrant and 10- and 12-mm. trocars are placed in the left lower quadrant.

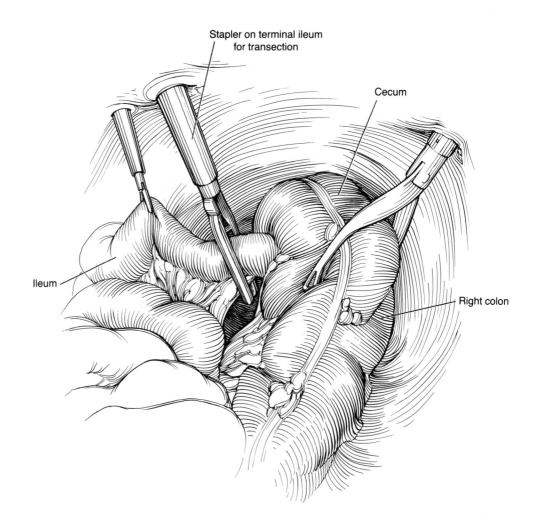

FIGURE 85–2. Mobilization of the right colon can be done by retracting it medially with an Endo-Babcock clamp. This allows sharp dissection of the retroperitoneal attachment of the right colon. An Endo-GIA stapler is shown passing through the 12-mm. trocar, transecting the terminal ileum after a small window is made in the mesentery. This allows the right colon to be further mobilized.

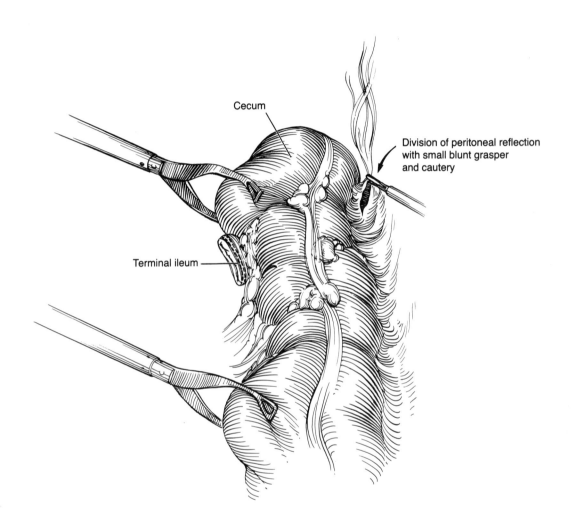

Cecum

Division of peritoneal reflection
with small blunt grasper
and cautery

Terminal ileum

FIGURE 85–3. This figure demonstrates the further mobilization of the right colon by placing the camera superiorly and incising the line of Toldt. This view is obtained by placing the camera in the right upper quadrant trocar.

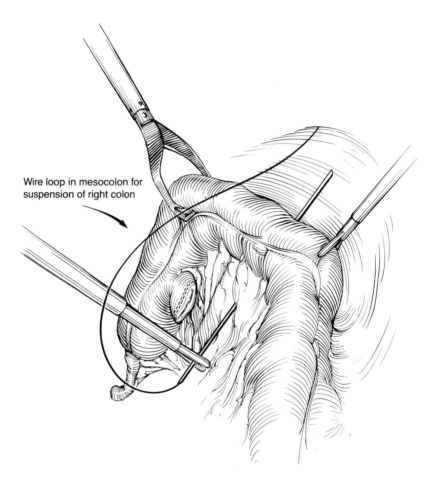

Wire loop in mesocolon for
suspension of right colon

FIGURE 85–4. The camera is again placed in the umbilical trocar, and a Keith needle is placed transabdominally through the colonic mesentery and passed out through the abdomen for retraction. A window is then created in the midright colonic mesentery to prepare the bowel for division with the Endo-GIA.

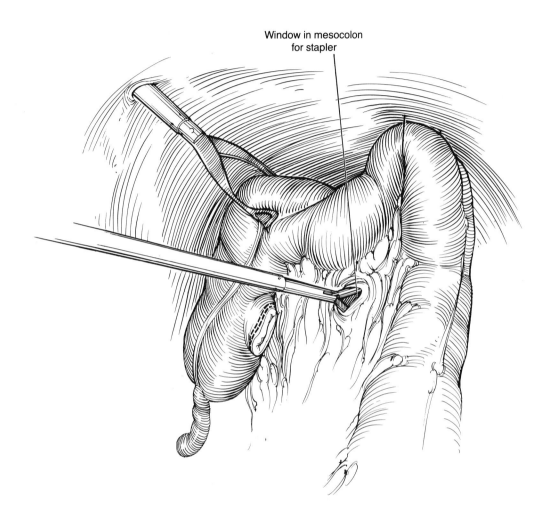

Window in mesocolon
for stapler

FIGURE 85–5. The 30-mm. Endo-GIA is passed through the left lower quadrant 12-mm. trocar, and the colon is divided with two firings of the stapler. This leaves the colon, a small piece of terminal ileum, and the appendix on a vascular pedicle only.

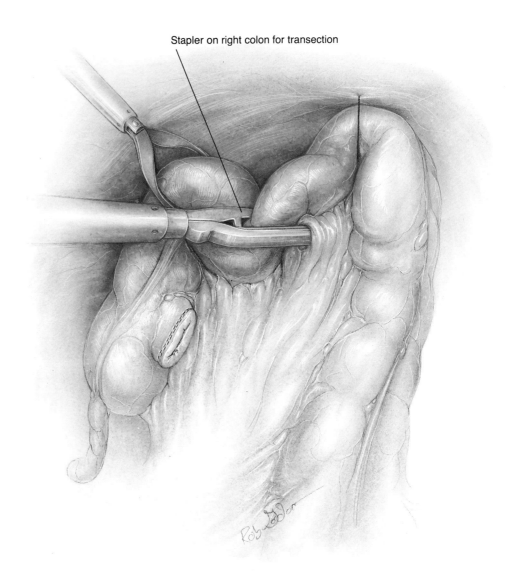

Stapler on right colon for transection

FIGURE 85–6

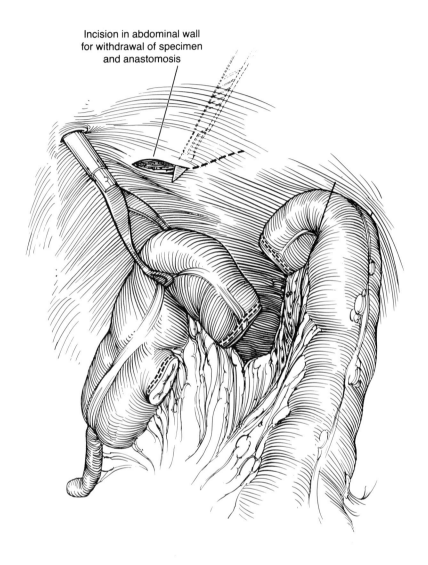

Incision in abdominal wall
for withdrawal of specimen
and anastomosis

FIGURE 85–7. At this point, the vascular pedicle is divided with a vascular cartridge of the Endo-GIA or, as in this case, a small incision is made and the specimen is easily mobilized through this incision.

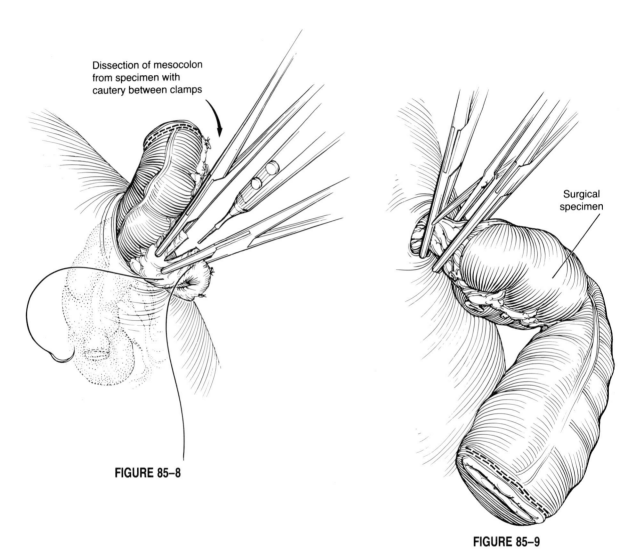

Dissection of mesocolon
from specimen with
cautery between clamps

FIGURE 85–8

Surgical
specimen

FIGURE 85–9

FIGURES 85–8 and 85–9. The blood supply is transected between Kelly clamps outside of the abdomen as the specimen is mobilized and the tissue is tied with 2-0 silk sutures. The specimen is completely removed, and the laparoscope is replaced, allowing mobilization of the two ends of bowel (the terminal ileum and right colon) up into the incision.

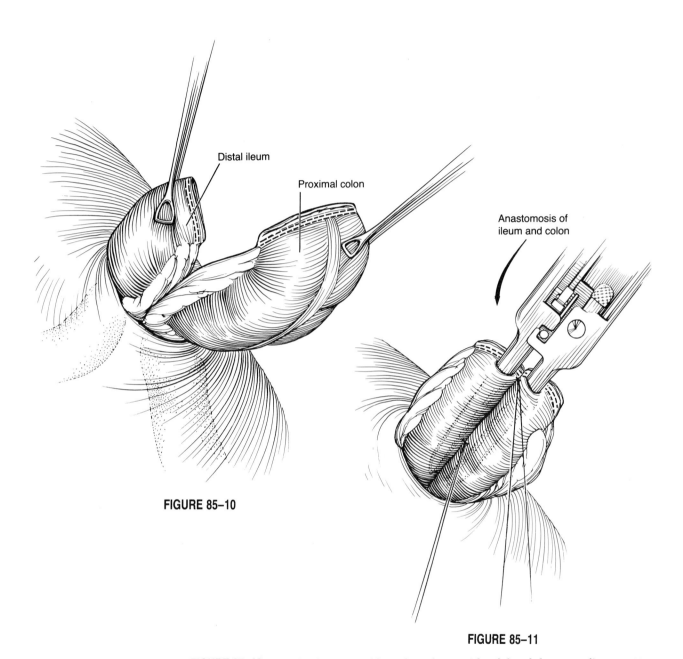

Distal ileum

Proximal colon

Anastomosis of
ileum and colon

FIGURE 85–10

FIGURE 85–11

FIGURE 85–10. With both pieces of bowel on the outside of the abdomen, a linear cutter and linear stapler (3.5-mm. staples) are used to staple the ileocolonic anastomosis.

FIGURE 85–11. Once the anastomosis is complete, it is replaced into the abdomen, and the mesentery is laparoscopically closed with hernia-type staples.

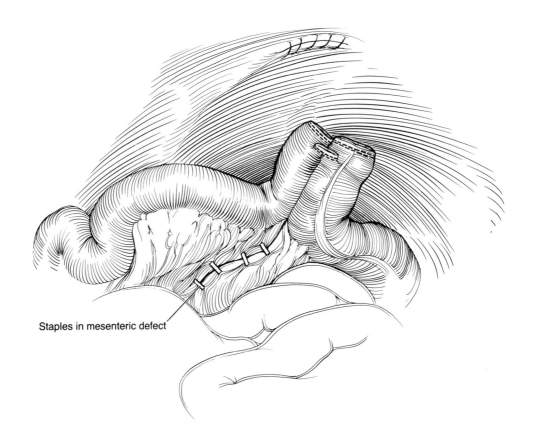

Staples in mesenteric defect

FIGURE 85–12. The abdominal incision is closed in the usual manner, as an appendectomy incision might be, with running or interrupted polyglycolic acid sutures.

SECTION VII

Rectum

86

Correction of Rectal Prolapse

R. RANDAL BOLLINGER, M.D., Ph.D.

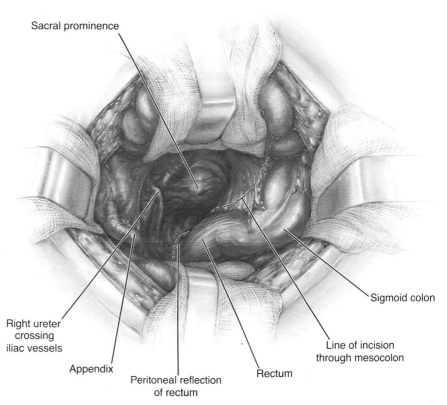

Sacral prominence

Right ureter
crossing
iliac vessels

Appendix

Peritoneal reflection
of rectum

Rectum

Sigmoid colon

Line of incision
through mesocolon

FIGURE 86–1. The lower abdomen and pelvis are exposed through either a lower midline incision or a Pfannenstiel incision. After routine exploration of the abdomen, the sigmoid colon is mobilized and the left ureter is identified. The right ureter is evident well away from the operative field. The peritoneum over the sigmoid mesentery is divided, but the primary blood supply to the sigmoid colon and proximal rectum is preserved. The peritoneal incision is continued distally around the peritoneal reflection so that the rectum can be mobilized circumferentially. The sacral prominence is identified.

Ligation of lateral stalks

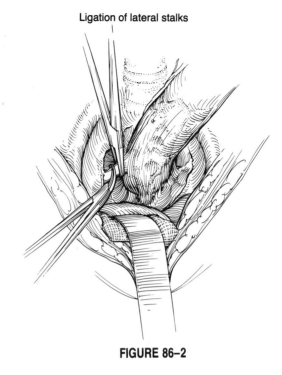

FIGURE 86–2

Blunt dissection of rectum

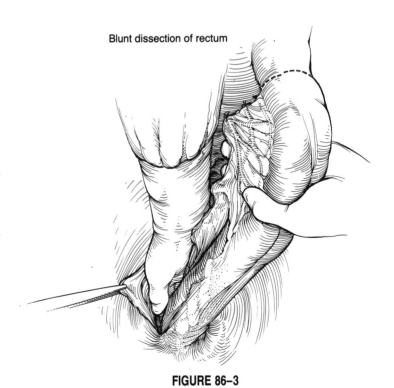

FIGURE 86–3

FIGURES 86–2 and 86–3. Any middle sacral vessels crossing the sacrum are avoided or ligated and divided. The rectum is mobilized out of the pelvis by dissection adjacent to the longitudinal muscles, with care taken to preserve the proximal blood supply.

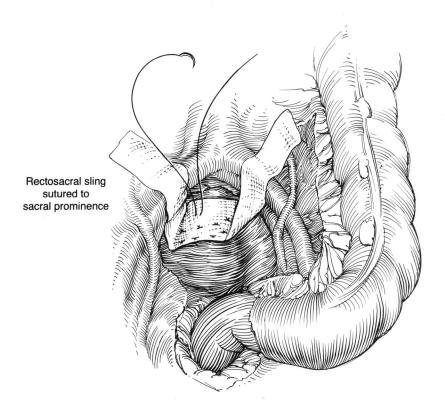

Rectosacral sling
sutured to
sacral prominence

FIGURE 86–4. Once the rectum has been mobilized sufficiently to reduce the prolapse entirely, a sling is fashioned to resuspend the rectum higher in the pelvis. A nonabsorbable Mersilene mesh is sutured to the presacral fascia with multiple interrupted sutures of soft, nonabsorbable material such as Mersilene. Three rows of interrupted sutures are placed, and long free ends are left on the sling for subsequent attachment to the rectum. The rectal sling is designed so that a 1-cm. strip of rectum is left free of mesh anteriorly. The Mersilene mesh is trimmed to the appropriate length so that no permanent constricting band is created that might subsequently cause bowel obstruction.

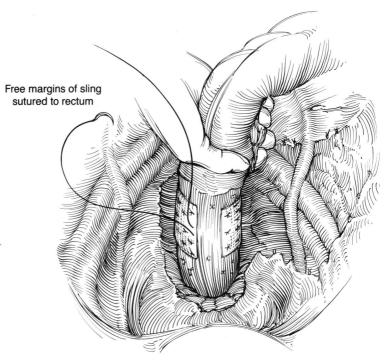

Free margins of sling
sutured to rectum

FIGURE 86–5. Multiple interrupted seromuscular sutures are placed while the assistant holds traction on the resuspended rectosigmoid segment. The sutures are placed through the Mersilene mesh and tied to fix the rectum high in the pelvis.

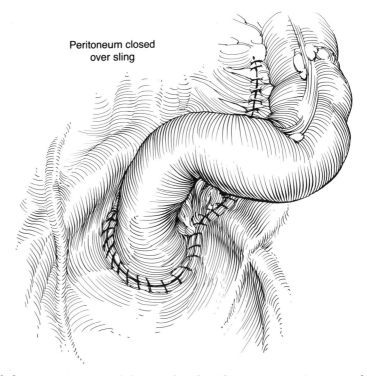

Peritoneum closed
over sling

FIGURE 86–6. The mesenteric defect is closed with running or interrupted chromic sutures. If a large, redundant descending and sigmoid colon has contributed to the prolapse, a segmental resection may be added to prevent volvulus, decrease pressure at the repair, and improve the function of the resuspended rectum. Stool softeners are continued for several months after the procedure.

87

Hemorrhoidectomy

JOSEPH A. MOYLAN, M.D.

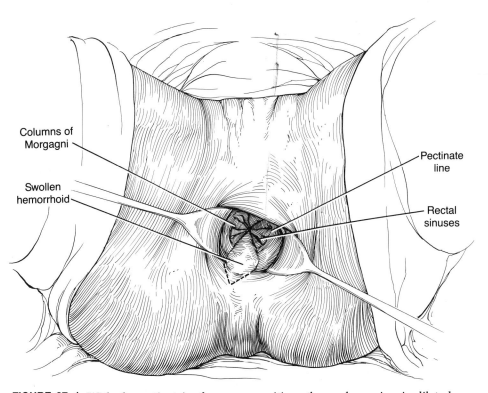

Columns of
Morgagni

Swollen
hemorrhoid

Pectinate
line

Rectal
sinuses

FIGURE 87–1. With the patient in the prone position, the anal opening is dilated up. The internal/external hemorrhoid is identified.

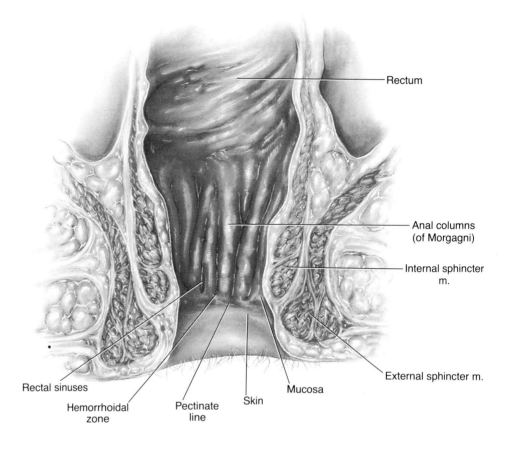

Rectum

Anal columns
(of Morgagni)

Internal sphincter
m.

External sphincter m.

Rectal sinuses

Hemorrhoidal
zone

Pectinate
line

Skin

Mucosa

FIGURE 87–2. The anatomy of the rectum. External hemorrhoids occur outside the pectinate line, and internal hemorrhoids occur internal to the pectinate line. Combined internal/external hemorrhoids cross this area. The goal of this operation is to preserve the sphincter mechanism.

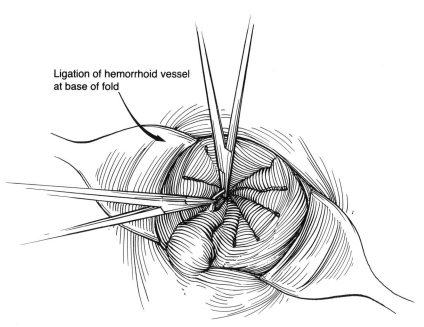

Ligation of hemorrhoid vessel
at base of fold

FIGURE 87–3. After the internal extent of the hemorrhoid is defined, the base of the hemorrhoid is ligated with an absorbable suture such as Vicryl or chromic catgut. Beginning at the external segment, a V-like incision is made.

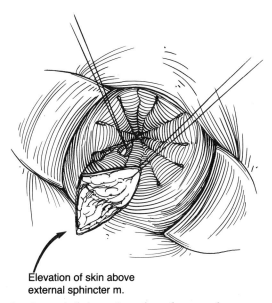

Elevation of skin above
external sphincter m.

FIGURE 87–4. Dissection is carried down into the submucosal space, and the hemorrhoid is excised.

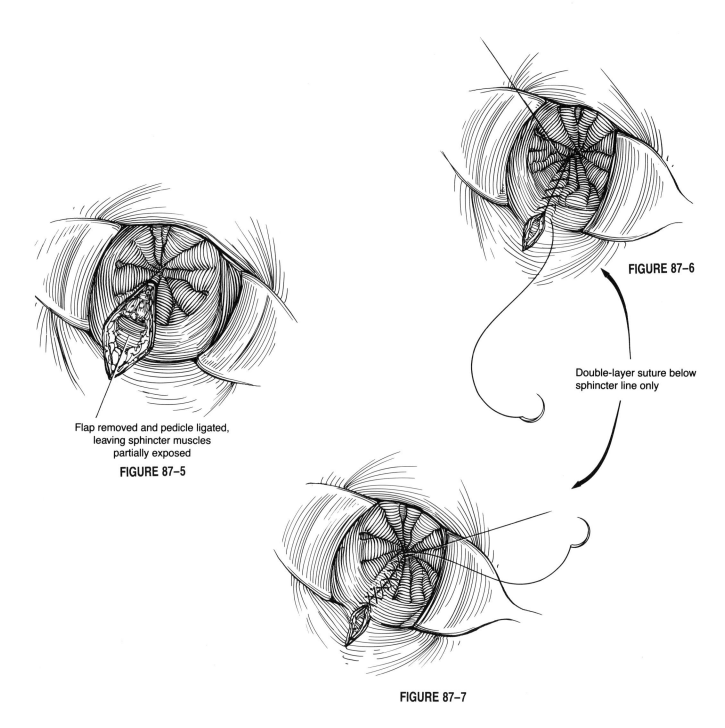

Flap removed and pedicle ligated,
leaving sphincter muscles
partially exposed

FIGURE 87–5

FIGURE 87–6

Double-layer suture below
sphincter line only

FIGURE 87–7

FIGURE 87–5. The incision is extended to the base internal hemorrhoid, dissecting it from the submucosal space and then excising it.

FIGURE 87–6. The excised area is closed with a running locking suture down to the pectinate line.

FIGURE 87–7. The suture is then returned to the base to prevent pursestringing. An absorbable topical hemostatic agent such as Surgicel is placed into the rectal opening. This is removed in the immediate postoperative period.

88

Drainage of Rectal Abscess

JOSEPH A. MOYLAN, M.D.

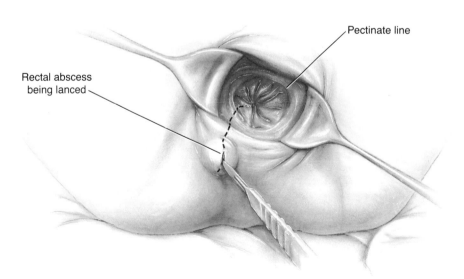

FIGURE 88–1. The patient with a rectal abscess presents with a painful mass outside the external sphincter. Because of communication to an internal tract, it is important at the time of initial drainage to define the tract and open it. With the patient in the lithotomy position, the anal opening is dilated up. The abscess is identified and, using a linear incision, is drained.

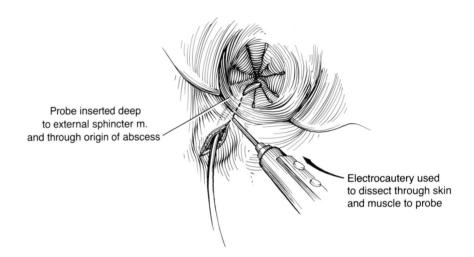

Probe inserted deep
to external sphincter m.
and through origin of abscess

Electrocautery used
to dissect through skin
and muscle to probe

FIGURE 88–2. A probe is placed into the abscess cavity, and the internal opening, which lies above the pectinate line, is identified. With cautery for hemostasis and the probe to identify the tract, this area is opened and packed. The packing is usually removed in 24 hours, and sitz baths are used to keep the area clean.

89

Excision of Fissure-in-Ano

JOSEPH A. MOYLAN, M.D.

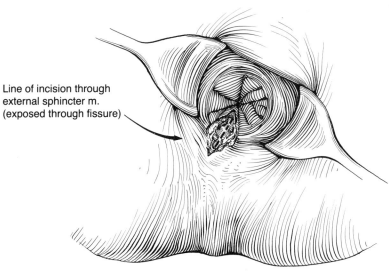

FIGURE 89–1. With the patient in the lithotomy position, the rectum is dilated and the fissure identified. The goal of this surgical procedure is to excise the fibrous tissue of the tract and to allow natural healing. A probe is placed between the external fistula opening and the internal tract.

Line of incision through external sphincter m. (exposed through fissure)

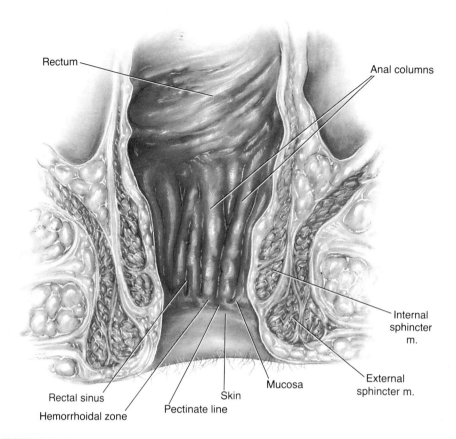

Rectum

Anal columns

Internal sphincter m.

Rectal sinus

Hemorrhoidal zone

Pectinate line

Skin

Mucosa

External sphincter m.

FIGURE 89–2. With cautery, the tract is exposed, which usually involves dividing the external sphincter.

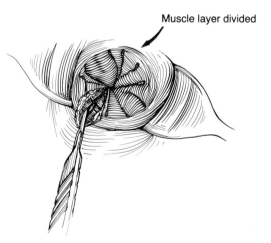

Muscle layer divided

FIGURE 89–3. With an elliptical incision, which usually extends through the external muscle, the fissure is excised back to normal tissue. Hemostasis is obtained by electrocautery, and a hemostatic pack is placed into the rectal opening with an absorbable agent such as Surgicel.

90

Incision of Fistula-in-Ano

JOSEPH A. MOYLAN, M.D.

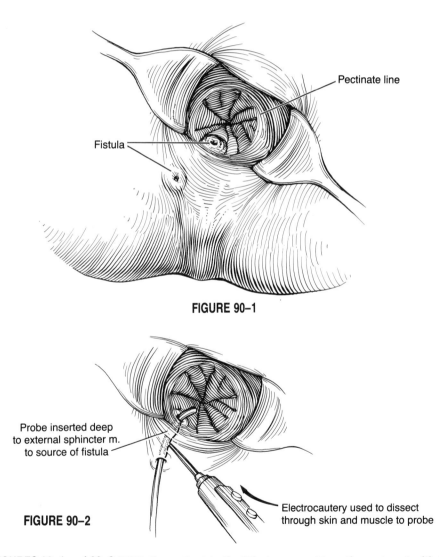

FIGURE 90–1

FIGURE 90–2

Pectinate line

Fistula

Probe inserted deep to external sphincter m. to source of fistula

Electrocautery used to dissect through skin and muscle to probe

FIGURES 90–1 and 90–2. With the patient in the lithotomy position, the rectum is dilated and a probe is placed between the external fistula opening and the internal tract. With cautery, the tract is exposed. This usually involves dividing the external sphincter. The base of the fistula tract is excised to normal tissue, and wound hemostasis is obtained by use of electrocautery. Topical hemostatic material is placed into the sinus tract.

Gallbladder

91

Laparoscopic Cholecystectomy

THEODORE N. PAPPAS, M.D.

Laparoscopic cholecystectomy involves the same principles as open cholecystectomy, except access to the abdomen is gained transabdominally, with video laparoscopic techniques used for dissection.

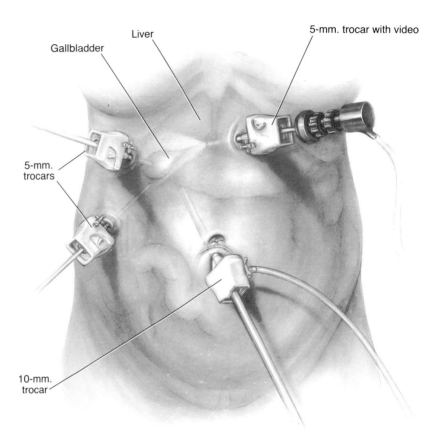

Liver

Gallbladder

5-mm. trocar with video

5-mm. trocars

10-mm. trocar

FIGURE 91–1. The trocars are placed in the abdomen. With a nasogastric tube and Foley catheter in place and the patient in the Trendelenburg position, a small umbilical incision is made. A Veress needle is placed in the abdomen for insufflation of carbon dioxide; care should be taken in placement of the needle to avoid intra-abdominal injury. A combination of the Trendelenburg position and upward retraction on the abdominal fascia assists in placement of the needle. Careful observation of the insufflation pressures aids in creation of the intrapneumoperitoneum. The initial .inflation pressures should be under 10 mm. Hg and usually near 5 mm. Hg. Insufflation flow should be approximately 1 liter per minute through the Veress needle.

An alternative technique involves an incision on the peritoneal cavity with placement of a pursestring suture at the fascial level and use of the Hasson trocar. This avoids blind puncture into the abdomen and obviates the occasional intra-abdominal injury with placement of the Veress needle.

A 10-mm. trocar is placed in the umbilical incision and in the upper midline. Two 5-mm. trocars are placed in the right side of the abdomen. With the high-flow insufflator maintaining a pneumoperitoneum, the video laparoscope is placed in the umbilical port. The right-sided trocars are used for retraction of the gallbladder. The most superior trocar on the right is used to retract the dome of the gallbladder over the liver. This distracts the portal structures and aids in dissection. The second right-sided abdominal retractor can be used to retract the infundibulum of the gallbladder laterally. The upper midline trocar is used by the surgeon for dissection.

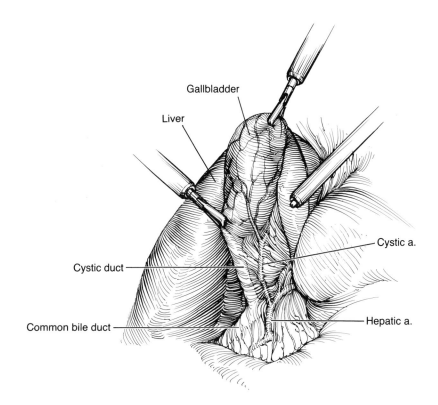

FIGURE 91–2. When the retractors are placed on the gallbladder, it is retracted cephalad and laterally. Any adhesions to the gallbladder are removed by blunt dissection. All dissection is done in the direction of the gallbladder down to the common duct. At this point, a decision concerning cholangiography is made. Cholangiograms are obtained either routinely for anatomic purposes or as indicated based on the preoperative and intraoperative assessment. A cholecystocholangiogram can be taken by the percutaneous placement of a 14-gauge angiocatheter into the gallbladder under direct vision. Bile is then aspirated, and full-strength Renografin is reinfused to a volume of 30 ml. plus the volume of aspirated bile. The angiocatheter is then removed, and an x-ray film is obtained. This can also be done under fluoroscopic control.

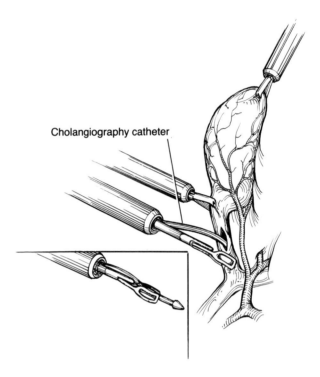

Cholangiography catheter

FIGURE 91-3. An alternative method for cholangiography is to place a clip at the cystic duct–gallbladder junction and make a small incision in the cystic duct. A cholangiography catheter is then threaded into the cystic duct, and the cholangiogram is taken. In either situation, following completion of the cholangiogram, the cystic duct and cystic artery are completely dissected.

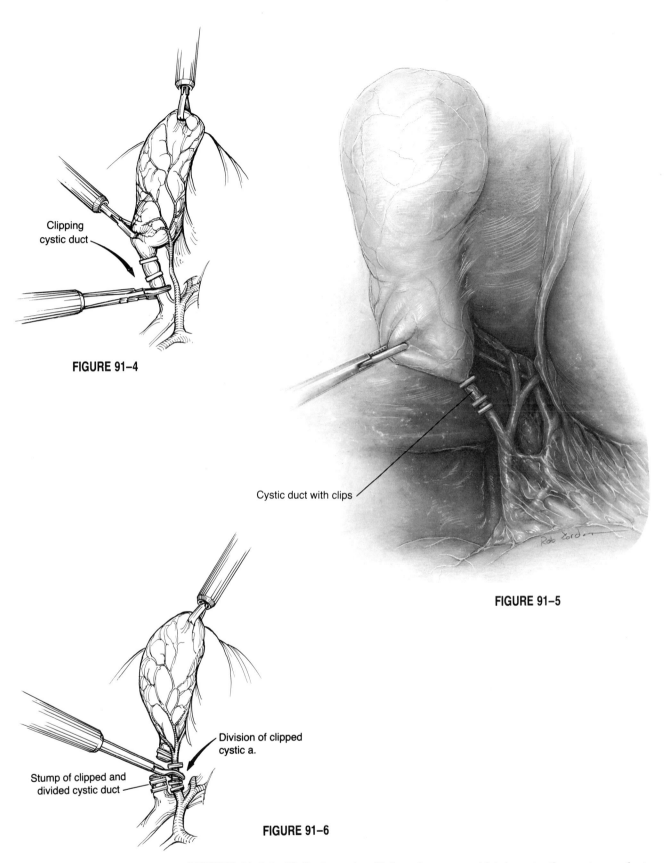

FIGURE 91–4

Clipping cystic duct

Cystic duct with clips

FIGURE 91–5

Division of clipped cystic a.

Stump of clipped and divided cystic duct

FIGURE 91–6

FIGURES 91–4 to 91–6. Care should be taken to avoid injury to the common duct, particularly because maximal retraction is often required and causes tenting of the common duct. Two clips are placed on the cystic duct stump, and one clip is placed on the cystic duct–gallbladder junction. The cystic duct is then divided. The cystic artery is controlled in a similar manner and divided. When the cystic duct and cystic artery have been divided, the gallbladder is removed from the liver bed with electrocautery.

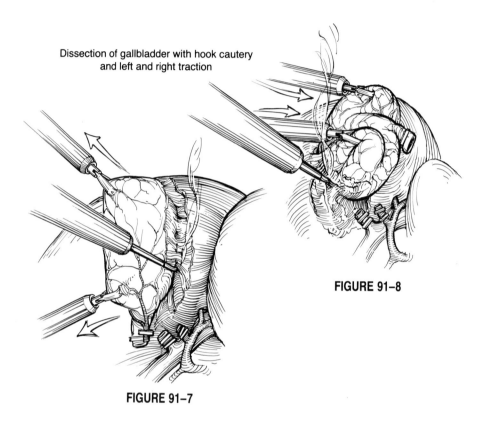

Dissection of gallbladder with hook cautery
and left and right traction

FIGURE 91–8

FIGURE 91–7

FIGURES 91–7 and 91–8. Removal of the gallbladder is accomplished by retracting it maximally to the left or right in an effort to apply tension to the tissues and to facilitate the use of the electrocautery. When the dissection is nearly complete, the gallbladder bed is fully inspected to ensure that there is no persistent bleeding. The gallbladder is then removed and extracted from the umbilical port. Removal of the gallbladder through the umbilical incision is facilitated by aspiration of the bile in it, removal or crushing of the stones, or occasionally extending the umbilical incision slightly. The right upper quadrant is then irrigated and inspected, and closure is accomplished by approximating the umbilical fascia with an absorbable suture with Steri-Strips for the skin.

92

Cholecystectomy and Exploration of Common Duct

THEODORE N. PAPPAS, M.D.

Elective surgery for cholelithiasis is the most common abdominal operation performed. A careful history characterizing the patient's pain is important to be certain that the symptoms are referable to the biliary tract. In most patients, gallstones are documented by ultrasonography; liver function tests, including alkaline phosphatase and bilirubin, are required preoperatively. A preoperative upper gastrointestinal series is occasionally necessary to distinguish duodenal ulcer disease from gallbladder disease. In most patients, the decision to obtain an intraoperative cholangiogram is made preoperatively on the basis of the history, physical examination, and laboratory tests. Patients who do not require an intraoperative cholangiogram include those with a normal-sized bile duct on ultrasonography, no history of bile duct obstruction or jaundice, and normal liver function tests. In addition, intraoperative assessment of the size of the gallstones can assist in the decision of whether to obtain an intraoperative cholangiogram.

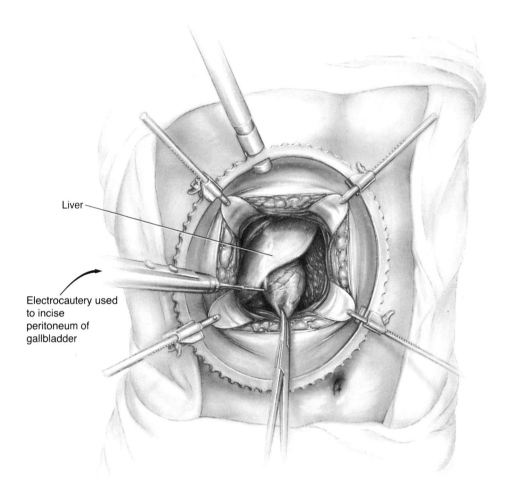

Liver

Electrocautery used
to incise
peritoneum of
gallbladder

FIGURE 92–1. A right subcostal incision is usually made for cholecystectomy and common
duct exploration, or a midline incision can be used in most patients. The abdomen is
explored, and a self-retaining retractor is placed for most cholecystectomies. Both
retrograde and antegrade removal of the gallbladder is possible, although the antegrade
technique is most common. The dome of the gallbladder is initially scored with
electrocautery, and a tonsil clamp is used to establish a plane in the thickened gallbladder
in proximity to the gallbladder wall itself. The cautery is then used to incise the
peritoneal surface of the entire dome.

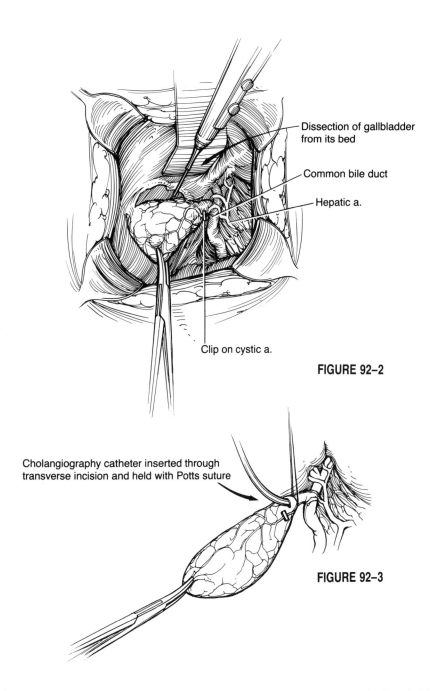

Dissection of gallbladder
from its bed

Common bile duct

Hepatic a.

Clip on cystic a.

FIGURE 92-2

Cholangiography catheter inserted through
transverse incision and held with Potts suture

FIGURE 92-3

FIGURE 92-2. The fundus of the gallbladder is removed from the liver bed with blunt and sharp dissection. Care should be taken in mobilizing the infundibulum of the gallbladder to be certain that it is not adherent to the common bile duct. The cystic artery and its extension are usually encountered on the medial surface of the gallbladder. The cystic artery can be temporarily controlled with a silver clip on the surface of the gallbladder prior to its formal ligation. The gallbladder is then completely mobilized from the liver bed until it is attached only by the cystic duct.

FIGURE 92-3. At this point, the final decision should be made concerning the need for intraoperative cholangiography. The cholangiogram is taken by making a transverse incision at the junction between the gallbladder and the cystic duct. The cholangiography catheter is introduced into the cystic duct stump, and bile is usually aspirated from the catheter. A Potts suture of 3–0 silk is placed around the neck of the gallbladder and tied, and a silver clip is placed on the suture to secure the catheter in the cystic duct.

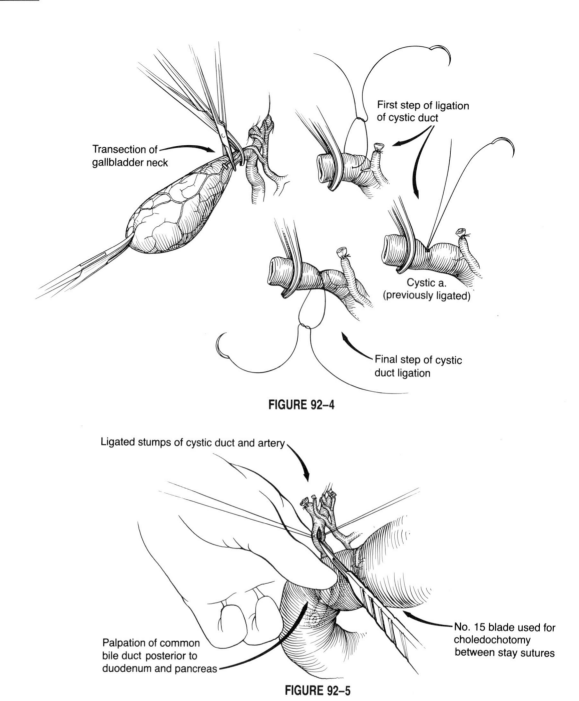

Transection of gallbladder neck

First step of ligation of cystic duct

Cystic a. (previously ligated)

Final step of cystic duct ligation

FIGURE 92–4

Ligated stumps of cystic duct and artery

Palpation of common bile duct posterior to duodenum and pancreas

No. 15 blade used for choledochotomy between stay sutures

FIGURE 92–5

FIGURE 92–4. The quality of the cholangiogram can be optimized by rolling the patient slightly to the right, which shifts the common duct off the spine to improve the intraoperative images. Two films should be obtained with half-strength radiograffin, 5 and 15 ml. each. While waiting for the cholangiogram to be processed, the cystic duct–common duct junction should be dissected. Care should be taken to expose the common duct and bifurcation of the hepatic ducts completely to be certain that there is no abnormal anatomy in this area. The cholangiogram not only determines the presence of biliary stones but also assists in determining the presence of abnormal anatomy. If the cholangiogram confirms normal anatomy, the cystic duct can be taken by placing a right-angle clamp on the cystic duct and dividing it with removal of the specimen. The gallbladder is usually opened intraoperatively to reconfirm the type of stones in the gallbladder. The cystic duct stump is then ligated with a 2–0 silk ligature placed through the cystic duct stump and tied.

FIGURE 92–5. *See legend on opposite page*

FIGURE 92–5. Exploration of the common duct should be reserved for patients who have jaundice, cholangitis, palpable stones in the common bile duct, or an abnormal cholangiogram. When the decision to explore the common duct has been made, a Kocher maneuver is performed by incising the peritoneal surface on the second portion of the duodenum with Metzenbaum scissors. The duodenum is then mobilized upward by blunt dissection. This allows complete palpation of the common duct posteriorly as it enters the pancreas and duodenum. A 3-cm. portion of the common bile duct is then carefully exposed on its anterior surface. Stay sutures of 4–0 silk are placed on either side of the common bile duct, and a choledochotomy is made with a No. 15 blade. This choledochotomy is extended with Potts scissors in both directions. On exploration of the common bile duct, a 10 French red rubber catheter is used to irrigate the duct proximally into the liver and distally as well. Stones that are retrieved are sent for pathologic examination. Irrigation should continue until no further stones are retrieved. At this point, an attempt is made to pass the red rubber catheter into the duodenum with minimal force.

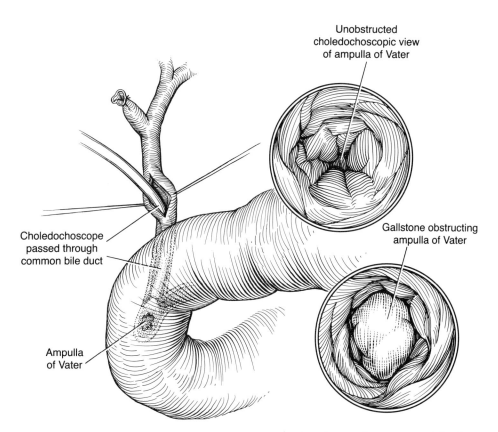

Unobstructed
choledochoscopic view
of ampulla of Vater

Gallstone obstructing
ampulla of Vater

Choledochoscope
passed through
common bile duct

Ampulla
of Vater

FIGURE 92–6. The flexible choledochoscope is introduced into the common bile duct, and the hepatic side of the common bile duct is visualized. The choledochoscope is usually easily passed to the bifurcation and occasionally it can be passed more proximally. The choledochoscope is then passed distally into the common bile duct until the ampulla is visualized. At this point, a clear view of the ampulla of Vater from within should be noted and the presence or absence of stones again determined. If no stones are encountered on complete visualization of the biliary tract by the choledochoscope, the exploration is then completed.

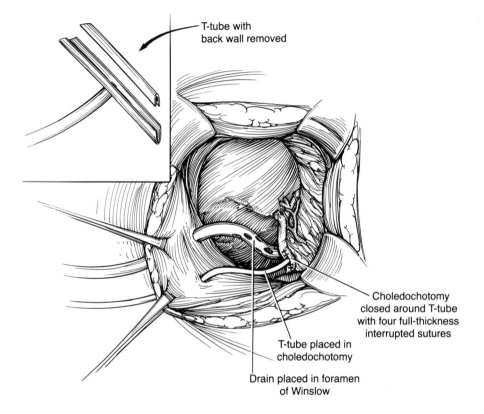

T-tube with
back wall removed

Choledochotomy
closed around T-tube
with four full-thickness
interrupted sutures

T-tube placed in
choledochotomy

Drain placed in foramen
of Winslow

FIGURE 92–7. A T-tube is placed in the common bile duct. The T-tube is cut by removing the back wall of the tube. The size of the tube is determined on the basis of the size of the common bile duct. Except for unusual cases, the minimal size used is a 16 French tube. The T-tube is placed and is secured by approximating the common bile duct over the T-tube with 4–0 PDS. When the T-tube is secured, saline is infused into the T-tube to ensure that a water-tight seal is present. The T-tube is brought through a separate stab wound in the skin, and a T-tube cholangiogram is obtained to confirm its location in the bile duct and to confirm that there are no residual bile duct stones. A closed-suction drain is placed in the foramen of Winslow and is brought out through a separate stab wound in the abdomen. The nasogastric tube is removed in the recovery room, and the patient may be placed on a clear liquid diet as early as the evening of the operation. The drain is removed on the second or third postoperative day if there is no bile leaking around the T-tube. A T-tube cholangiogram is obtained on the fifth day and, if normal, the T-tube can be clamped prior to discharge. An alternative approach is to have the patient discharged on the third or fourth postoperative day and to obtain an outpatient cholangiogram on the seventh day.

93

Excision of Ampulla of Vater and Bile Duct

WILLIAM C. MEYERS, M.D.

A local resection of the periampullary region is generally performed for small benign tumors accessible to resection by that method. Local resection of malignant tumors is limited to patients unfit for the Whipple procedure because of the high incidence of recurrence.

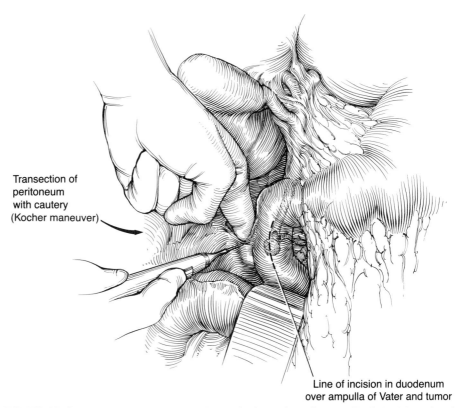

Transection of peritoneum with cautery (Kocher maneuver)

Line of incision in duodenum over ampulla of Vater and tumor

FIGURE 93–1. The procedure is performed through a longitudinal incision in the duodenum over the ampulla of Vater, and the site for incision is selected after a generous Kocher maneuver and attempt at external palpation of the tumor or papillae. A search has already been conducted for evidence of metastatic disease because generally there is no certainty that the lesion is, indeed, benign.

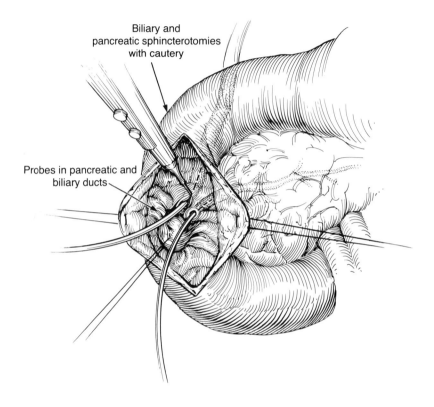

Biliary and
pancreatic sphincterotomies
with cautery

Probes in pancreatic and
biliary ducts

FIGURE 93–2. After the duodenum is opened and the tumor inspected, a margin of normal tissue is identified around the tumor and the site is selected for incision. Sometimes, the bile and pancreatic ducts can be cannulated through the tumor, although it may be easier to perform a "precut" such as is sometimes performed with endoscopic sphincterotomy, i.e., incision into the biliary or pancreatic system without prior cannulation.

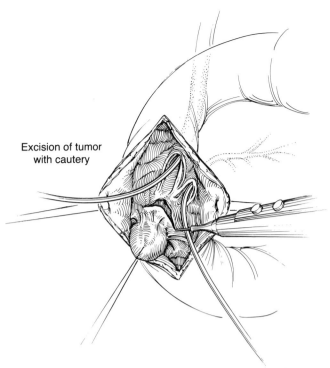

Excision of tumor
with cautery

FIGURE 93–3. Excision of the lesion is performed submucosally. However, deeper tissue may be included in the specimen, including a portion of the pancreas. Vessels are cauterized or ligated as they are encountered. The Cavitron ultrasonic aspirator (CUSA) may be helpful in deeper resections. The primary instrument used for dissection is a sharp-pointed cautery.

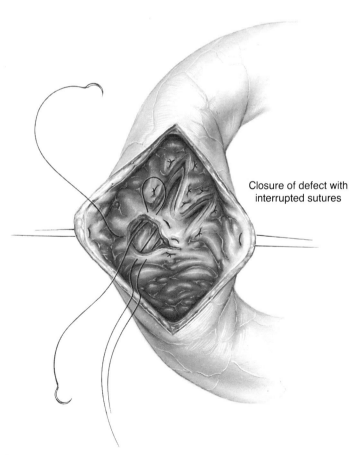

Closure of defect with
interrupted sutures

FIGURE 93–4. The defect is closed following removal of the tumor with interrupted or running 4–0 chromic sutures.

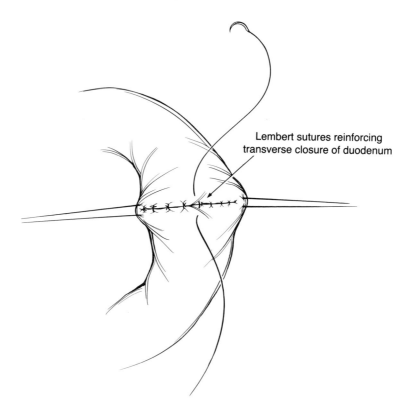

Lembert sutures reinforcing
transverse closure of duodenum

FIGURE 93–5. After confirmation of hemostasis, the duodenum is closed in a transverse manner, as in a Heineke-Mikulicz pyloroplasty.

SECTION IX

Liver

94

Surgical Management of Hepatic Trauma

R. LAWRENCE REED II, M.D.

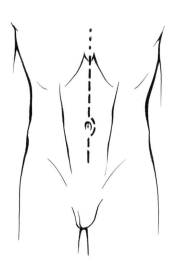

Midline incision
with optional sternotomy

FIGURE 94–1. Surgical procedures for abdominal trauma are best approached through a midline laparotomy incision. Occasionally, severe liver wounds may necessitate extension of the incision into the chest for additional exposure and may be accomplished by extending the midline laparotomy with a right anterolateral thoracotomy. This exposure can sometimes be limited, and the placement of a right atrial catheter for volume infusion is best accomplished with a midline sternotomy. A median sternotomy, as an extension of the midline laparotomy incision, offers the best exposure of the retrohepatic vena cava. It also allows access to the right atrium should an atriocaval shunt be elected.

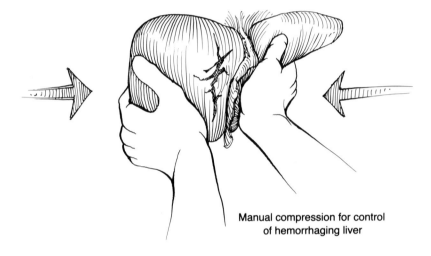

Manual compression for control
of hemorrhaging liver

FIGURE 94–2. Most bleeding from the liver is venous in origin, owing to its dual venous blood supply and the low hydrostatic pressure. Intraoperative manual compression of the liver is usually effective in achieving temporary hemostasis.

While the operator evacuates blood and clots in a search for other bleeding sites, the assistant can apply the *left* hand over the right lobe of the liver, the *right* hand over the left lobe and hilum, and compress the hepatic substance between the two hands. Padding to avoid capsular tears by the fingers can usually be provided with gauze laparotomy pads between the hands and the liver. Positioning of the hands is adjusted as necessary until temporary control of bleeding is achieved, and care should be taken not to compress the underlying inferior vena cava. If such control can be achieved, resuscitation with infusion of crystalloid solutions and packed red blood cells should be aggressively pursued. Surgical procedures should not be performed until the patient is adequately resuscitated unless uncontrolled bleeding persists. Attempts to perform surgical repairs during hemorrhage in the underresuscitated patient are likely to result in exsanguination.

Monitoring of filling pressures, heart rate, pulse pressure, and urinary output should be routine to assess the success of control of hemorrhage and resuscitation.

Index finger and jaw of clamp in
epiploic foramen in preparation for occlusion
of porta hepatis (Pringle maneuver)

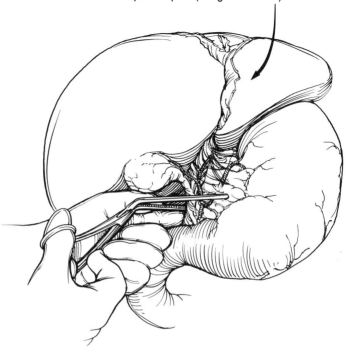

FIGURE 94–3. Temporary vascular occlusion can be obtained by compressing the hepatoduodenal ligament with the fingers or by a vascular clamp (Pringle maneuver). The safe hepatic ischemic time is difficult to determine under the variable conditions of shock, hypovolemia, and hypothermia. Therefore, periodic release of the occluded portal triad should best be done every 15 to 30 minutes for hepatic perfusion. Control of the hemorrhage is initially sought by manual compression and the Pringle maneuver. Selective ligation of vessels with hepatotomy and finger fracture, where necessary, is then performed to identify and control the major bleeding sites. Resection is limited to debridement of clearly devascularized tissue.

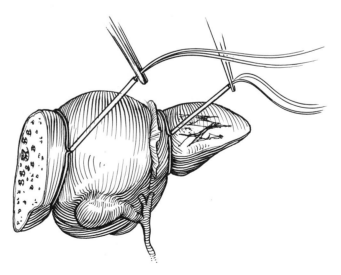

Tourniquets used intraoperatively
while hemostasis is achieved through
resection and/or ligation

FIGURE 94–4. Tourniquet control of bleeding from the hepatic margins and raw surfaces can provide temporary control while resuscitation is continued and more definitive hemostatic techniques are undertaken. Penrose drains or Rumel tourniquets may be used for this purpose.

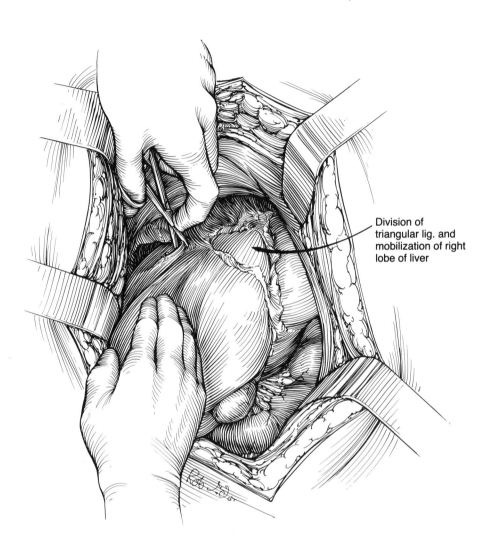

Division of
triangular lig. and
mobilization of right
lobe of liver

FIGURE 94–5. If temporary control cannot be achieved and blood continues to surround the liver, early consideration should be given to the possibility of injury to a hepatic vein. The greatest likelihood of achieving survival in patients with these injuries is early identification and control. Access to this area is achieved through rapid mobilization of the right lobe of the liver by division of the triangular ligament. The triangular ligament is sharply divided over the right and left lobes of the liver. Care should be taken to dissect near the liver capsule during this division, as large phrenic veins often course between the leaves of the peritoneal reflection. These can be injured during the division of the triangular ligaments, producing a rapid loss of blood that further obscures the operative field. Care must also be taken as this mobilization proceeds, because the inferior vena cava can often be retracted out of position and inadvertently injured.

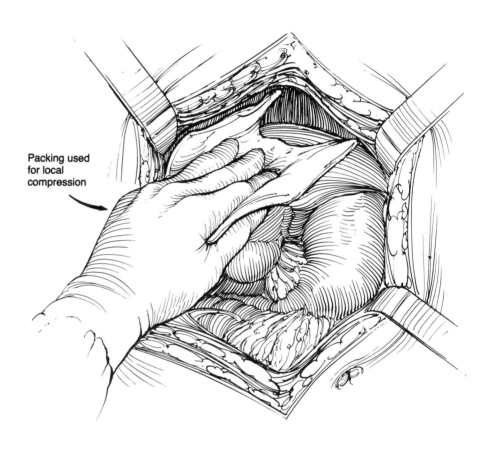

Packing used
for local
compression

FIGURE 94–6. Temporary gauze packing is used in some patients to assist in compression of the bleeding, and it may control retrohepatic caval bleeding as well.

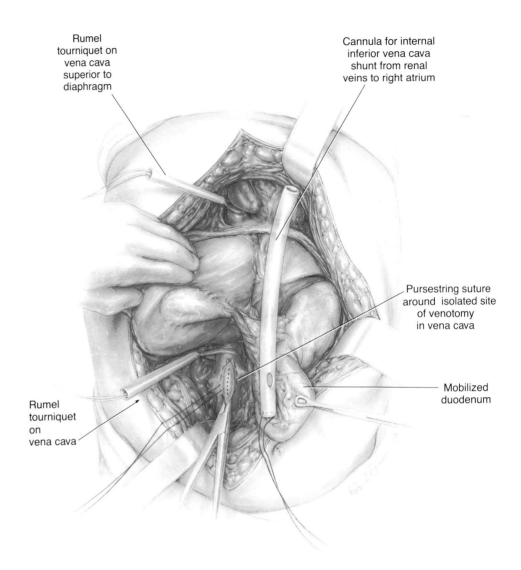

Rumel
tourniquet on
vena cava
superior to
diaphragm

Cannula for internal
inferior vena cava
shunt from renal
veins to right atrium

Pursestring suture
around isolated site
of venotomy
in vena cava

Rumel
tourniquet
on
vena cava

Mobilized
duodenum

FIGURE 94–7. If bleeding from the hepatic veins or the retrohepatic vena cava is identified, temporary control can often be achieved by gentle digital pressure over the tear in the vessel and, when larger, by compression with a gauze sponge. If the bleeding site can be identified and controlled easily, repair can usually be accomplished by simple venous suture or occasionally by oversewing when the hepatic vein is avulsed. However, if the bleeding point cannot be identified and blood continues to flow from the retrohepatic area, early consideration must be given to increased exposure via a thoracotomy. Injuries of the retrohepatic vena cava and large juxtacaval liver wounds can be very difficult to control. These often bleed massively, and attempts to visualize the injured areas for repair often worsen the bleeding by further tearing the torn vessels and parenchyma by retraction of the liver.

Total vascular isolation of the liver can be achieved by a clamp or Rumel tourniquet occlusion of the suprahepatic and infrahepatic inferior vena cava, the hepatoduodenal ligament, and the supraceliac aorta. However, this maneuver can produce a severe reduction in venous return and cause a low cardiac output with subsequent cardiac arrest. Thus, an alternative approach is to provide a temporary shunt for blood to flow through the inferior vena cava while still occluding blood flow into and from the liver. A large chest tube or endotracheal tube may be used for such a shunt and may be inserted retrograde from the right atrium or antegrade from the infrahepatic inferior vena cava, as shown in the figure. A large silk suture is placed on the inferior end of the shunt to permit easy removal. A pursestring suture in the inferior vena cava is tightened to secure the shunt in place.

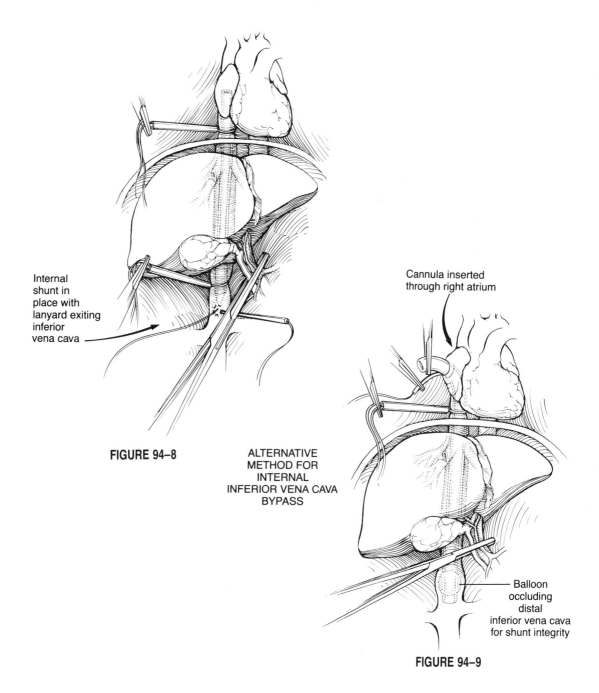

Internal
shunt in
place with
lanyard exiting
inferior
vena cava

FIGURE 94–8

ALTERNATIVE
METHOD FOR
INTERNAL
INFERIOR VENA CAVA
BYPASS

Cannula inserted
through right atrium

Balloon
occluding
distal
inferior vena cava
for shunt integrity

FIGURE 94–9

FIGURE 94–8. Injury to a hepatic vein or the retrohepatic cava often necessitates hepatic vascular isolation for control while allowing for venous return to the heart. An infrahepatic atriocaval shunt is inserted through a venotomy in the infrahepatic inferior vena cava. The shunt is secured in position, and venous blood loss is prevented with Rumel tourniquets placed around the inferior vena cava above and below the liver. The Pringle maneuver is applied to prevent vascular inflow to the liver while the venous repair is undertaken, and the pursestring suture in the inferior vena cava is loosened and the shunt removed. The venotomy is then closed by tying the pursestring suture.

FIGURE 94–9. An alternative placement of an atriocaval shunt is *retrograde* from the right atrium with a large endotracheal tube. An advantage of this variation is that the balloon on the endotracheal tube may be inflated to provide venous occlusion around the shunt. This helps to prevent venous bleeding from the site of injury while allowing blood to flow into the right atrium without the need for an inferior Rumel tourniquet.

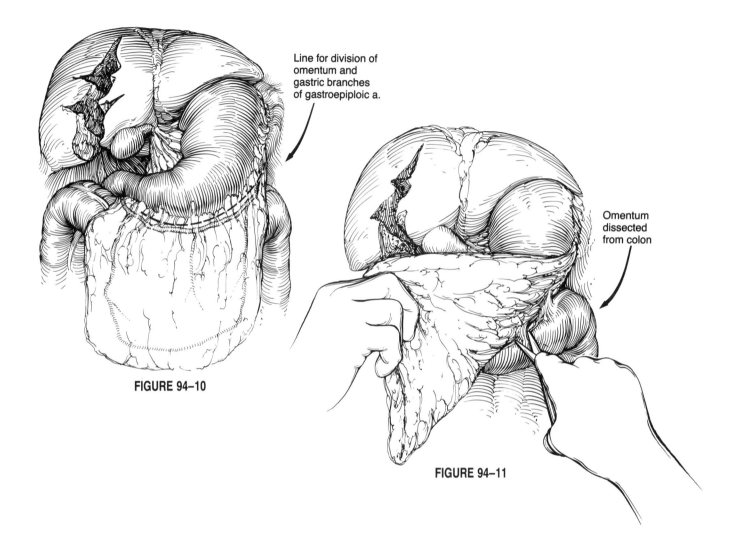

Line for division of
omentum and
gastric branches
of gastroepiploic a.

FIGURE 94-10

Omentum
dissected
from colon

FIGURE 94-11

FIGURE 94-10. Occasionally, large defects in the liver parenchyma may be packed with a portion of the omentum with its blood supply intact. Viability of the omental pack is based on the right gastroepiploic artery, and severe associated injuries of the stomach or celiac axis may preclude this technique because of compromise of the blood supply to the greater curvature.

FIGURE 94-11. The greater omentum is quickly dissected from the transverse colon in an avascular plane.

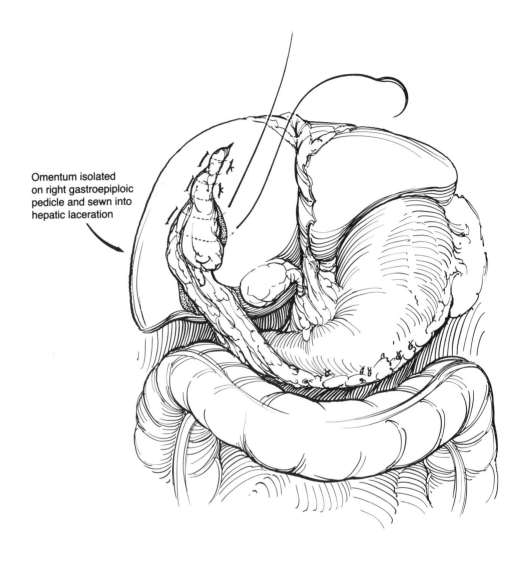

Omentum isolated
on right gastroepiploic
pedicle and sewn into
hepatic laceration

FIGURE 94–12. The omental pack is rotated and placed into the liver laceration and secured in position with large mattress sutures with a large, curved blunt-tipped needle.

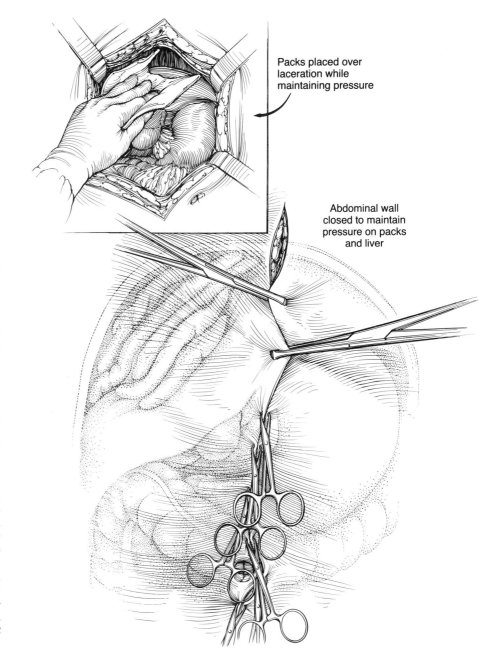

Packs placed over
laceration while
maintaining pressure

Abdominal wall
closed to maintain
pressure on packs
and liver

FIGURE 94–13. If uncontrolled hemorrhage continues, the problem becomes one of coagulopathy, and, at this point, effective hemostatic control cannot be achieved until the clotting abnormalities are corrected. Frequently, this necessitates rewarming the patient, aggressive resuscitation, and administration of clotting factors, including platelets. Rewarming is usually best accomplished with the abdomen closed. Temporary closure of the abdomen can be quickly performed by the use of multiple towel clips applied to the skin. Gauze packs are left in place both above and below the area of hepatic injury to tamponade the bleeding site. The packs are removed at a second laparotomy, usually 1 to 3 days later, when the coagulopathy is controlled and the patient is normothermic and hemodynamically stable.

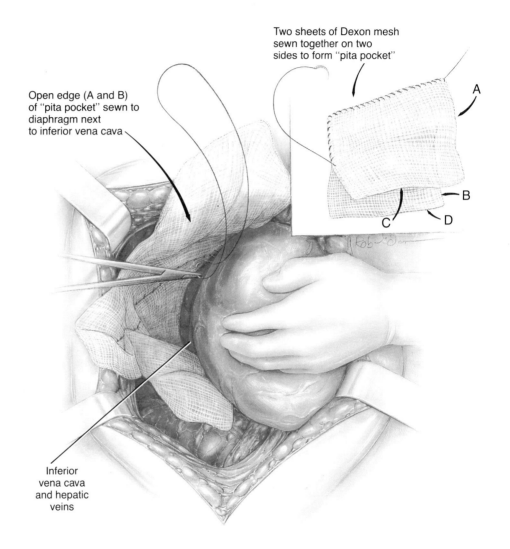

Two sheets of Dexon mesh sewn together on two sides to form "pita pocket"

Open edge (A and B) of "pita pocket" sewn to diaphragm next to inferior vena cava

A

B

C   D

Inferior vena cava and hepatic veins

FIGURE 94–14. Compression and tamponade of severe hepatic bleeding can also be achieved by wrapping one lobe at a time with absorbable synthetic mesh (polyglycolic acid or polyglactin mesh) and using the falciform ligament as a point of attachment for the mesh. A hepatorrhaphy of the right lobe with mesh is depicted. A cholecystectomy is often performed prior to such a hepatorrhaphy of the right lobe, as the gallbladder would otherwise be enveloped within the wrap. Two sheets of mesh are sutured together on two contiguous sides to create a "pita pocket" *(insert)*. The posterior suture line is extended from the diaphragm, over the dome of the right lobe of the liver, and downward along the lateral border of the inferior vena cava using the edge labeled B.

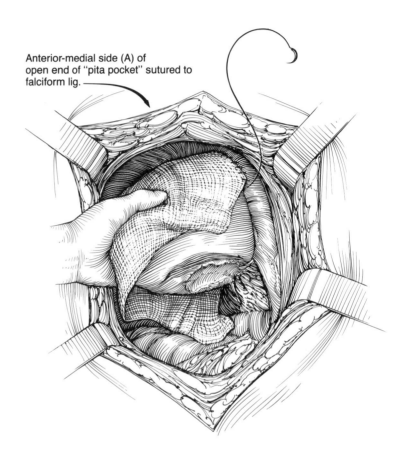

Anterior-medial side (A) of
open end of "pita pocket" sutured to
falciform lig.

FIGURE 94–15. Anteriorly, the mesh is fixed (using the edge labeled A) to the falciform ligament anteriorly or to the left anterior abdominal wall if the falciform ligament has been divided in the initial process of exploring and mobilizing the liver.

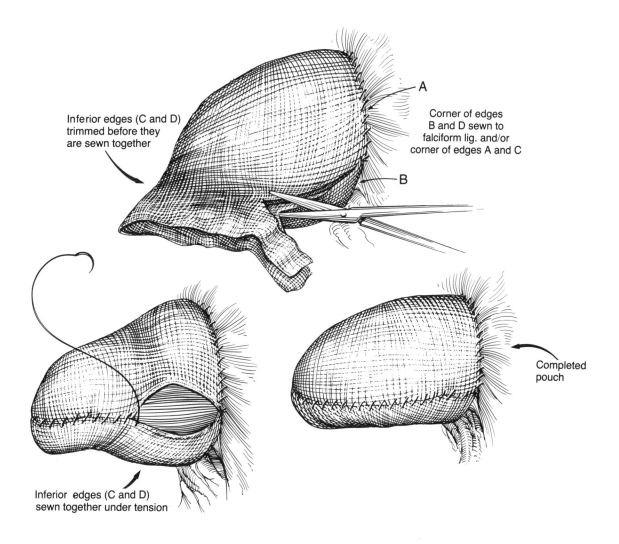

Inferior edges (C and D)
trimmed before they
are sewn together

Corner of edges
B and D sewn to
falciform lig. and/or
corner of edges A and C

A

B

Inferior edges (C and D)
sewn together under tension

Completed
pouch

FIGURE 94–16. The inferior edges of the anterior and posterior leaflets of mesh are attached to each other and to the falciform ligament on the inferior and medial aspect of the wrap. The inferior edge of the wrap remains open, and the edge is stretched by retracting inferiorly on its lateral and medial points, with trimming of the redundant mesh.

FIGURE 94–17. The inferior edges of the mesh are approximated snugly with a continuous suture line. The mesh can be gathered with sutures or continuously trimmed such that the wrap provides a tight compressive fit to the liver substance.

FIGURE 94–18. The completed wrap should be sufficiently tight to stop hemorrhage but not produce ischemia. Focal areas of bleeding can be controlled with simple or figure-of-eight sutures through the mesh.

95

Segmental Hepatic Resection

WILLIAM C. MEYERS, M.D.

Most metastatic tumors of the liver arise from malignant cells lodging principally in a hepatic segment via the portal vein. Primary hepatic tumors also metastasize *locally* along portal routes, providing a rational basis for segmental resection of these tumors as well. The French segments, as described by Couinaud and others, are determined by the portal and hepatic venous branching systems.

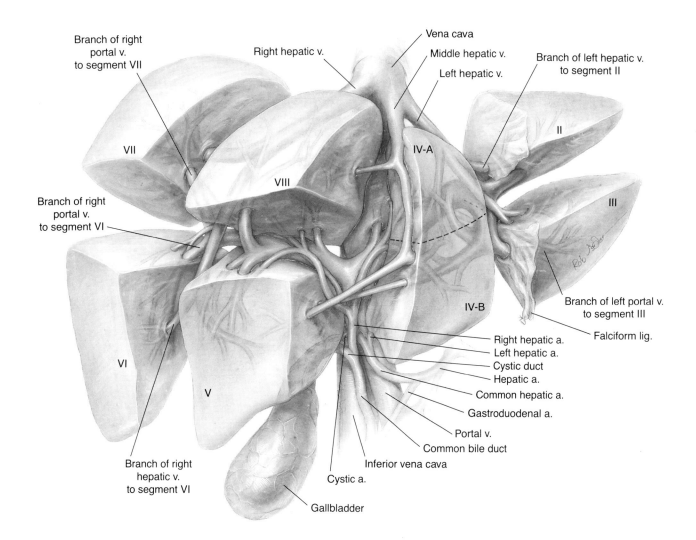

Branch of right
portal v.
to segment VII

Right hepatic v.

Vena cava

Middle hepatic v.

Left hepatic v.

Branch of left hepatic v.
to segment II

VII

VIII

IV-A

II

Branch of right
portal v.
to segment VI

III

Branch of right
hepatic v.
to segment VI

VI

V

IV-B

Branch of left portal v.
to segment III

Falciform lig.

Right hepatic a.
Left hepatic a.
Cystic duct
Hepatic a.
Common hepatic a.
Gastroduodenal a.
Portal v.
Common bile duct
Inferior vena cava
Cystic a.

Gallbladder

FIGURE 95–1. The following logic can be employed to remember the segmental sections:
The caudate lobe is its own segment (segment I) and is located posteriorly. In a *clockwise*
order beginning from the top, segments II and III determine the tissue left of the
falciform ligament (i.e., the left lateral segment in the American system). Segment IV
corresponds to the tissue between the falciform ligament and Cantlie's line or the middle
hepatic vein (and corresponds to the left medial segment). Segment IV is sometimes
divided into part A, a superior part, and part B, an inferior part. Segments V, VI, VII,
and VIII continue according to this clockwise labeling. The gallbladder fossa lies between
segments IV and V. The figure depicts the internal vascular skeleton, which is confirmed
with intraoperative ultrasonography.

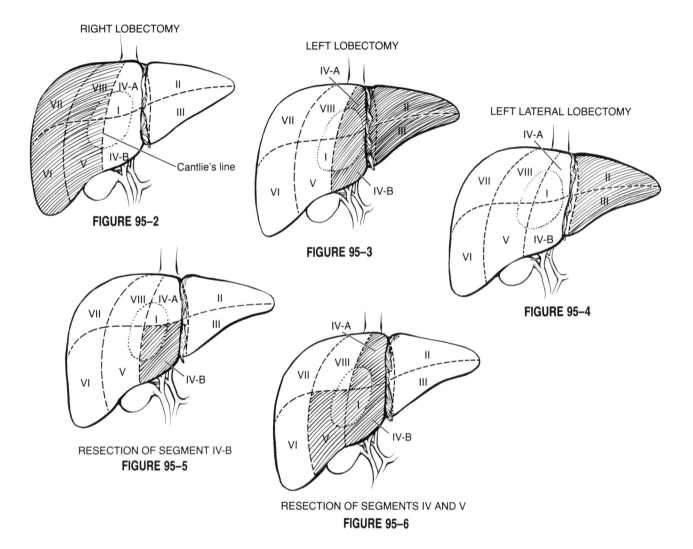

RIGHT LOBECTOMY

Cantlie's line

FIGURE 95–2

LEFT LOBECTOMY

FIGURE 95–3

LEFT LATERAL LOBECTOMY

FIGURE 95–4

RESECTION OF SEGMENT IV-B
FIGURE 95–5

RESECTION OF SEGMENTS IV AND V
FIGURE 95–6

FIGURES 95–2 to 95–6. Several types of hepatic resections are shown schematically. The classic *right hepatic lobectomy* consists of removal of segments V, VI, VII, and VIII (Fig. 95–2). The classic *left hepatic lobectomy* consists of removal of segments II, III, and IV (Fig. 95–3). The classic *left lateral segmentectomy* consists of removal of segments II and III (Fig. 95–4). The classic *right trisegmentectomy* is not depicted except as the converse of Figure 95–4—that is, only segments II and III are preserved. One of the eight or nine types of standard *segmental* resections is the removal of segment IV, as shown in Figure 95–5. Usually, removal of segment IV includes only the inferior half (segment IVB), although the entire segment may be more formally resected as well. Removal of *multiple* segments is depicted in Figure 95–6 (segments IV and V). This particular multiple segmentectomy might be used for a central lesion or for hepatic resection of a carcinoma of the gallbladder or bile duct. Some surgeons advocate routine removal of segment I in addition to segments IV and V for these neoplasms. In our experience, segment VI is probably the simplest segment to resect, followed by a combination of segments II and III or segment V. With proper mobilization of the liver, resection of segment VII can also be relatively easy; whereas resection of segments IV and VIII is generally more difficult.

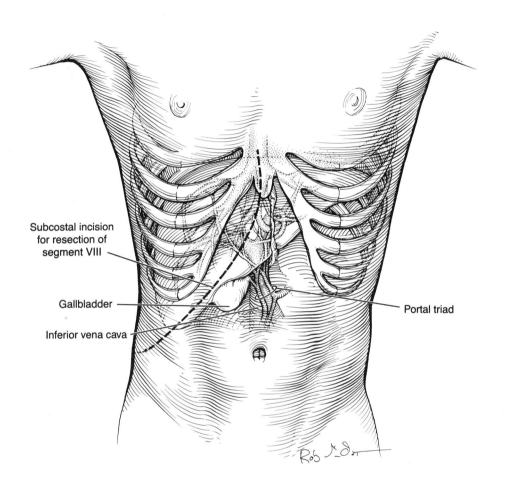

Subcostal incision
for resection of
segment VIII

Gallbladder

Inferior vena cava

Portal triad

FIGURE 95–7. The standard approach for segmental resection is a *generous* subcostal incision beginning an inch or two *above* the tip of the xiphoid process and extending posteriorly to the limit of the drapes. The most common mistake made in initiating the procedure is limiting the length of the incision. The anatomic relationships of the structures encountered during the remainder of the exposure are shown in Figure 95–1. Note the position of the liver when the patient is asleep, supine, and relaxed. It extends just below the rib cage, extending to allow the left lobe to be seen clearly below the ribs. The superior extent of the liver lies immediately beneath the upper point of the incision, and a thoracic extension is rarely necessary. In more than 300 resections performed by the author, the only indication for thoracic extension has been for removal of tumors that extended above the diaphragm.

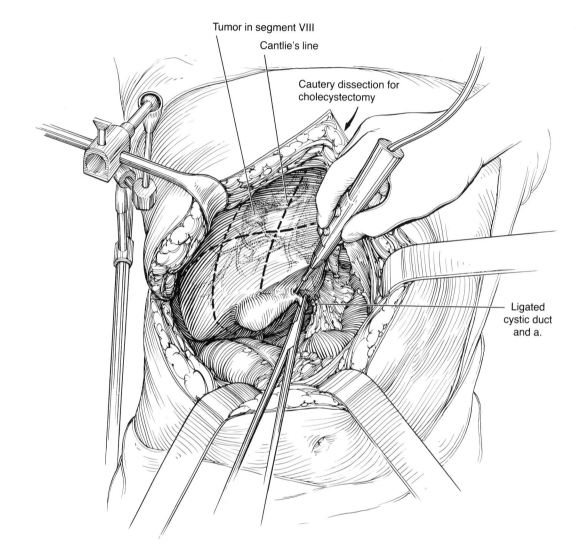

Tumor in segment VIII

Cantlie's line

Cautery dissection for
cholecystectomy

Ligated
cystic duct
and a.

FIGURE 95–8. After the incision is made and the presence of extrahepatic tumor is excluded, appropriate retractors are placed to permit optimal mobilization of the liver. It is usually preferable to mobilize the liver partially prior to the use of stationary retractors to reduce the necessity of frequent repositioning. The best retractor for this is the Elmed type, which is a triple-jointed arm retractor capable of holding any common instrument and retracting tissue in any direction by simply screwing and unscrewing one part. The drawback of this retractor is its fragility. Even one attempt at moving a hinge without untightening the screw could damage the instrument permanently. In other words, one should *untighten* the screw compulsively each time prior to repositioning the retractor. It is also important to remind the assistants how appreciative they should be of this retractor because it almost does much of their work.

Even when a hilar dissection is not needed, one usually removes the gallbladder as an initial maneuver. Cholecystectomy serves two purposes: (1) it provides easy, quick access to the portal hilum should it be necessary, and (2) it prevents the possibility of a second operation for cholecystectomy in a scarred right upper quadrant. However, cholecystectomy is not anatomically necessary for removal of several segments, such as segment VIII, unless hilar control is needed.

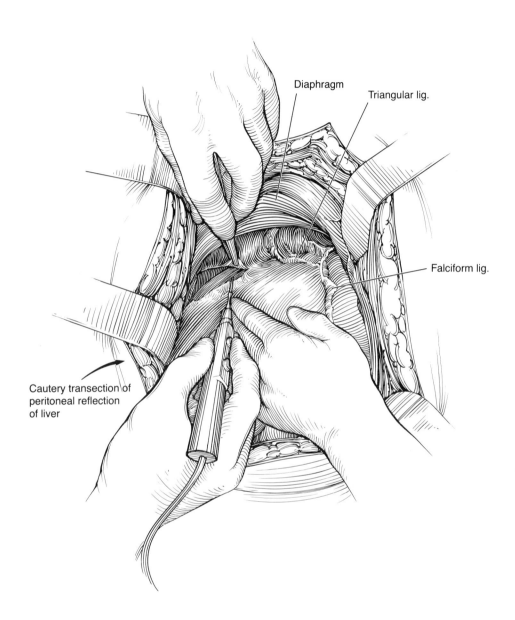

Diaphragm

Triangular lig.

Falciform lig.

Cautery transection of
peritoneal reflection
of liver

FIGURE 95–9. For nearly every segmental resection, the avascular ligaments of the liver are nearly completely divided to provide maximal mobilization of the liver. This begins with the division of the falciform ligament and mobilization of the right lobe of the liver with separation of the liver and triangular ligament from the diaphragm and should require only about 10 minutes. Full mobilization means freeing the liver posteriorly to the vena cava, thus providing easy venous control should it become necessary. For full mobilization, it is usually *not* necessary to ligate and divide any venous branches, including the right adrenal vein and caudate lobe branches to the vena cava. It is necessary to divide the inferior attachment of the vena cava as well as the ligament of the left lateral segment. During the mobilization of the latter, the gastrohepatic ligament is properly visualized to exclude a large left hepatic artery originating from the left gastric artery.

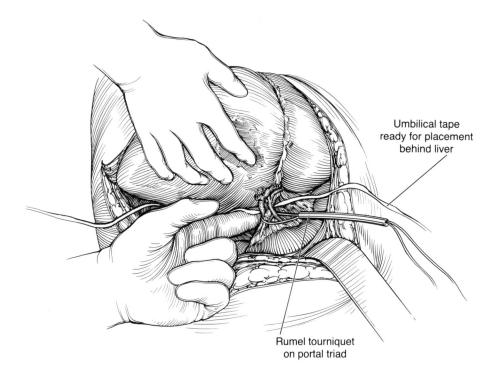

Umbilical tape
ready for placement
behind liver

Rumel tourniquet
on portal triad

FIGURE 95–10. Two easily achieved maneuvers for potential vascular isolation can be performed and are generally applicable to most hepatic resections. The first, *portal* isolation, is well known and provides access for the Pringle maneuver. The second maneuver is not previously described but is equally easy and is quite useful, particularly if temporary total occlusion of the right part of the liver becomes necessary. This is termed a right *hepatic venous tourniquet*. A similar procedure can be performed for the left side by reversing the relationship of the umbilical tape with respect to the portal triad and the inferior vena cava. Essential for this hepatic venous tourniquet maneuver is complete right hepatic mobilization.

Isolation of the *portal* triad is a *simple* maneuver. One cannot stress too strongly how simple it is even in the presence of massive portal collaterals. If there is difficulty in accomplishing the isolation, it is usually owing to dissection in the improper plane. At this point, one stops and seeks the foramen of Winslow again and surrounds the *portal* triad by placing a finger in the foramen of Winslow (i.e., the space above the vena cava to the right and inferior to the triad). Without encountering any resistance, one can encircle the thick, firm structure by dividing only a small film of peritoneum on the gastrohepatic side. Total portal occlusion can be accomplished with a Rumel tourniquet prepared for later use if necessary.

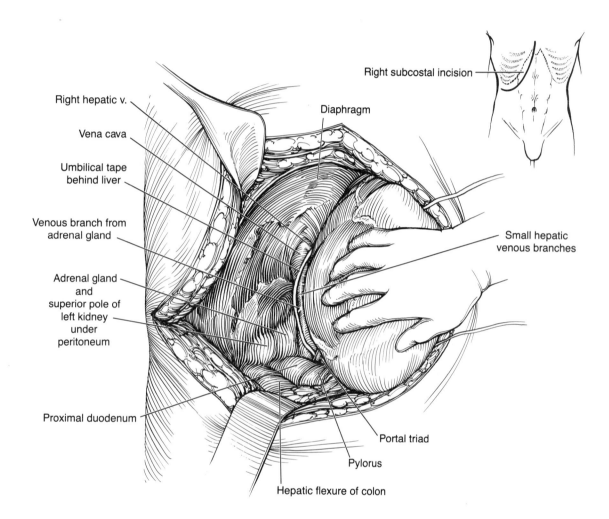

Right subcostal incision

Right hepatic v.

Vena cava

Umbilical tape
behind liver

Venous branch from
adrenal gland

Adrenal gland
and
superior pole of
left kidney
under
peritoneum

Proximal duodenum

Diaphragm

Small hepatic
venous branches

Portal triad

Pylorus

Hepatic flexure of colon

FIGURE 95–11. A similar maneuver is performed for the right hepatic venous tourniquet. An umbilical tape is placed behind the portal triad and then behind the entire right lobe of the liver. The tape is retrieved anteriorly, to the right of the suprahepatic vena cava, and a clamp or Rumel tourniquet is prepared for later use if necessary. The hepatic venous tourniquet is used *after* application of the portal tourniquet for severe hemorrhage and is *not* applied without portal occlusion. Application of both tourniquets usually means total occlusion of the right lobe of the liver, and their use should be limited to 15 to 20 minutes and employed only if necessary. The relationship of the hepatic venous tourniquet to the hepatic venous branches is shown.

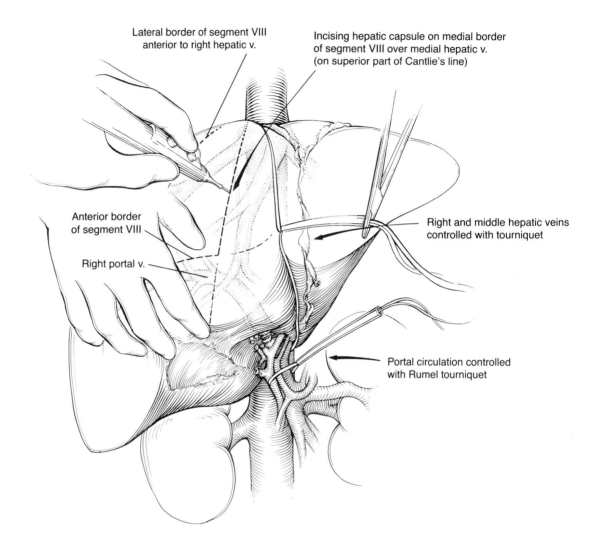

Lateral border of segment VIII
anterior to right hepatic v.

Incising hepatic capsule on medial border
of segment VIII over medial hepatic v.
(on superior part of Cantlie's line)

Anterior border
of segment VIII

Right portal v.

Right and middle hepatic veins
controlled with tourniquet

Portal circulation controlled
with Rumel tourniquet

FIGURE 95–12. The initiation of resection for segment VIII is shown and is identified by intraoperative ultrasonography. The portal branch to this segment may be injected or occluded, but this is usually not necessary for a segmental resection. An incision is made with the cautery through Glisson's capsule along the anticipated borders of the segment.

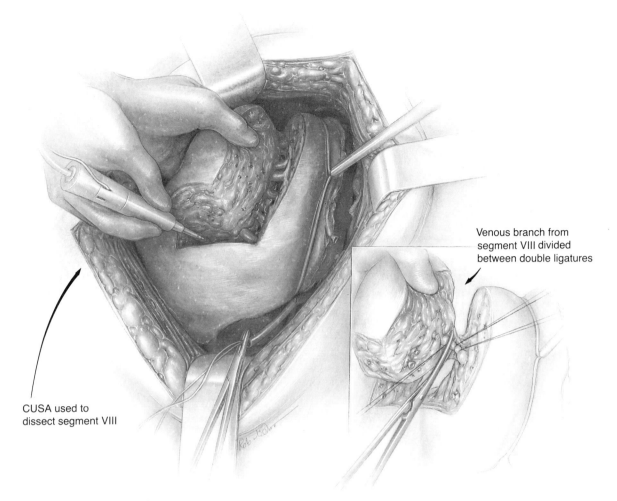

CUSA used to dissect segment VIII

Venous branch from segment VIII divided between double ligatures

FIGURES 95–13 and 95–14. The dissection is performed through the hepatic parenchyma, using ultrasonography intermittently. Segmental resection of this type is usually best performed without extrahepatic hilar control. It does require meticulous dissection and usually takes about 2 hours. Temporary portal venous occlusion is used as necessary, but a venous tourniquet is seldom required. The individual vessels lie in a portal direction, the segmental biliary duct is usually closely bound to the main hepatic arterial branch, and the portal branch is somewhat separate. The right hepatic vein or a major branch lies 90 degrees to the portal branches and forms another border of the resection and is usually ligated and divided intraparenchymally. Several other major tributaries are usually encountered during this dissection. If tumor is present in the line of dissection, adjacent tissue should be removed to provide an appropriate margin of resection. This may necessitate removal of an adjacent segment or simply several centimeters of additional tissue.

Considerable practice is required for proper use of the ultrasonic aspirator. The novice may be frustrated and judge this instrument to be unsatisfactory. The usual frustrations relate to the false expectation that the instrument is capable of controlling bleeding. Instead, the instrument only aspirates the tissue around the vessel so that it can be ligated or cauterized. The instrument causes sinusoidal bleeding and also *major* bleeding if applied to a vessel for an excessive time.

Another frustration relates to lack of awareness of the necessity for *slow* and *meticulous* dissection. Although the parenchymal dissection may necessitate slightly more time initially than that needed to perform a classic lobectomy with hilar control, the procedure is often shorter than the other methods because the operation is essentially finished when the specimen is removed. Nearly all the vessels are *ligated* during the dissection, whereas with classic resection by finger fracture, much time is spent obtaining homeostasis. During the dissection, particular care is taken to ligate, or doubly ligate, the vessels that remain. Often, the ends of the vessels in the specimen are left unligated until after division. Otherwise, the ligatures on the specimen hinder exposure. Bleeding from the vessels in the specimen is easily controlled prior to deeper dissection.

With segmental resection, one works deeper and deeper into a hole. The art of the procedure involves adequate exposure deep within this hole so that important vessels can be ligated safely. Therefore, ligature of important vessels often occurs near the end of the procedure, after most peripheral tissue has been dissected.

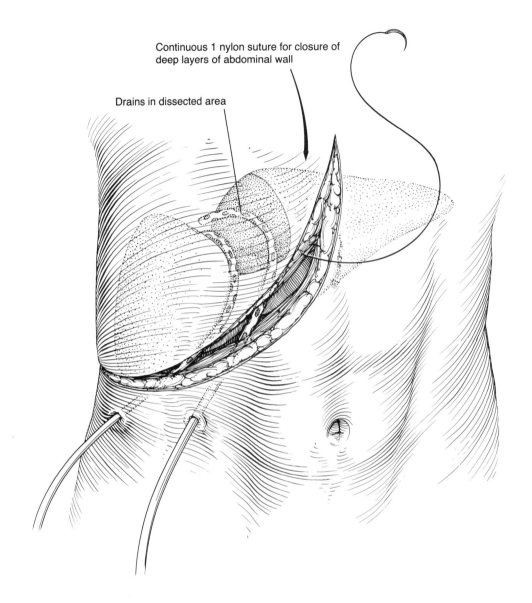

Continuous 1 nylon suture for closure of
deep layers of abdominal wall

Drains in dissected area

FIGURE 95–15. The incision is closed and appropriate drains are placed without the use
of omentum or excessive application of hemostatic agents. Care should be taken not to
cauterize or suction the cut edge of the liver vigorously for fear of disturbing important
ligatures or cauterized vessels. After identification and control of mechanical bleeding,
a careful search for obvious bile leakage is important. Blake-type drains are preferred
because they provide an effective combination of internal and external drainage. These
drains usually remain patent longer than the Jackson-Pratt type and also serve well as
external drains in the presence of prolonged bile leakage, which is the principal reason
for drainage as well as bleeding. Some biliary leakage from the cut surface is unavoidable
and may not be detected at operation. Severe bile leakage is generally due to an
unligated segmental duct with an intact distal system, and usually only patience is
required for control; therefore, the drain should not be removed too soon. A significant
biliary fistula may not become apparent until after the patient is taking a regular diet.

The essentials of postoperative care after hepatic resection are the same as with
limited resections. These include surveillance for hypoglycemia and hypoalbuminemia.
Hepatic failure may occur even with limited resection for a week or more, and the
primary problems are the neurologic consequences of hypoglycemia and fluid balance
related to hypoalbuminemia. Therefore, albumin and glucose solutions are generally
administered for the first week after operation. Postoperative hemorrhage is infrequent,
occurring in some 3 per cent of patients.

96

Right Hepatic Lobectomy

WILLIAM C. MEYERS, M.D.

A standard right hepatic lobectomy is performed in a manner similar to segmental resection. A formal extrahepatic hilar dissection may not be necessary, depending on the patient's anatomy. However, in most patients, a hilar dissection is preferred primarily to save time.

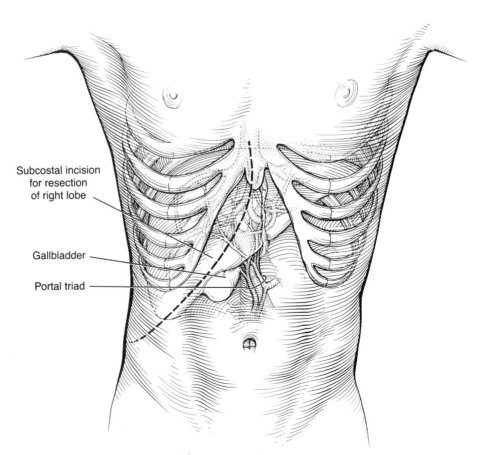

Subcostal incision for resection of right lobe

Gallbladder

Portal triad

FIGURE 96–1. A *generous* subcostal incision is made such as that for a segmental resection.

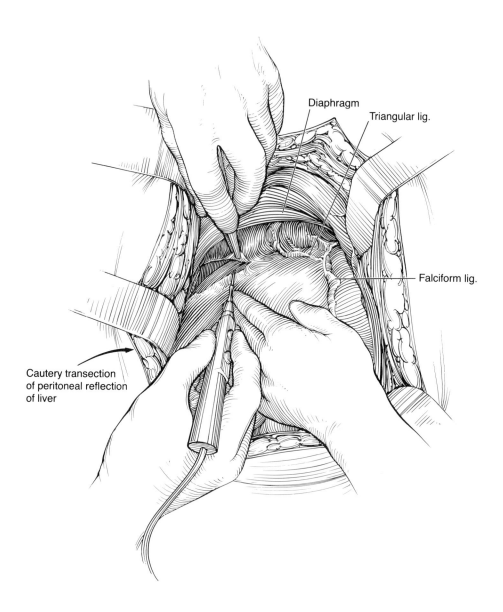

FIGURE 96–2. The liver is exposed and mobilized as described for a segmental resection.

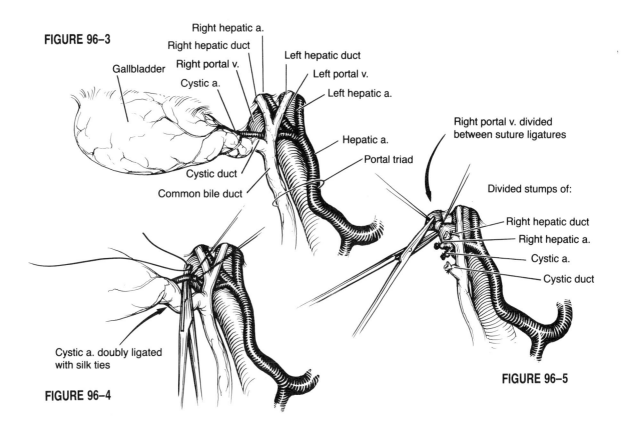

FIGURE 96–3

Gallbladder

Right hepatic a.

Right hepatic duct

Right portal v.

Cystic a.

Cystic duct

Common bile duct

Left hepatic duct

Left portal v.

Left hepatic a.

Hepatic a.

Portal triad

Right portal v. divided
between suture ligatures

Divided stumps of:

Right hepatic duct

Right hepatic a.

Cystic a.

Cystic duct

FIGURE 96–5

Cystic a. doubly ligated
with silk ties

FIGURE 96–4

FIGURES 96–3 to 96–5. The gallbladder is removed in a prograde manner to expose the right aspect of the portal triad. The right hepatic artery is usually identified first and ligated. An additional branch may supply the right side in the central superior aspect of the hilum and should also be ligated. One must be certain that the left hepatic artery remains intact, by assessing the pulse or by dissecting the bifurcation of the main hepatic artery, if the patient's anatomy is unusual. It is important to know that the right bile duct and right portal vein do not have to be divided during this portion of the hilar dissection. If difficult to locate, these can be found easily during the parenchymal dissection. The right portal vein is found after the right hepatic artery is divided. This dissection is approached from the right lateral aspect of the triad, and a thin layer of peritoneum overlying the main trunk is divided. One should identify the bifurcation and left portal vein prior to ligature to exclude this trunk, which, if included, would lead to disaster. Simple ligation of the right portal vein without division is safest at this stage, especially if there is question about adequate length. Similarly, it may be best simply to place a 4-0 Prolene suture ligature around the right bile duct rather than to dissect it from its posterior branches, which are easily torn. In about half of patients, extraparenchymal ligation and division of all three major segmental vessels are achieved with minimal difficulty.

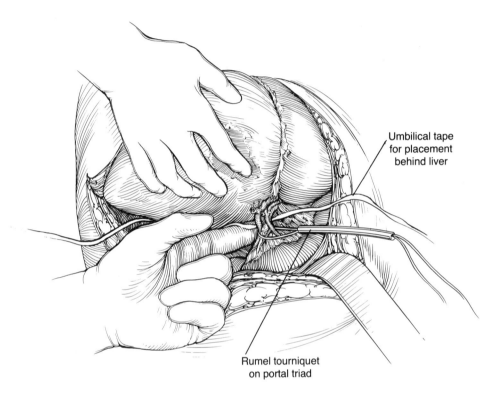

Umbilical tape
for placement
behind liver

Rumel tourniquet
on portal triad

FIGURE 96–6

FIGURES 96–6 and 96–7. Prior to dissection of the portal triad or even to the cholecystectomy, portal and hepatic venous tourniquets are placed in position. Division into Cantlie's plane is begun with the cautery. Cantlie's line extends from slightly to the left side of the gallbladder fossa to the inferior vena cava. It is preferable to leave some parenchyma along the superior aspect near the junction of the hepatic vein and vena cava to maximize the length of the right hepatic venous stump for control if necessary. The amount of parenchyma remaining depends on the location of the tumor and the indication for removal.

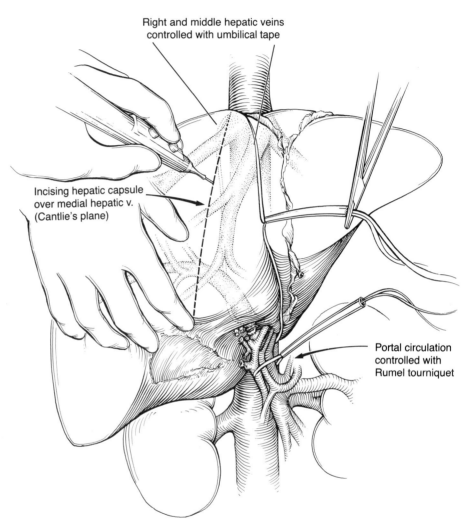

Right and middle hepatic veins
controlled with umbilical tape

Incising hepatic capsule
over medial hepatic v.
(Cantlie's plane)

Portal circulation
controlled with
Rumel tourniquet

FIGURE 96–7

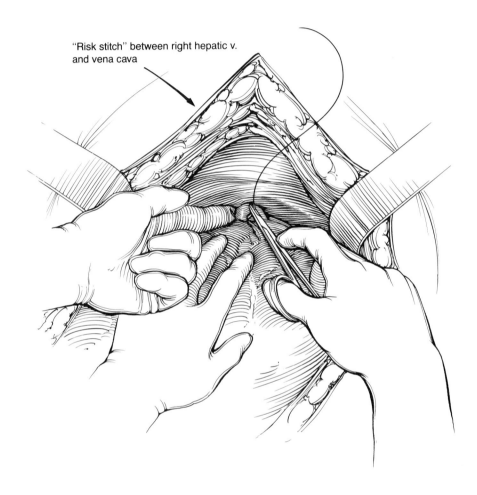

"Risk stitch" between right hepatic v.
and vena cava

FIGURE 96–8. At this stage, a "risk" suture is placed around the right hepatic vein. This completes the occlusion of the primary vessels to this side of the liver and can be accomplished quite safely with experience. The bifurcation of the right hepatic vein is barely dissected. With the left index finger placed behind the liver and with excellent assistance, a single 3-0 Prolene suture on a large (e.g., MH) needle can be secured around the vein. The vein should not be divided at this point nor the liver further mobilized, as this may cause tearing and hemorrhage. Only rarely should the hepatic vein be ligated and divided at this stage.

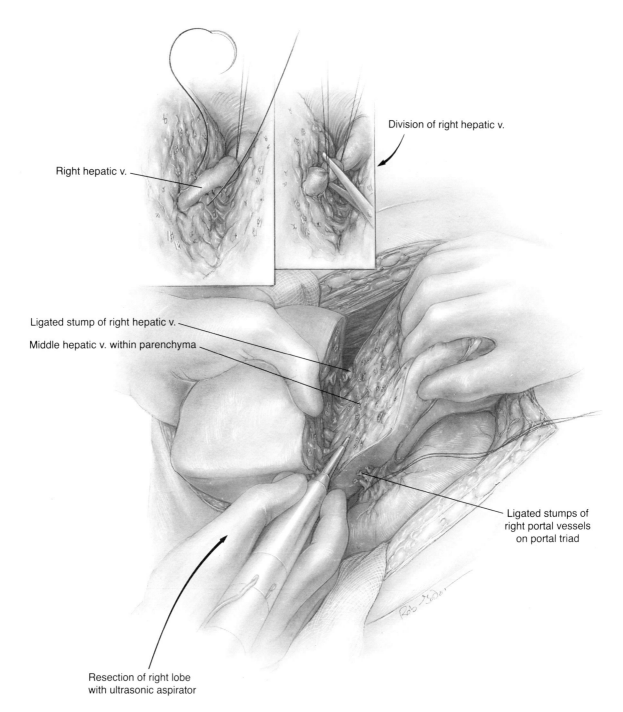

Right hepatic v.

Division of right hepatic v.

Ligated stump of right hepatic v.

Middle hepatic v. within parenchyma

Ligated stumps of
right portal vessels
on portal triad

Resection of right lobe
with ultrasonic aspirator

FIGURES 96–9 to 96–11. If one thoroughly understands the suprahepatic anatomy, the term "risk" stitch is easily appreciated. It is actually quite a safe suture and reduces the risk of hemorrhage during the latter part of the parenchymal dissection. The important feature is not to perform heroic dissection of the right hepatic venous system from the extrahepatic side. This was definitely the primary reason for a number of fatalities prior to modern resectional techniques. Instead, the right hepatic vein is safely secured intraparenchymally later in the dissection, as shown.

The plane of dissection shown in Figure 96–11 is appropriate for most dissections. After good mobilization, one should be able to place the left hand behind the specimen and dissect toward the tip of the fingers rather than more centrally toward the inferior vena cava. Maintaining this direction provides adequate exposure throughout the dissection. Usually, the right hepatic vein is sutured in continuity before dividing it. It is easy to control the side of the specimen after dividing the vein.

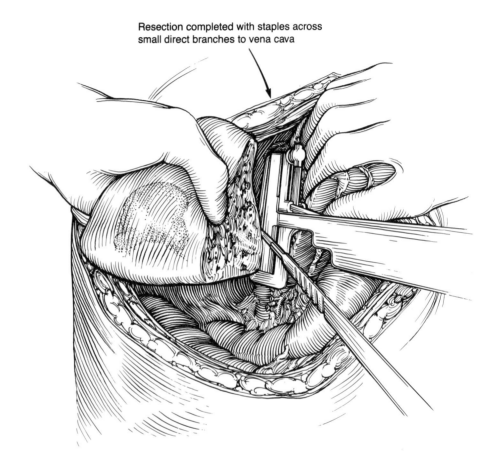

Resection completed with staples across small direct branches to vena cava

FIGURE 96–12. After division of the major vessels, including the right hepatic vein, numerous smaller vessels communicating directly to the vena cava or left side of the liver remain. In most patients, the dissection is completed at this point by simple application of a TA-90 or TA-55 stapler and a No. 10 blade on a long handle. However, there should be no loss of pride by completing the dissection in a more standard manner. Parenchymal dissection during a right hepatic lobectomy can be performed in a variety of ways. Use of the ultrasonic aspirator, direct finger fracture, a fine-tipped Crile clamp, or a combination of these techniques is preferred. Others use a water jet, laser, argon beam, or other instruments with success.

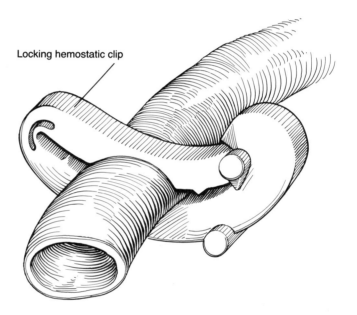

Locking hemostatic clip

FIGURE 96–13. One important but seemingly simple technical advance that is frequently used is a locking clip (''Hemolock-Weck''). It is available in various sizes but basically is a barrette-type of clip that does not disengage with use of suction or vigorous instrumentation. It can be used for most vessels and saves much time, but it does have limitations in that the vessel must be completely free and the clip must fit well around it. Following the dissection, the areas should be sponged with gauze, taking care not to let the cloth fibers pull on the clips and tear the vessels.

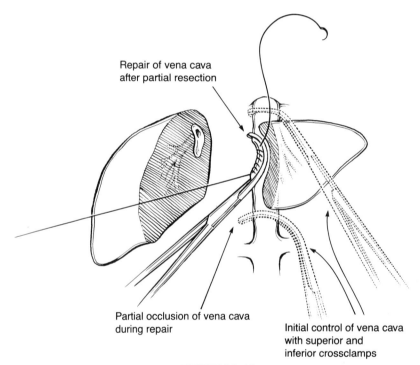

Repair of vena cava
after partial resection

Partial occlusion of vena cava
during repair

Initial control of vena cava
with superior and
inferior crossclamps

FIGURE 96–14

FIGURES 96–14 and 96–15. The abdomen is closed in the manner previously described with continuous or interrupted nylon sutures after placement of drains. Cryoprecipitate glue or hemostatic agents are often applied to the exposed surface of the liver. A careful search for bile leakage is also accomplished as previously described. The classic right trisegmentectomy is accomplished in a manner similar to that used for right hepatic lobectomy except that more care is given to dissection of the small branches to the medial segment of the left lobe prior to parenchymal dissection. The portal tourniquet is applied as necessary.

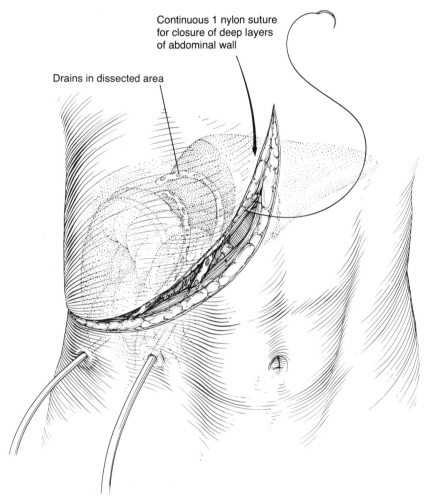

Continuous 1 nylon suture
for closure of deep layers
of abdominal wall

Drains in dissected area

FIGURE 96–15

A tumor may involve a portion of the right hepatic vein or the inferior vena cava and necessitate resection of a portion of the vena cava. A wedge resection of the inferior vena cava can be relatively easily accomplished by first surrounding the superior and inferior hepatic vena cava for total hepatic venous control. The ultrasonic aspirator is used to expose a portion of normal vena cava around the point of tumor invasion, and a partially occluding clamp is applied. Excision can also be accomplished directly without a partial clamp if necessary. The vena cava is repaired directly with a continuous 3-0 Prolene suture. Care should be taken not to narrow the vena cava, and a more precise plastic surgical repair may be necessary. At times, a saphenous or even femoral venous patch is needed. Such a repair is usually done during an autotransplantation resection, in which the liver is removed with the patient on venovenous bypass, with resection of the hepatic tumor on a back table. The portion of the liver to be saved is reinserted with a patch on the intrahepatic vena cava.

97

Left Hepatic Lobectomy

WILLIAM C. MEYERS, M.D.

The classic left hepatic lobectomy in most patients is performed in a similar manner to the right hepatic lobectomy with a few important differences.

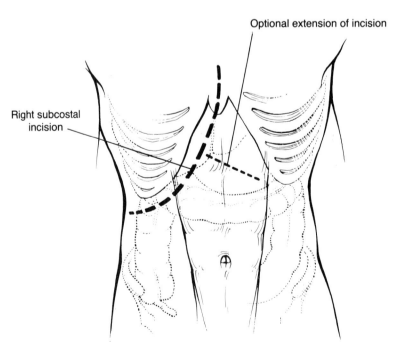

FIGURE 97–1. A similar incision is made, but an "asymmetric T" extension is more apt to be necessary for exposure (the incision as for liver transplantation). The liver is extensively mobilized, paying greater attention to the site of the left hepatic veins.

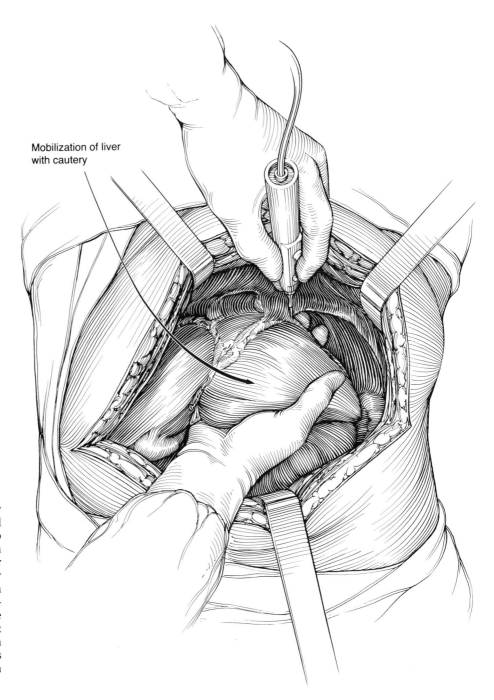

Mobilization of liver with cautery

FIGURE 97–2. The easiest way to mobilize the left lateral segment of the liver is to place the right hand beneath it and incise the avascular plane above the liver. Ability to use the opposite hand in many cases in liver procedures is often helpful. A safe way to learn to use the left hand is during mobilization of the left lateral segment as performed in correction of a hiatal hernia.

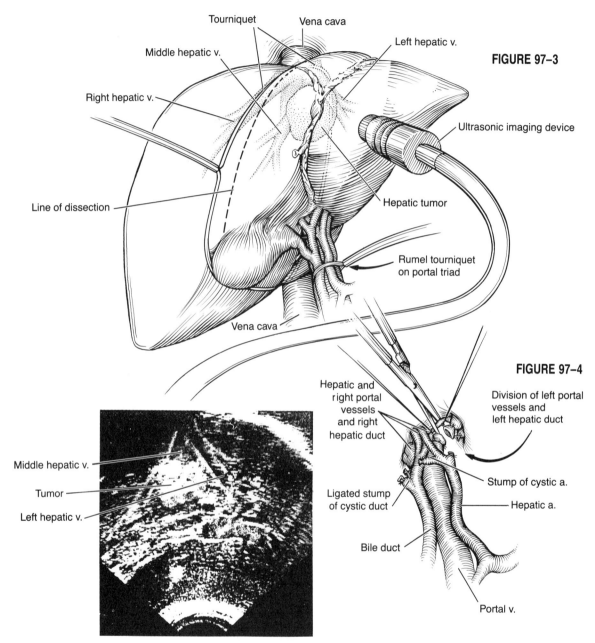

FIGURE 97–3

Tourniquet

Vena cava

Middle hepatic v.

Left hepatic v.

Right hepatic v.

Ultrasonic imaging device

Line of dissection

Hepatic tumor

Rumel tourniquet
on portal triad

Vena cava

FIGURE 97–4

Hepatic and
right portal
vessels
and right
hepatic duct

Division of left portal
vessels and
left hepatic duct

Middle hepatic v.

Tumor

Left hepatic v.

Stump of cystic a.

Ligated stump
of cystic duct

Hepatic a.

Bile duct

Portal v.

ULTRASOUND OF LIVER DEMONSTRATING TUMOR

FIGURES 97–3 and 97–4. A tumor in a difficult location involving both the left and the middle hepatic veins is shown. Removal of this particular tumor actually necessitates slightly more than a left hepatic lobectomy, with inclusion of some parenchyma from segment VIII of the right side. The inverted ultrasound nicely depicts the location of the tumor and its relationship to the left and middle hepatic veins. The left portal branches are ligated and divided. The left portal vein is usually longer than the right, and adequate length is usually achieved so that it can be divided.

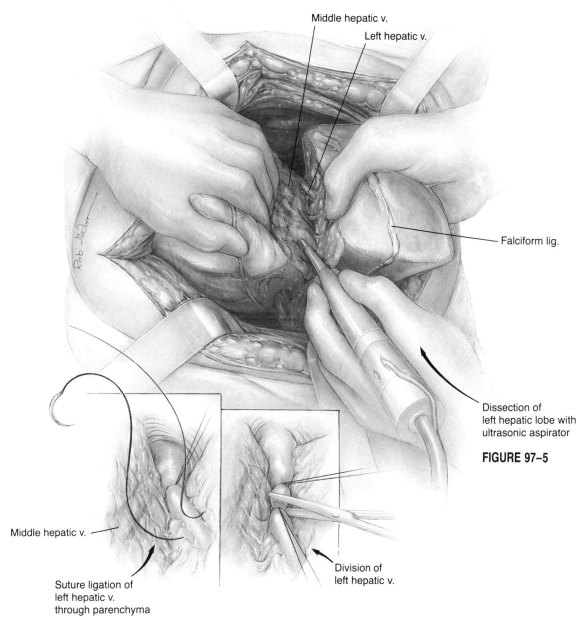

Middle hepatic v.

Left hepatic v.

Falciform lig.

Dissection of
left hepatic lobe with
ultrasonic aspirator

FIGURE 97–5

Middle hepatic v.

Suture ligation of
left hepatic v.
through parenchyma

Division of
left hepatic v.

FIGURE 97–6   **FIGURE 97–7**

FIGURE 97–5. The assistant provides adequate retraction of the right side of the liver to expose a good plane for exposure throughout the dissection. This resection is often more easily accomplished from the left side of the table, using the left hand for the primary dissection.

FIGURES 97–6 and 97–7. The middle and left hepatic veins are treated in a manner similar to the right hepatic vein. A "risk" stitch can be placed but is generally more difficult at this stage than later. The left and middle hepatic veins usually join for a very short distance prior to junction with the suprahepatic vena cava.

It is important to recognize that the above dissection refers to a formal left hepatic lobectomy and *not* to a left lateral segmentectomy. For the latter procedure, a formal hilar dissection is usually unnecessary and predisposes the patient to unnecessary risk.

Pancreas

98

Partial Pancreatectomy (DISTAL)

THEODORE N. PAPPAS, M.D.

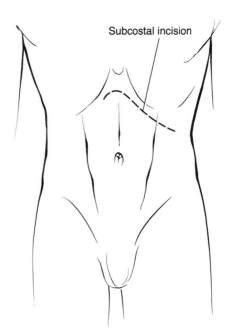

FIGURE 98–1. The abdomen is explored through a left subcostal incision with extension to the right. On exploration, the entire lesser sac is exposed by incising the gastrocolic ligament.

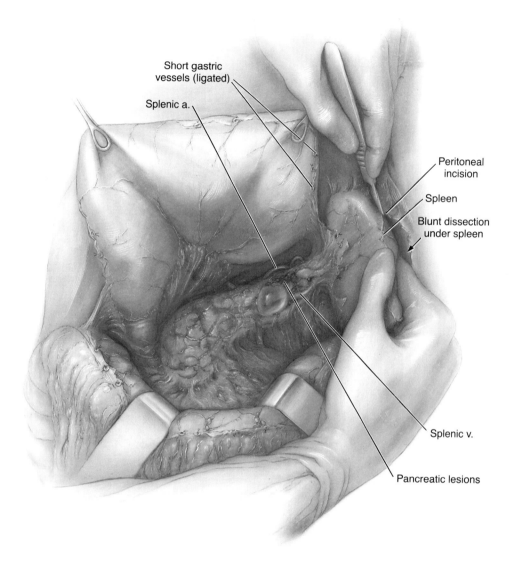

FIGURE 98–2. The stomach is reflected upward, and the transverse colon is reflected inferiorly. The entire surface of the pancreas is palpated in an effort to localize the mass. Once it is localized, the extent of the resection is determined. The resection of the tail is best begun by mobilization of the spleen. The tail of the pancreas can be resected leaving the spleen *in situ*, but it requires a lengthy and tedious dissection that has no proven benefit in adult patients. The short gastric vessels are divided between the stomach and the spleen with Kelly clamps and 2–0 silk sutures. Once the stomach is completely separated from the spleen, the spleen is mobilized by incising the lateral attachments to the retroperitoneum.

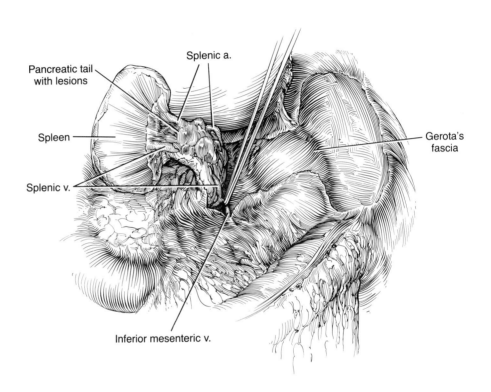

FIGURE 98–3. A plane is developed between the spleen and the tail of the pancreas and Gerota's fascia. It is usually avascular, and the spleen can be mobilized and brought into the wound without difficulty. After the spleen is exposed, the tail of the pancreas is mobilized by incising the peritoneal reflection on the inferior border of the pancreas with electrocautery. Care should be taken to identify the inferior mesenteric vein, which joins the splenic vein in the midtail region, and it is divided with Kelly clamps and 2–0 silk sutures. Similarly, the superior border of the pancreas is incised with the electrocautery, and care should be taken to preserve the splenic artery, which courses on the superior border.

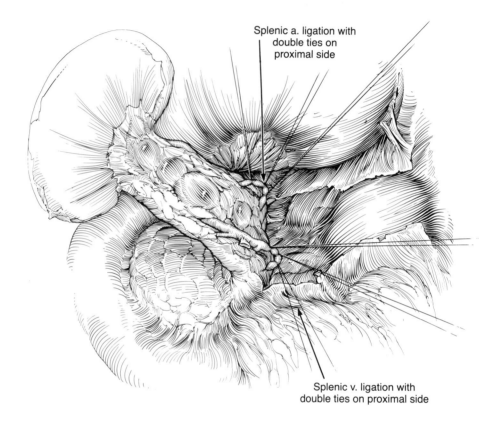

Splenic a. ligation with
double ties on
proximal side

Splenic v. ligation with
double ties on proximal side

FIGURE 98–4. The pancreas is mobilized to a sufficient length to allow at least a 2-cm. margin on the pancreatic mass. The splenic artery and vein are localized on the undersurface of the gland. A right-angle clamp is passed around the splenic artery on the undersurface of the gland. The splenic artery is tied with 2–0 silk triple ligatures in continuity. The splenic artery is then divided. Similarly, the splenic vein is dissected on the inferior border of the pancreas, encircled with 0 silk, and ligated. When intense inflammation in the retroperitoneum due to chronic pancreatitis or pancreatic pseudocyst is encountered, it may be difficult to obtain a safe plane beneath the pancreas. In this case, Gerota's fascia can be entered, and a safe plane is usually encountered on the surface of the kidney.

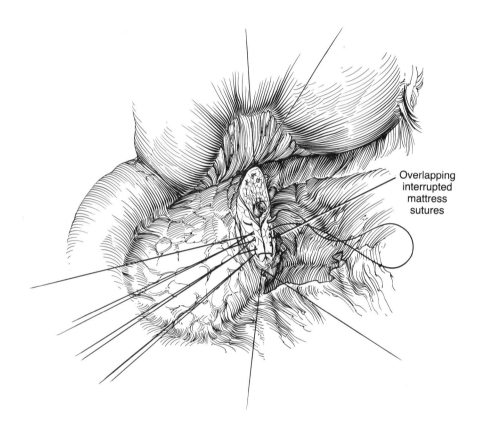

Overlapping
interrupted
mattress
sutures

FIGURE 98–5. Once the splenic artery and vein have been divided, the pancreas can be dissected proximal to the mass. If the gland is soft, it is often easier to transect it with a linear stapling device. A firm gland in the presence of chronic pancreatitis may be difficult to transect with a stapling device, and it is often easier to transect with electrocautery. After transection of the gland, the specimen is removed, and hemostasis on the open end of the gland is obtained. Bleeding is usually encountered on the superior and inferior margins of the gland, which can be controlled with 3–0 silk ligatures. Whether the gland is stapled or not, the end of the gland should be resecured with a row of interrupted, interlocking horizontal mattress sutures of 2–0 Prolene. The sutures are interlocked to be certain that every aspect of pancreatic vessel tissue has been oversewn to prevent lateral pancreatic fistula. If the pancreatic duct is easily visualized, it should be separately ligated with 2–0 Prolene suture. Once the tail of the pancreas is oversewn, the bed of the wound is inspected for bleeding, and a closed suction drain is placed in the bed of the tail of the pancreas.

99

Drainage of Pancreatic Pseudocyst: Cystogastrostomy

THEODORE N. PAPPAS, M.D.

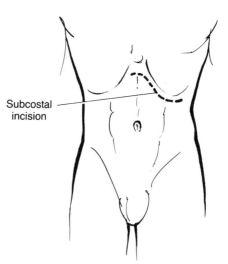

FIGURE 99–1. A variety of incisions can be made for drainage of pseudocysts. The choice primarily depends on the location of the pseudocyst. For most cysts behind the stomach midline, a bucket-handle or left subcostal incision that extends across the midline to the right is preferable.

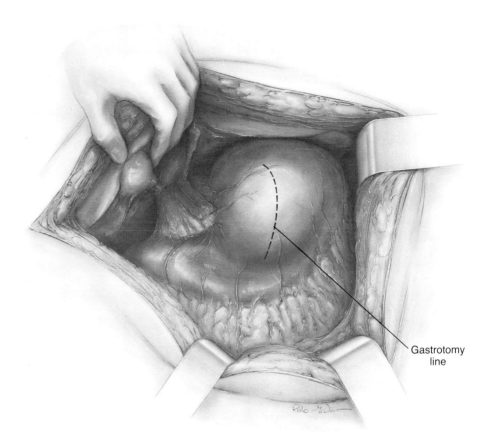

Gastrotomy
line

FIGURE 99-2. On exploration of the abdomen, the pseudocyst is usually encountered protruding behind the stomach. After thorough exploration, the anterior wall of the stomach is opened longitudinally. A transverse incision may be necessary in the antrum to avoid narrowing the gastric outlet during closure and to prevent antral denervating and subsequent delayed gastric emptying. The gastrotomy should be positioned directly over the palpable pseudocyst.

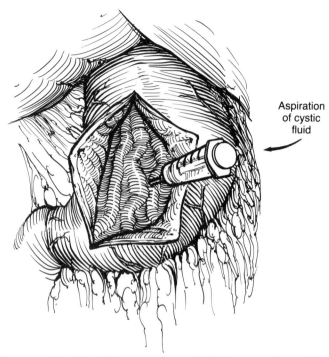

FIGURE 99–3. Upon examination of the posterior wall of the stomach, an 18-gauge needle is placed through the posterior wall, and fluid is aspirated.

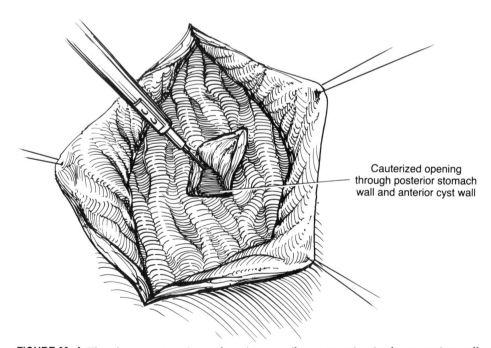

FIGURE 99–4. The electrocautery is used to circumscribe an opening in the posterior wall of the stomach approximately 3 cm. in length. Some bleeding is occasionally encountered during this procedure because of the vascularity of the stomach and the wall of the pseudocyst. Once the pseudocyst is entered, the fluid is evacuated with a suction device. A complete circle of tissue, including stomach wall and pseudocyst, is removed and sent for frozen section diagnosis to exclude malignancy.

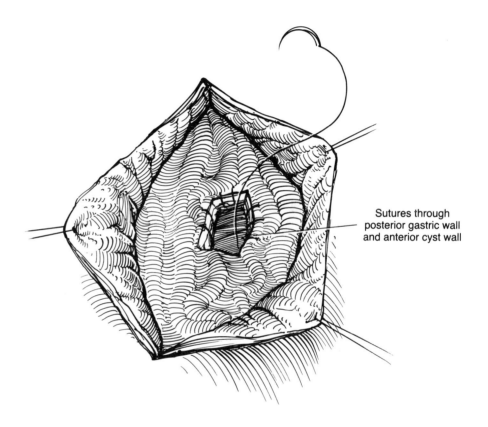

Sutures through
posterior gastric wall
and anterior cyst wall

FIGURE 99–5. At this point, the interior surface of the cyst is inspected. If it appears smooth and the fluid is relatively translucent, this small aperture is considered adequate for drainage of a simple pseudocyst. In contrast, if the cyst wall is lined with necrotic pancreas and the cyst fluid is green or opaque, the opening in the posterior stomach is enlarged to approximately 5 to 6 cm. in diameter and a gentle debridement of the liquefied pancreatic phlegmon is undertaken. Care should be taken to prevent inadvertent disruption of the splenic artery or vein.

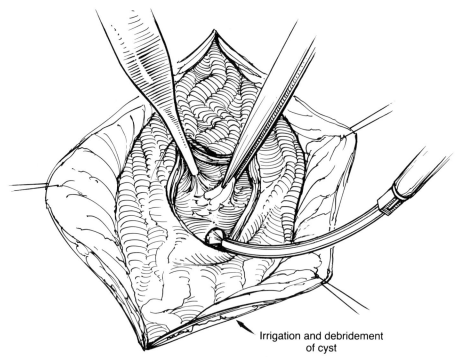

Irrigation and debridement
of cyst

FIGURE 99–6. The edge of the cystogastrostomy site is sutured with a continuous locked
0 Vicryl suture. This is a hemostatic suture to prevent late hemorrhage from the cyst or
stomach wall.

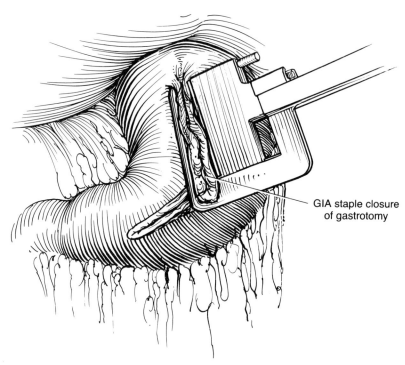

GIA staple closure
of gastrotomy

FIGURE 99–7. The gastrostomy is closed with a 55-mm. linear stapler. For simple
pancreatic pseudocysts and cystogastrostomies, no gastrostomy tube is placed. The
abdomen is closed. If the patient has a liquefied pancreatic phlegmon with necrotic
pancreas in the pseudocyst, the gastrostomy tube is placed through a separate gastrostomy site, the stomach is tacked to the peritoneum, and the tube is brought out through
a lateral stab wound. The gastrostomy tube is placed in these cases because of high
incidence of postoperative gastric paresis.

100

Pancreaticojejunostomy (PUESTOW)

THEODORE N. PAPPAS, M.D.

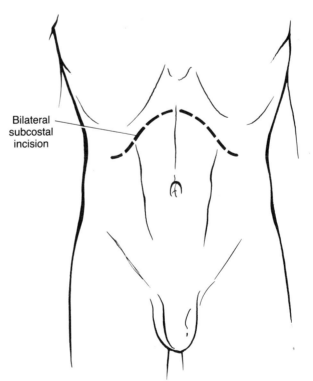

FIGURE 100–1. The abdomen is explored through a bucket-handle incision. In patients with narrow costal angles, an upper midline incision will also suffice.

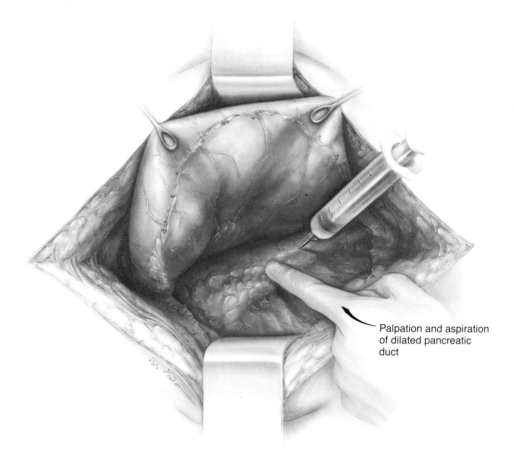

Palpation and aspiration
of dilated pancreatic
duct

FIGURE 100–2. After thorough exploration of the abdomen, the lesser sac is entered by dividing the gastrocolic ligament between clamps. The colon is then packed into the lower abdomen, and the stomach is retracted upward. This exposure should allow visualization of the ventral surface of the pancreas from the uncinate to within 3 cm. of the tail. A 19-gauge needle and a syringe are used to locate the dilated pancreatic duct. The ventral surface of the pancreas is palpated to locate pancreatic duct stones or a distended pancreatic duct. If the duct cannot be localized by palpation, aspiration through the surface of the gland is begun in transverse fashion at the neck. The gland is often atrophied; therefore, deep aspiration is usually not necessary. Clear fluid will be aspirated from the duct when it is encountered. At this point, needle-tip cautery is used to mark the site where the duct was aspirated, and a small transverse opening in the surface of the pancreas is accomplished with electrocautery to confirm the location of the pancreatic duct. Occasionally, needle aspiration is not successful in locating the duct, in which case a transverse incision should be made in the neck of the pancreas until the dilated duct is found.

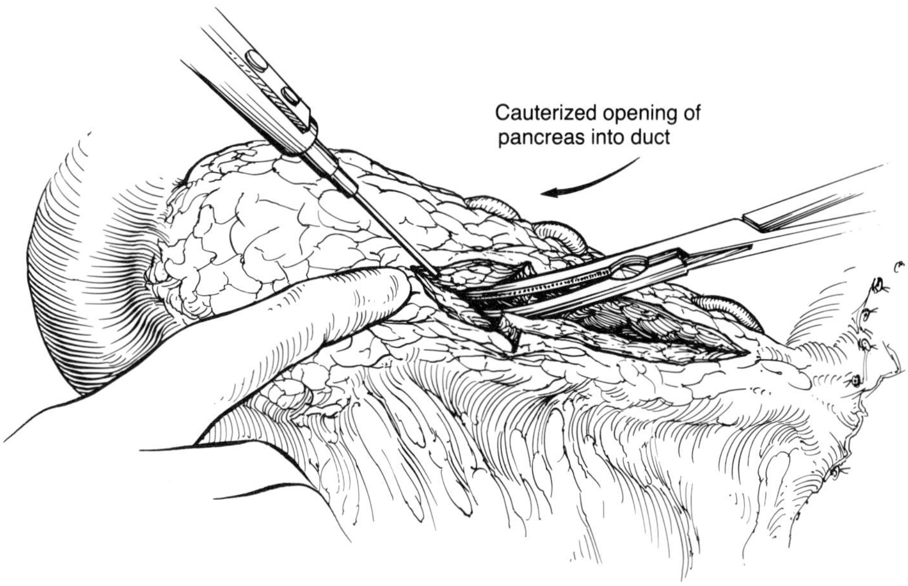

Cauterized opening of
pancreas into duct

FIGURE 100–3. When the pancreatic duct is found, a long longitudinal opening in the duct is made with the help of a tonsil clamp and needle-tip electrocautery. The duct is opened in its entirety from the uncinate process to the tail. The extent of the lateral opening in the duct is particularly important if multiple areas of stenosis of the main pancreatic duct are encountered (chain-of-lakes configuration).

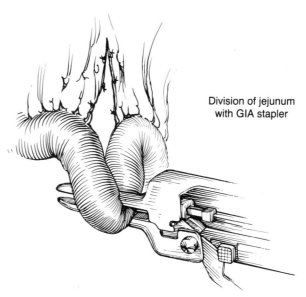

Division of jejunum
with GIA stapler

FIGURE 100–4. Once the pancreatic duct has been completely opened, a 40-cm. Roux-en-Y limb of small bowel is created. This is fashioned by dividing the mesentery with suture and dividing the bowel with a linear cutting stapler or linear stapler and a bowel clamp.

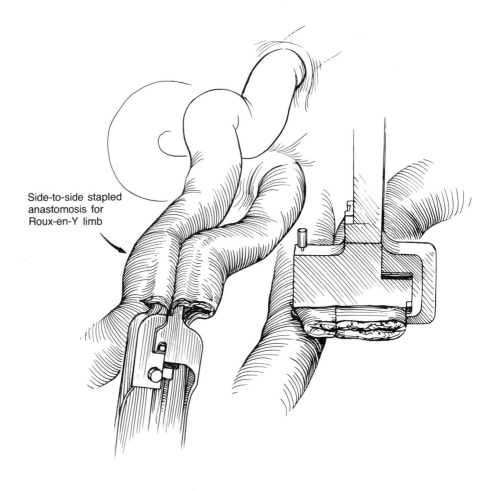

Side-to-side stapled
anastomosis for
Roux-en-Y limb

FIGURE 100–5. The continuity of the distal small bowel is recreated with a linear cutting
stapler, and the ends of small bowel are closed with a linear stapler.

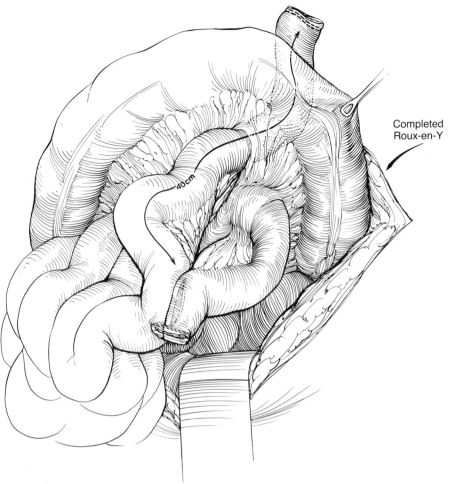

Completed
Roux-en-Y

FIGURE 100–6. The 40-cm. Roux limb is brought through the Roux to the transverse mesocolon and laid next to the lateral opening of the pancreatic duct.

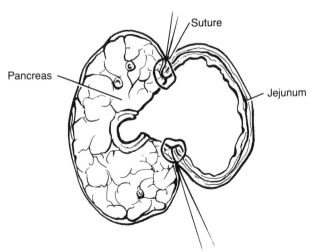

Suture

Pancreas

Jejunum

FIGURE 100–7. Small bowel is opened longitudinally to a length similar to that of the pancreatic duct. Anastomosis is accomplished as a single layer between the pancreatic duct and small bowel. The anastomosis is made with 4–0 PDS suture, and the knots can be left on the inside of the pancreatic duct on the posterior layer if it is easier technically.

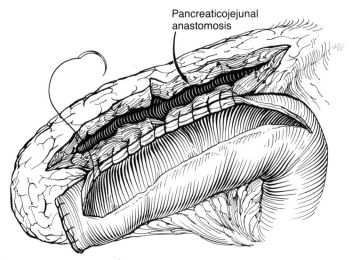

Pancreaticojejunal
anastomosis

FIGURE 100–8. If the pancreatic duct is sufficiently dilated, direct anastomosis can be made between small bowel and pancreatic duct, which would include pancreatic parenchyma. Fortunately, in patients who require Puestow procedures, the pancreas is indurated, allowing sutures to pass through the pancreas alone without including pancreatic duct. These sutures are often technically easier and equally successful in achieving chronic lateral pancreatic drainage.

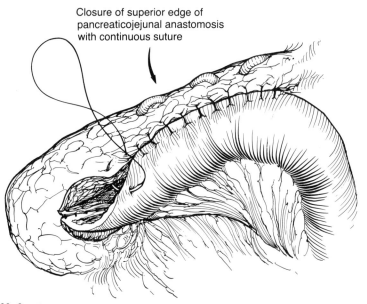

Closure of superior edge of
pancreaticojejunal anastomosis
with continuous suture

FIGURE 100–9. The anterior suture line is completed with 4–0 PDS, either running or interrupted, with the knots outside the lumen. A single Jackson-Pratt drain is placed in the lesser sac and brought out through a lateral stab wound prior to closure.

101

Pancreaticoduodenectomy: Whipple Procedure

THEODORE N. PAPPAS, M.D.

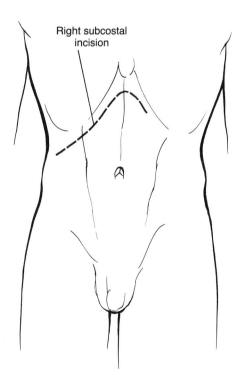

FIGURE 101–1. Exploration for a Whipple resection should begin with a right subcostal incision. If the initial exploration reveals resectable disease, the incision can be extended farther into the left subcostal region.

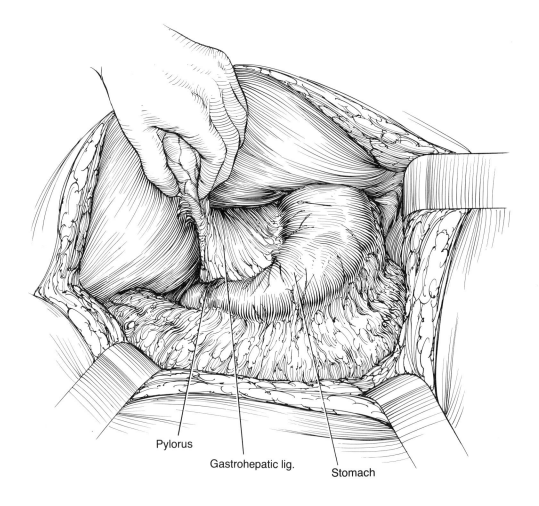

Pylorus

Gastrohepatic lig.

Stomach

FIGURE 101–2. Extensive exploration is done initially for ruling out other pathology and confirming preoperative staging. Intraoperative staging is done by manual palpation, wide kocherization, complete exposure of the lesser sac by dividing the gastrocolic ligament, and biopsy of any available nodes. Specifically, adenopathy should be sought posterior to the common bile duct near the cystic artery at the root of the colonic and transverse mesocolon just to the left of the portal vein at the superior border of the pancreas and along the lesser curvature of the stomach. Histologic confirmation of the tumor type can be made at the time of exploration if this information has not been obtained preoperatively.

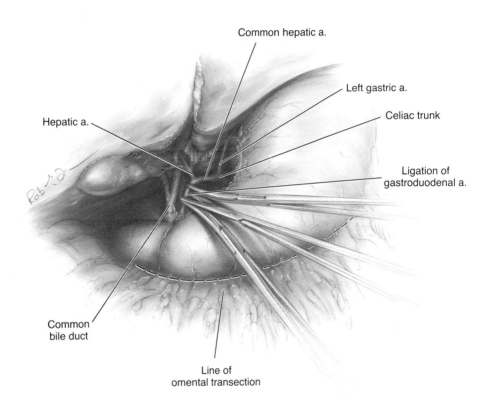

Common hepatic a.

Left gastric a.

Celiac trunk

Hepatic a.

Ligation of
gastroduodenal a.

Common
bile duct

Line of
omental transection

FIGURE 101–3. Resection is begun by exploring the region of the gastroduodenal artery just superior to the duodenal artery. In this region, care is taken to identify the junction between the hepatic artery and gastroduodenal artery accurately. The surgeon must be certain that there is no abnormal arterial anatomy in this region (if a preoperative arteriogram has not been obtained). Aberrant hepatic arteries can course through this region and would cause liver ischemia if ligated. If normal anatomy of the hepatic and gastroduodenal arteries is defined, the gastroduodenal artery is doubly ligated.

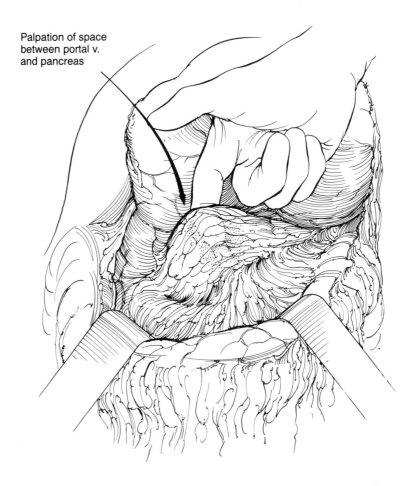

Palpation of space
between portal v.
and pancreas

FIGURE 101–4. A plane is created between the pancreas and the portal vein just beneath the takeoff of the ligated gastroduodenal artery. At this point, the portal vein courses behind the pancreas to join the splenic and superior mesenteric veins. The plane between the pancreas and the portal vein has no vascular attachments. Therefore, a finger can pass from superior to inferior along this plane to ensure that the tumor has not invaded the portal vein. The surgeon's finger can be seen protruding from beneath the inferior margin of the pancreas directly over the superior mesenteric vein.

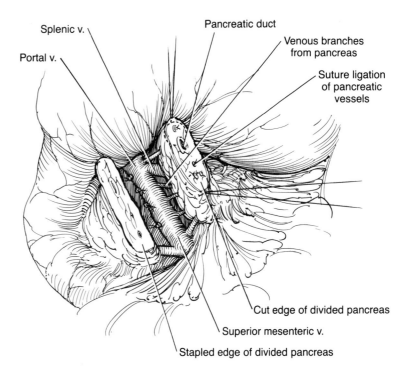

Splenic v.

Portal v.

Pancreatic duct

Venous branches
from pancreas

Suture ligation
of pancreatic
vessels

Cut edge of divided pancreas

Superior mesenteric v.

Stapled edge of divided pancreas

FIGURE 101–5. If this plane can be negotiated without difficulty, the pancreas can be divided at this level. The pancreas is divided by passing a linear stapling device across the proximal portion of the pancreas for hemostasis on the specimen. A No. 15 blade is used to divide the pancreas, and the staple gun is removed. Bleeding points are usually immediately noticed on the superior and inferior margins of the pancreatic body, and they should be controlled with 3–0 silk ligatures. Even if no bleeding is encountered in these regions, 3–0 silk ligatures should still be placed to ensure that bleeding does not occur later.

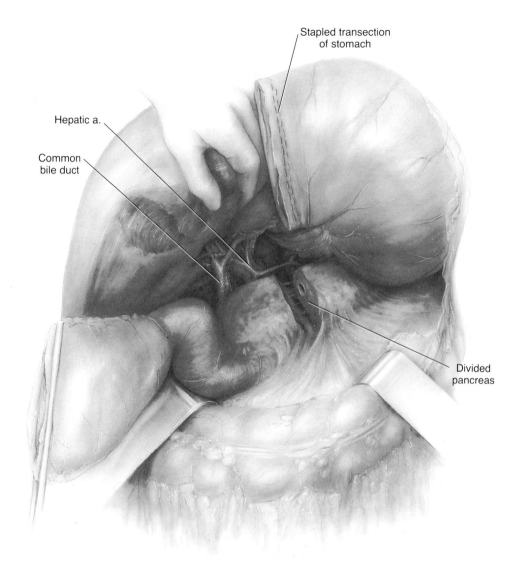

Hepatic a.

Common bile duct

Stapled transection of stomach

Divided pancreas

FIGURE 101–6. At this point, the stomach is divided. This is done by placing a 90-mm. linear stapler across the stomach at the upper border of the antrum. Staples are left on the proximal stomach side, and a large bowel clamp is placed across the open end of the antrum. The lesser curvature of the stomach and the upper border of the duodenum are mobilized by blunt dissection, and the right hepatic artery is divided between tonsil clamps and secured with 2–0 silk sutures. Alternate techniques include transection of the stomach just proximal to the pylorus for gastric preservation, and transection of the duodenum with its blood supply intact 3 to 4 cm. beyond the pylorus to ensure pyloric preservation. The common duct is then encircled with a right-angle clamp, and a No. 15 blade is used to incise the duct. A small bulldog clamp is placed in the proximal common bile duct to prevent a continued bile leakage into the field during the rest of the procedure. The pancreatic head and uncinate process are gently mobilized off the portal vein with blunt dissection. Small vessels are encountered that drain to the uncinate process into the portal vein, and they should be clipped and divided. Care should be taken that these hemoclips are not accidentally removed during the rest of the procedure. A large vein between the uncinate and the portal vein is encountered on the superior aspect of the uncinate process and another between the uncinate process branching toward the superior mesenteric vein. These should be controlled with 2–0 silk ligatures.

Transection of
lig. of Treitz

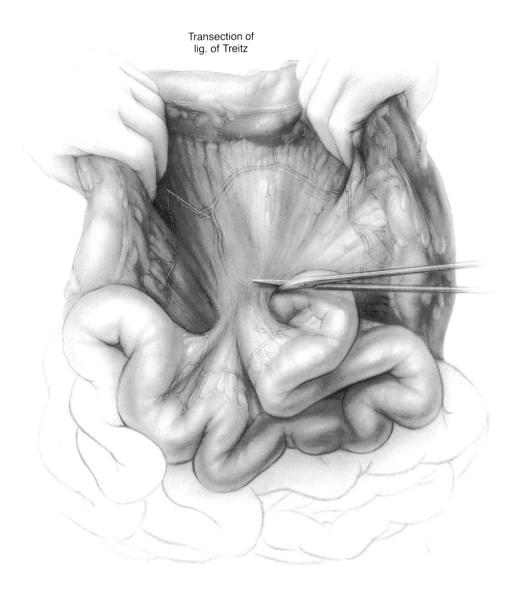

FIGURE 101–7. The ligament of Treitz should be mobilized by incising an avascular plane between the third portion of the duodenum and the aorta from the right side of the abdomen and then incising the attachments of the fourth portion of the duodenum at the ligament itself.

Proximal jejunum being advanced,
transected, and stapled

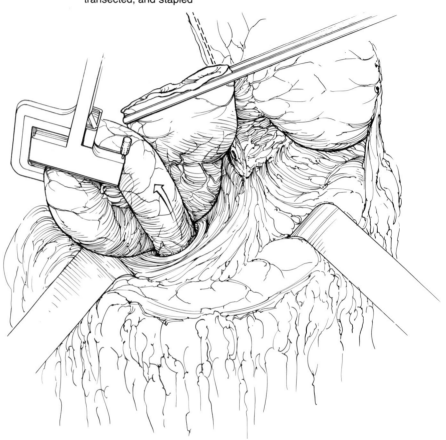

FIGURE 101–8. Once the duodenum is mobilized the entire small intestine can be pivoted into the right upper quadrant underneath the root of the mesentery. The duodenojejunal junction is divided with the linear stapler. At this point, the entire specimen is anchored only by the uncinate process to the retroperitoneum and the short duodenal mesentery. This short mesentery of the third and fourth portions of the duodenum is divided between Crile clamps, which are tied with 3–0 silk ligatures.

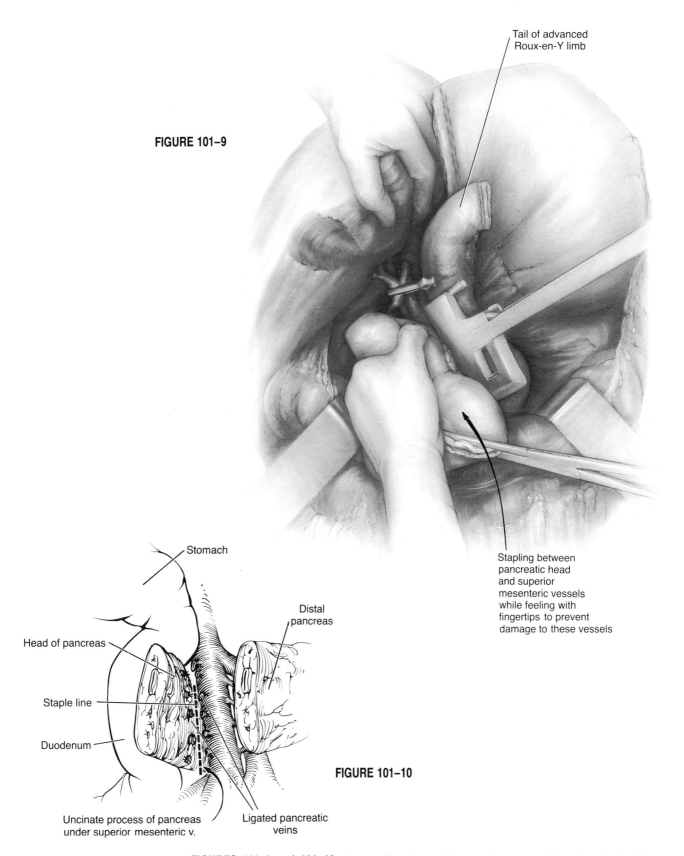

FIGURE 101-9

Tail of advanced
Roux-en-Y limb

Stapling between
pancreatic head
and superior
mesenteric vessels
while feeling with
fingertips to prevent
damage to these vessels

Stomach

Distal
pancreas

Head of pancreas

Staple line

Duodenum

Uncinate process of pancreas
under superior mesenteric v.

Ligated pancreatic
veins

FIGURE 101-10

FIGURES 101-9 and 101-10. Eventually, the entire specimen is anchored only by the uncinate process. At this point, a 55-mm. linear stapler can be used to transect the uncinate process from the retroperitoneum. Extreme care must be taken to be certain that neither the superior mesenteric artery nor the portal vein is pulled into the staple line. The staple gun is placed and fired, and the specimen is removed from the field. The staple line on the retroperitoneum usually requires 3–0 silk ligatures to control several bleeding points.

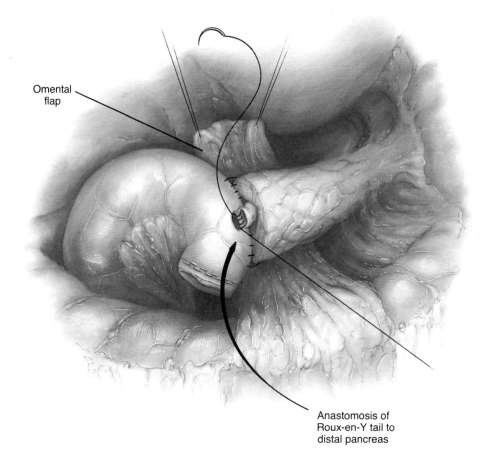

Omental
flap

Anastomosis of
Roux-en-Y tail to
distal pancreas

FIGURE 101–11. The reconstruction is accomplished by rotating the stapled end of the small bowel into the right upper quadrant and placing it directly over the portal vein. Prior to creating the pancreaticojejunal anastomosis, a vascularized tongue of greater omentum is mobilized off the transverse colon and is laid over the portal vein to lie beneath the pancreatic anastomosis. If the pancreatic duct is large, the anastomosis is accomplished with an outer layer of sutures (4–0 PDS) between the serosa of the small bowel and the capsule of the pancreas and an inner-layer mucosa-to-mucosa anastomosis. If the pancreatic duct is small (less than 5 mm.), a tonsil clamp is placed into the pancreatic duct, and needle-tip cautery is used to splay open the pancreatic duct and the pancreas approximately 2 cm.

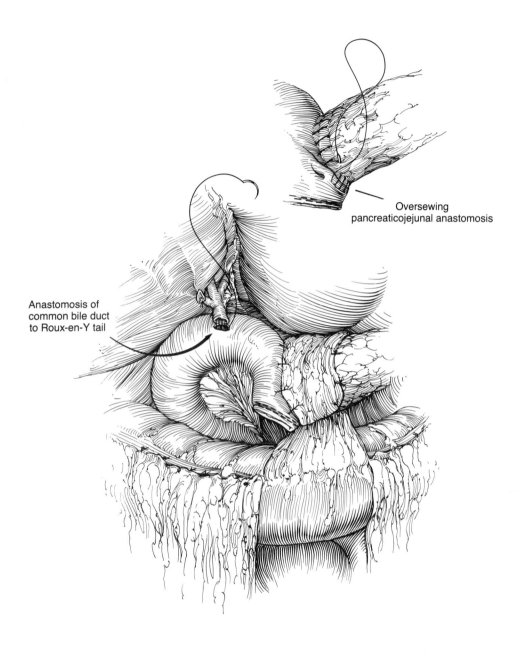

Oversewing
pancreaticojejunal anastomosis

Anastomosis of
common bile duct
to Roux-en-Y tail

FIGURE 101–12. This spatulated end of the pancreatic duct allows a double-layer anastomosis between bowel wall and pancreatic parenchyma, including a small margin of pancreatic duct. After the anastomosis is completed, the omentum "tongue" is used to complete a 360-degree wrap, which is secured with 3–0 silk sutures. No stent is used for the pancreatic anastomosis, whether it is dilated or not.

FIGURE 101–13. The biliary anastomosis is done end-to-side between the jejunum and the common bile duct. This is a single-layer anastomosis of 4–0 PDS suture. Absorbable suture is used here to allow placement of the knots inside of the bile duct for technical ease. No stent is used in this biliary anastomosis.

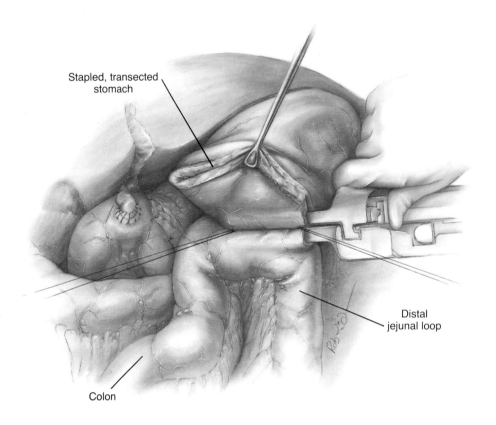

Stapled, transected stomach

Distal jejunal loop

Colon

FIGURE 101–14. The gastrojejunostomy is fashioned from the left side of the abdomen in an antecolic or retrocolic fashion to the underside of the stomach. This is done with a linear cutter and a linear stapling device. Multiple closed-suction drains are placed in the abdomen beneath the pancreatic and biliary anastomoses.

102

Pylorus-Saving Pancreaticoduodenectomy

ONYE E. AKWARI, M.D.

Pylorus-saving pancreaticoduodenectomy combines the Whipple concept of wide *en bloc* resection, when applicable, with preservation of an intact gastric reservoir. Advocates of this procedure reason that an intact stomach would eliminate the complications of a reduced gastric reservoir and improve the nutritional status of patients. Furthermore, they believe that this modification would decrease the postoperative incidence of jejunal ulceration, perforation, and bile reflux.

Although computed tomography, visceral arteriography, endoscopy, including cholangiopancreatography and, more recently, laparoscopy, have greatly improved preoperative evaluation of patients who are potential candidates for pancreaticoduodenectomy, intraoperative assessment remains the crucial final diagnostic step. Because gross disease is still overlooked in up to 10 per cent of patients who come to operation with the hope of curative resection based on clinical staging, careful intraoperative evaluation must be performed before radical resection is undertaken. First, gross distant metastasis to the liver, omentum, peritoneum surfaces, and periaortic lymph nodes must be excluded. Three groups of lymph nodes are routinely examined carefully: (1) nodes along the celiac and gastric arteries; (2) nodes in hepatoduodenal ligament and surrounding the hepatic artery, bile duct, and portal vein; and (3) nodes associated with the inferior pancreaticoduodenal artery, the superior mesenteric vessels, and vessels in the region of the ligament of Treitz. Involvement of the celiac axis, superior mesenteric vessels, or lymph nodes in the region of the ligament of Treitz indicates that the tumor has spread beyond the limits of resection. Tumor-bearing nodes in the hepatoduodenal ligament and distally along the gastroduodenal artery may be included in an *en bloc* dissection, so the lesion may still be resectable. The hepatic flexure of the colon must necessarily be widely mobilized, and the duodenum kocherized in order to obtain necessary evaluation in the right upper quadrant.

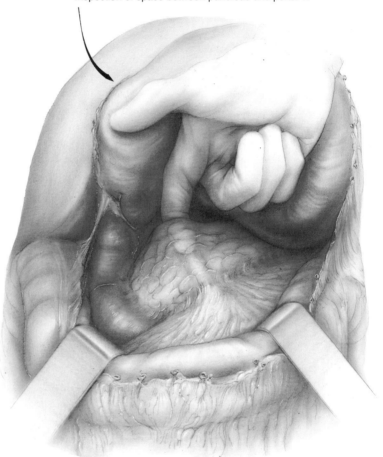

Inspection of space between pancreas and portal v.

FIGURE 102–1. Illustrated is the important final step of ensuring that the superior mesenteric and portal veins are free of tumor before committing to pancreaticoduodenectomy. The neck of the pancreas is carefully elevated off the anterior surface of the portal vein and demonstrates portal venous freedom from invasion superiorly. Obtaining access in this manner, by manual manipulation between the finger in the neck of the pancreas and the finger directed posteriorly behind the pancreas through the bed of the kocherized duodenum, ensures that invasion of the lateral aspect of the portal vein has not been overlooked.

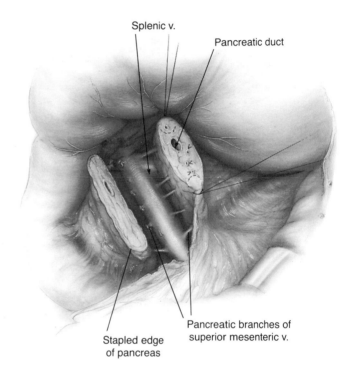

Splenic v.

Pancreatic duct

Stapled edge
of pancreas

Pancreatic branches of
superior mesenteric v.

FIGURE 102–2. The limits of resection for pylorus-saving pancreaticoduodenectomy are identical to those of the standard Whipple operation except for division of the proximal duodenum, which preserves continuity with the intact pylorus and stomach.

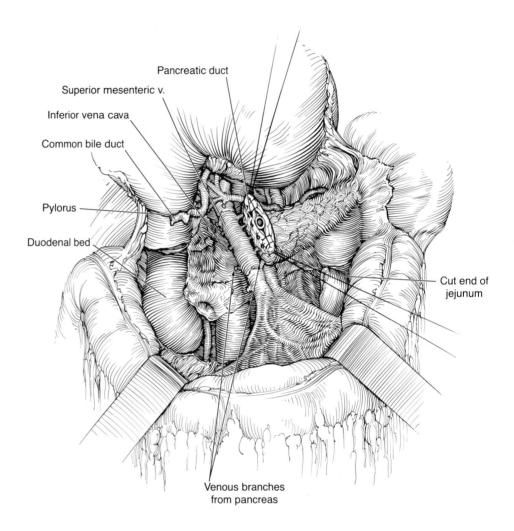

Pancreatic duct

Superior mesenteric v.

Inferior vena cava

Common bile duct

Pylorus

Duodenal bed

Cut end of
jejunum

Venous branches
from pancreas

FIGURE 102–3. Methods of managing the pancreatic remnant include (1) anastomosis of the pancreatic duct over a stent that is inserted through the side wall of the jejunum and (2) two-layer end-to-side pancreaticojejunostomy. The "dunking" or intussuscepting pancreaticojejunostomy, in which the end of the pancreas is inserted into the open end of the jejunum, is preferred. This is perhaps the easiest option when the gland is soft and the duct is normal in size. However, care must be exercised not to compromise the duct during placement of the pancreatic sutures. Pancreaticogastrostomy, occlusion of the pancreatic duct with solidifying agents, and ligation of the duct have been advocated.

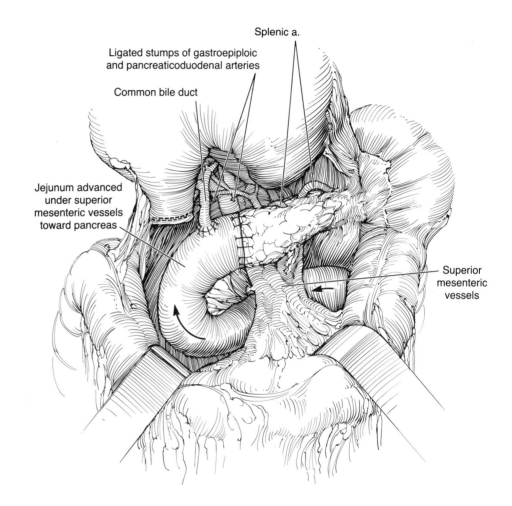

Splenic a.

Ligated stumps of gastroepiploic
and pancreaticoduodenal arteries

Common bile duct

Jejunum advanced
under superior
mesenteric vessels
toward pancreas

Superior
mesenteric
vessels

FIGURE 102–4. Most surgeons re-establish biliary-intestinal continuity by end-to-side
choledochojejunostomy. Side-to-side anastomosis may be preferred in patients in whom
the common bile duct is of normal caliber, as is often the case in the absence of
obstructive jaundice.

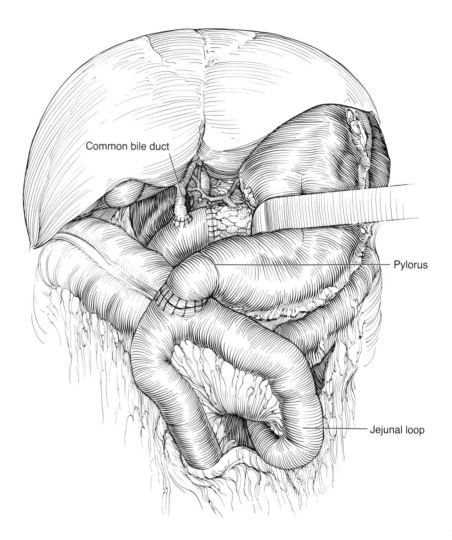

Common bile duct

Pylorus

Jejunal loop

FIGURE 102–5. Two techniques for duodenojejunostomy have been used. The first, reported by Traverso and Longmire, consists of an end-to-side anastomosis of the duodenal segment to a loop of jejunum passed dorsal to the mesenteric vessels in the bed of the resected duodenum. The second type of duodenojejunostomy, first performed by Watson, consists of an end-to-end anastomosis. Watson ligated the pancreatic duct and performed a cholecystojejunostomy distal to the duodenojejunostomy. End-to-end duodenojejunostomy has been performed in combination with pancreatic duct occlusion, pancreaticogastrostomy, and pancreaticogastrostomy with Roux-en-Y choledochojejunostomy.

Illustrated is an end-to-side duodenojejunostomy fashioned with an antecolic loop of jejunum after the pancreatic remnant and common bile duct have been anastomosed in sequence to the proximal jejunal limb passed through the bed of the resected duodenum.

SECTION XI

Spleen

103

Splenectomy, Including Elective and Traumatic

J. DIRK IGLEHART, M.D.
ONYE E. AKWARI, M.D.

Elective splenectomy is indicated for the treatment of a wide variety of benign and malignant disorders of the hematopoietic and lymphatic system. Two of the most common indications for splenectomy are Hodgkin's disease and immune thrombocytopenic purpura (ITP). However, the number of disorders that may be improved by splenectomy are many and include primary disease of the spleen, immune destruction of the formed elements of the blood, nonimmune destruction of formed blood elements, and hematopoietic malignancies. Special note is made regarding Hodgkin's disease when removal of the spleen accompanies a staging laparotomy. In this procedure, the operation includes biopsy of the liver and systematic biopsy of the major node-bearing areas of the abdomen.

Traumatic splenectomy is performed for damage to the spleen that causes an intra-abdominal hemorrhage. This procedure follows the outline for elective splenectomy and is combined with repair of other injuries as indicated at the time of emergency laparotomy.

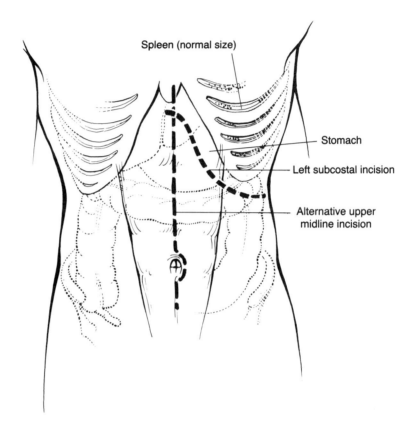

Spleen (normal size)

Stomach

Left subcostal incision

Alternative upper
midline incision

FIGURE 103–1. Splenectomy is performed with the patient in the supine position. Exposure of the spleen, which lies deep and under the left rib cage, is facilitated by placing the patient in a slight reverse Trendelenburg position and by tilting the right side of the table down. The surgeon usually stands on the right side of the table. A nasogastric tube, inserted into the stomach after intubation in elective cases, can be used to decompress the stomach and assist in exposure. In emergency splenectomy for trauma, insertion of the nasogastric tube may be accomplished prior to intubation to empty the stomach. Also in cases of trauma, preparation and draping of the entire abdomen and chest allow access to all injured structures if necessary.

For elective splenectomy when the spleen is normal in size or moderately enlarged, a left subcostal incision provides excellent exposure to the lateral peritoneal reflection along the left side of the spleen and to the inferior pole and its attachments to the splenic flexure of the colon. In patients with massive splenomegaly (in which the lower pole descends into the pelvis), in cases of abdominal trauma, or in cases in which splenectomy is combined with other intra-abdominal procedures such as staging laparotomy for Hodgkin's disease, it is best to use a long midline incision.

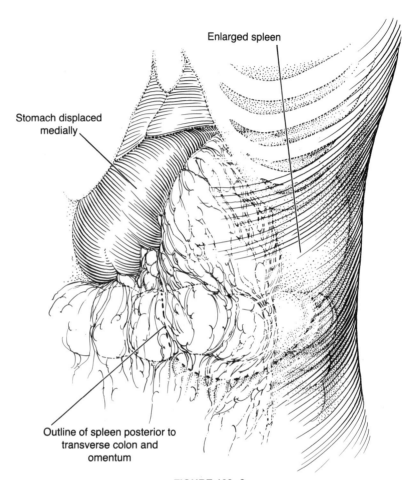

Enlarged spleen

Stomach displaced
medially

Outline of spleen posterior to
transverse colon and
omentum

FIGURE 103–2

FIGURES 103–2 and 103–3. Normally, the spleen lies to the left of the stomach and above
the splenic flexure of the colon. In cases in which the spleen is massively enlarged, the
lower pole descends under the transverse colon and stretches the attachments of the
splenic flexure. In this situation, the medial and anterior border of the spleen extends
over the anterior wall of the stomach to obscure the short gastric blood vessels, which
lie between the upper pole of the spleen and the upper aspect of the greater curvature
of the stomach.

Although a thoracoabdominal incision has been advocated by some surgeons in
cases of massive splenomegaly, we do not favor this approach. Extension of the incision
across the costal arch adds morbidity and is unnecessary because, in general, when the
spleen is massively enlarged, the splenic hilus is displaced inferiorly, making access to
the critical vessels paradoxically easier.

Illustration continued on following page

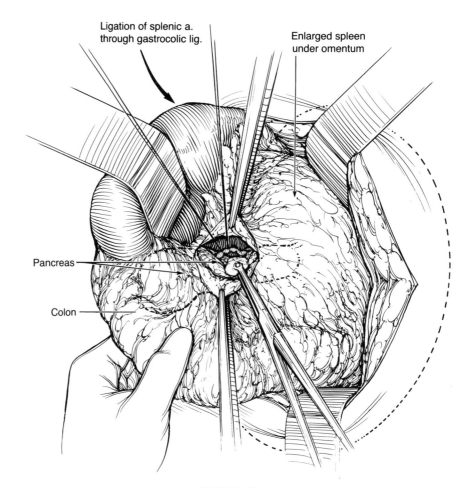

Ligation of splenic a.
through gastrocolic lig.

Enlarged spleen
under omentum

Pancreas

Colon

FIGURE 103–3

FIGURES 103–4 and 103–5. Complete mobilization of the spleen is essential for the ease and safety of the subsequent ligation of its vascular supply. This is particularly true for massive splenomegaly, in which the splenic artery and vein become greatly hypertrophied and conduct large amounts of blood. An appreciation of the relatively nonvascular attachments of the spleen is necessary for the initial mobilization. Although these attachments are referred to as "ligaments," they are in fact reflections of the parietal peritoneum as it sweeps up and over the spleen to fuse with its capsule. Three reflections are incised to allow mobilization of the spleen and its vascular mesenteries: (1) the splenophrenic; (2) the splenorenal, which is actually a posterolateral peritoneal reflection; and (3) the splenocolic, which is continuous with the splenic flexure of the colon.

With the spleen in its correct anatomic position, the attachments to the splenic flexure of the colon (the splenocolic ligament) are divided by incising the peritoneal reflections of the splenic flexure of the colon and passing a finger behind the tissues

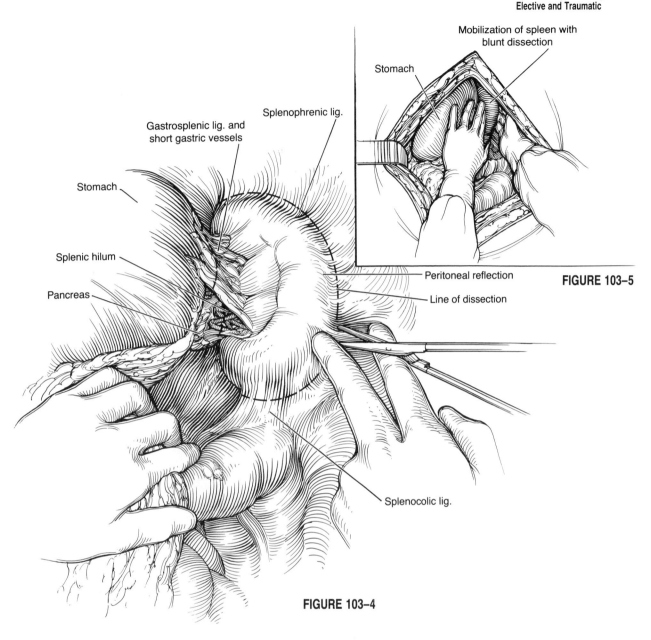

Gastrosplenic lig. and
short gastric vessels

Splenophrenic lig.

Stomach

Splenic hilum

Pancreas

Splenocolic lig.

FIGURE 103–4

Mobilization of spleen with
blunt dissection

Stomach

Peritoneal reflection

Line of dissection

FIGURE 103–5

running between the inferior pole of the spleen and the superior portion of the colon. This allows retraction of the colon away from the spleen. It is good policy to divide these tissues between one or two ligatures, particularly in cases of portal hypertension, massive splenomegaly, or when a coagulopathy is present. At this point, it may be convenient to divide branches of the splenic artery, which run in their own vascular mesentery and travel to the lower pole of the spleen. However, these are the only vessels in the hilum that should be divided prior to complete mobilization of the spleen.

By means of the defect created in the lateral peritoneal reflection, the splenorenal (lateral peritoneal) reflection is incised. The incision in this tissue is extended superiorly by bluntly dissecting behind the reflection close to the spleen and sharply dividing the elevated peritoneum with scissors or the electrocautery. This reflection is usually avascular except in cases of portal hypertension. By blunt dissection under the spleen, a space is created under the splenic mesentery and under the distal pancreas. With a hand around the spleen and under its mesentery, the organ is gently retracted inferiorly and medially up into the wound. This places the final ligament, the splenophrenic reflection, under tension and allows division of this avascular tissue. Care is taken at this point not to divide the uppermost short gastric blood vessels prematurely. However, the most superior short gastric vessels may be secured using a right-angle clamp and divided to allow complete mobilization.

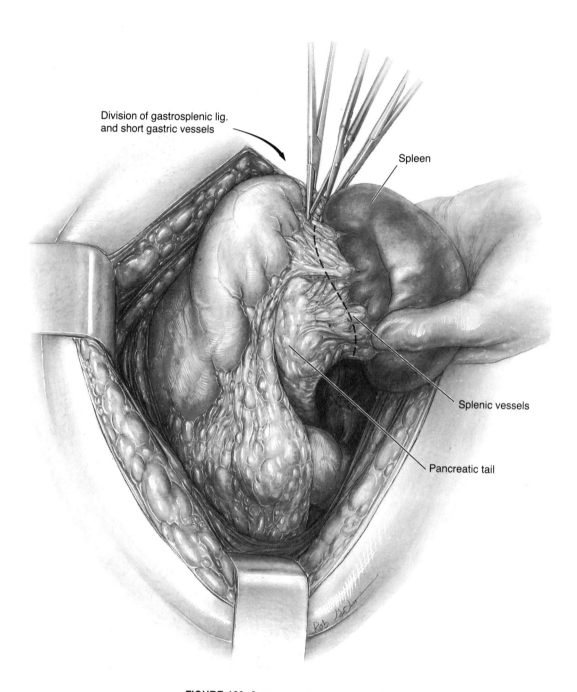

Division of gastrosplenic lig.
and short gastric vessels

Spleen

Splenic vessels

Pancreatic tail

FIGURE 103–6 *See legend on opposite page*

FIGURE 103–6. At this point, the spleen can be delivered onto the abdominal wall. If there is bleeding during the subsequent dissection, the surgeon's hand can easily control the hemorrhage while isolating and controlling the bleeding vessel. Attention is turned first to the short gastric vessels in the mesentery between the stomach and the spleen. Dissection is facilitated by careful incision of the peritoneal covering on the anterior side of this mesentery. The short gastric vessels, two or three in number, are sequentially divided between silk ties. These vessels are delicate structures and tear easily during mobilization of the spleen. The greater curvature of the stomach should be inspected carefully, and bleeding points controlled with figure-of-eight suture ligatures.

The final stage of splenectomy is ligation and division of the splenic arterial and venous blood vessels that lie inferior to the short gastric vessels. The splenic artery courses adjacent to the superior margin of the pancreas, and the splenic vein is located posteriorly and behind the pancreas. Division of these vessels is completed with the spleen delivered into the abdominal incision or, with massive spleens, onto the abdominal wall. It is wise to ligate individual branches of these vessels close to the spleen separately, thus lessening the chance of damage to the tail of the pancreas. Clamping the entire hilum within the jaws of a single instrument haphazardly should be avoided. The arterial and venous branches may be divided between right-angle or tonsil clamps and ligated with single ties of 2-0 silk. If the spleen is enlarged, it is wise to reinforce the ligation of arterial branches with additional suture ligatures. Also, if splenectomy is performed for Hodgkin's disease, large metallic hemoclips may be placed on the ligated ends to mark the distal extent of the splenic vessels for the radiation oncologist.

If splenectomy is performed for massive splenomegaly, particularly if there are adhesions around the spleen, the splenic artery can be ligated *in situ* as it courses along the superior aspect of the pancreas. The splenic artery is approached by dividing the gastrocolic omentum on the greater curvature of the stomach for a distance of several centimeters. This allows access to the lesser sac and to the posterior peritoneum overlying the pancreas and splenic artery. The artery is ligated in continuity, with a 1-0 silk ligature tied gently around the vessel to occlude blood flow.

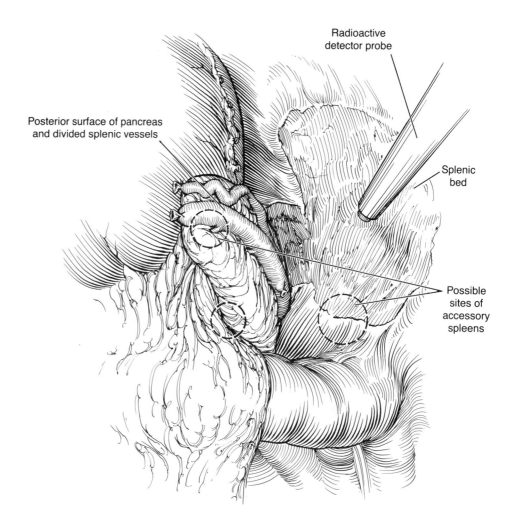

Radioactive
detector probe

Posterior surface of pancreas
and divided splenic vessels

Splenic
bed

Possible
sites of
accessory
spleens

FIGURE 103–7. At the conclusion of the procedure, it is necessary to reinspect the splenic bed and hilum for small uncontrolled bleeding points. This is best done by unrolling a large surgical sponge along the undersurface of the pancreas and into the splenic bed. If done from the right side of the table, the pancreas and stomach can be retracted toward the surgeon and the sponge slowly rolled upward to expose the critical areas. Also, the left upper quadrant is inspected for *accessory* splenic tissue, which is present in 10 to 15 per cent of cases. Accessory spleens are most commonly found in the splenic hilum along the course of the vascular supply, in the splenocolic reflection, or along the gastroepiploic branch of the splenic artery. Accessory spleens may occasionally be found in the greater omentum, in the lesser omentum along the lesser curve of the stomach, or in the mesentery of the large or small bowel.

It is not our practice to drain the splenic bed routinely, even after removal of very large spleens. The only routine indication for catheter drainage of the splenic bed is a recognized injury to the tail of the pancreas. If a catheter is left, a closed-system suction drain is preferable.

Retention of accessory splenic tissue is the most common cause for the recurrence of cytopenia, usually thrombocytopenia, after successful splenectomy. In cases of recurrent ITP, retention of accessory tissue can be preoperatively documented by injection of autologous platelets labeled with indium 111 followed by radionuclide scintigraphy. If an accessory spleen is detected, we have proceeded to laparotomy within 12 hours of the labeled platelet administration. With a hand-held isotope detector, shown wrapped in a sterile plastic bag, the area containing the suspected retained spleen is probed to detect accumulation of the indium 111–labeled platelets. After removal of the focus of activity, immediate pathologic confirmation of splenic tissue can be obtained by gross and microscopic examination.

104

Splenic Repair (PEDIATRIC)

ARTHUR J. ROSS, III, M.D.

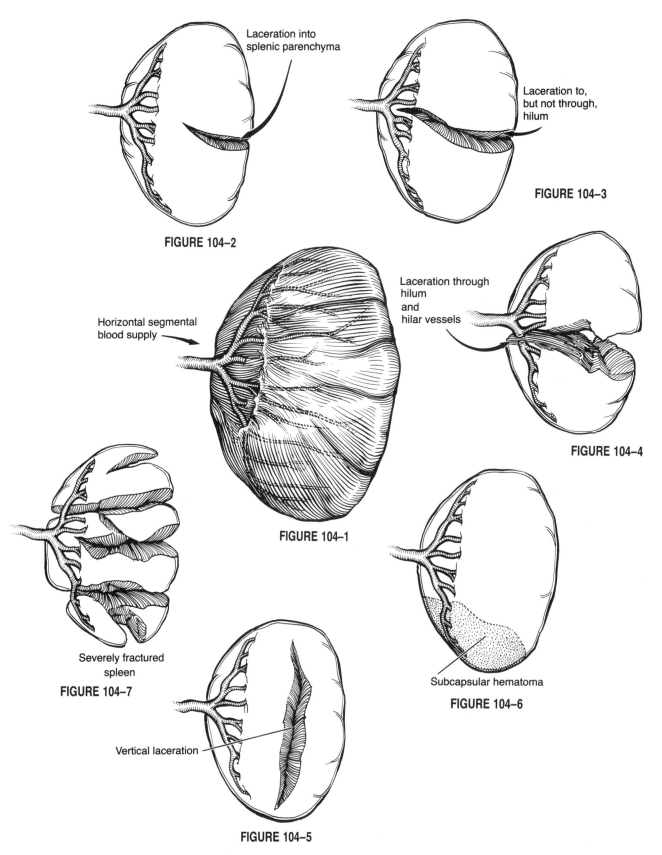

Laceration into
splenic parenchyma

FIGURE 104–2

Laceration to,
but not through,
hilum

FIGURE 104–3

Horizontal segmental
blood supply

FIGURE 104–1

Laceration through
hilum
and
hilar vessels

FIGURE 104–4

Severely fractured
spleen

FIGURE 104–7

Subcapsular hematoma

FIGURE 104–6

Vertical laceration

FIGURE 104–5

FIGURES 104–1 to 104–7. *See legend on opposite page*

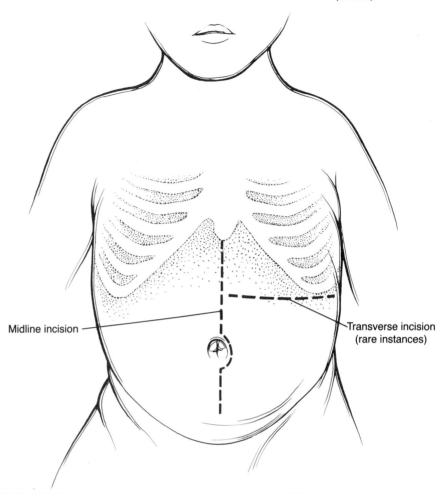

Midline incision

Transverse incision
(rare instances)

FIGURE 104–8. Many pediatric operations are performed through transverse incisions. However, in laparotomies for trauma in which thorough abdominal exploration is required, a vertical midline incision is often used. This incision extends from the xiphoid to a level below the umbilicus. There are uncommon instances in which the injury is known to be isolated to the spleen. In such patients, a long transverse incision extending from the tip of the eleventh rib in the midaxillary line to the midline can be employed with the child in a straight lateral position.

FIGURES 104–1 to 104–7. Splenorrhaphy is a technique commonly used in children who have sustained a traumatic injury to the spleen, and its success is strongly contingent on the surgeon's understanding of splenic anatomy. Critical in this regard is knowledge of the fact that the spleen has a horizontal segmental blood supply. Fortunately, most splenic injuries occur within the transverse plane and tend to consist of a spectrum of injuries, the least of which is a small incomplete transverse tear within the splenic parenchyma. Next in severity is a tear that goes to, but not through, the splenic hilum, followed by a tear that goes through the hilum itself but does not divide the hilar vessels. The most severe injury in this spectrum is the splenic tear, which goes through the hilus and also divides the hilar vasculature. Even the severely fractured spleen generally has sufficient fractures in a transverse plane such that splenorrhaphy and/or partial splenectomy can be accomplished. Difficult to manage, but fortunately rare, are the vertical lacerations of the spleen. Subcapsular hematomas of the spleen are very common injuries. Generally, these do not cause intra-abdominal hemorrhage and rarely require operative management.

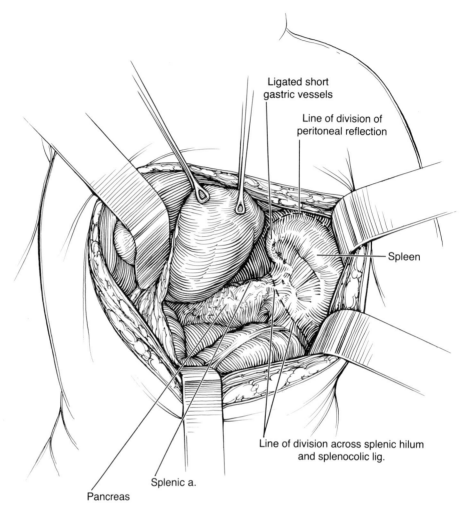

Ligated short
gastric vessels

Line of division of
peritoneal reflection

Spleen

Line of division across splenic hilum
and splenocolic lig.

Splenic a.

Pancreas

FIGURE 104–9

FIGURES 104–9 and 104–10. If optimal splenic repair is to be performed, it is imperative
that the spleen be completely mobilized from all of its attachments so that it can be very
closely inspected. This maneuver is required to obtain complete control of the segmental
vasculature to the spleen. To whatever degree is possible, care must be exercised in
mobilizing the spleen so that a capsular injury is not created or extended. In instances
in which bleeding is brisk, one is best advised to obtain control of the main splenic
artery promptly with a vessel loop. Temporary arterial occlusion with the vessel loop
as a tourniquet or with digital compression should allow mobilization of the injured
spleen without undue hemorrhage. Control of hemorrhage should allow the subsequent
division of the short gastric vessels as well as the splenic ligamentous attachments.
Once the spleen is mobilized, it is fully evaluated by gently removing the clotted blood
within damaged areas so that bleeding points deep within a splenic laceration can be
identified.

Illustration continued on following page

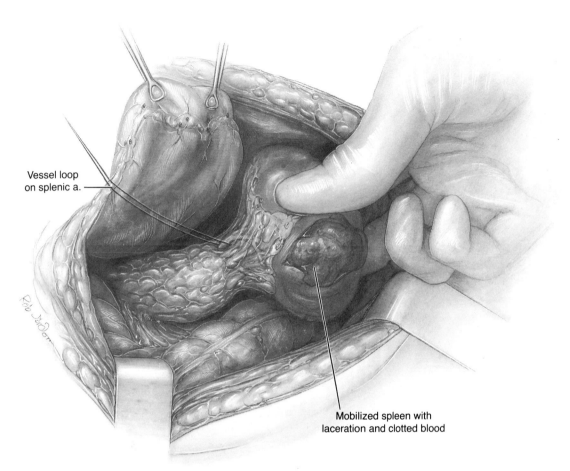

Vessel loop
on splenic a.

Mobilized spleen with
laceration and clotted blood

FIGURE 104–10

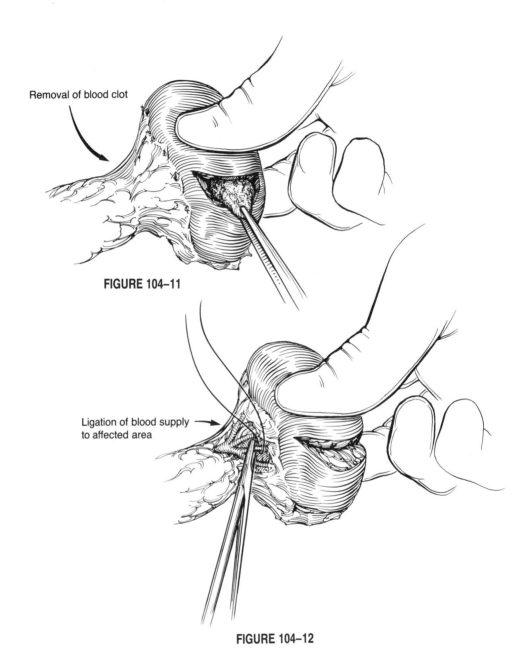

Removal of blood clot

FIGURE 104–11

Ligation of blood supply
to affected area

FIGURE 104–12

FIGURES 104–11 and 104–12. With the spleen fully mobilized, all damaged areas must first be completely evaluated. Clotted blood is removed in as gentle a manner as is possible so that bleeding points deep within a laceration can be identified.

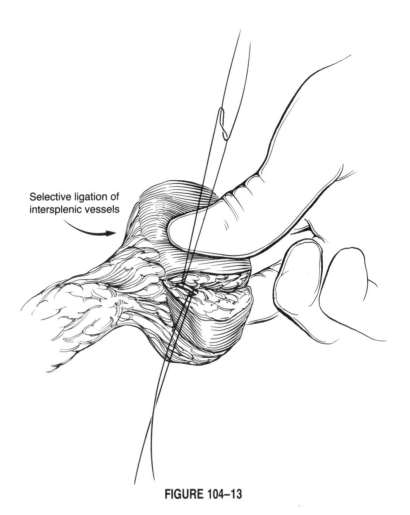

Selective ligation of
intersplenic vessels

FIGURE 104–13

FIGURES 104–13 to 104–15. Once the totality of the injury has been assessed, selective ligation of the appropriate segmental hilar vessels is undertaken. In addition, it is best to suture-ligate the individual intrasplenic vessels as is appropriate. Fine sutures as well as hemoclips are both useful for this purpose. At this point, the decision is made as to whether a formal partial splenectomy will be required or whether the splenorrhaphy can be completed with suture closure of the splenic parenchyma and capsule. Chromic catgut sutures are used for this purpose. The surgeon's judgment dictates whether these sutures are placed in a simple, mattress, or running manner. We have not found the need for pledgets.

Illustration continued on following page

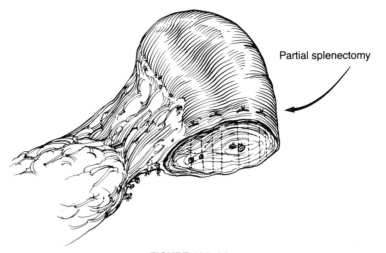

FIGURE 104–14

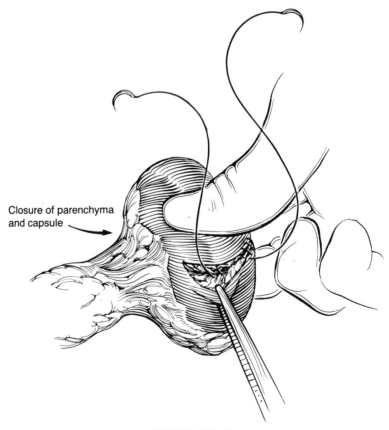

FIGURE 104–15

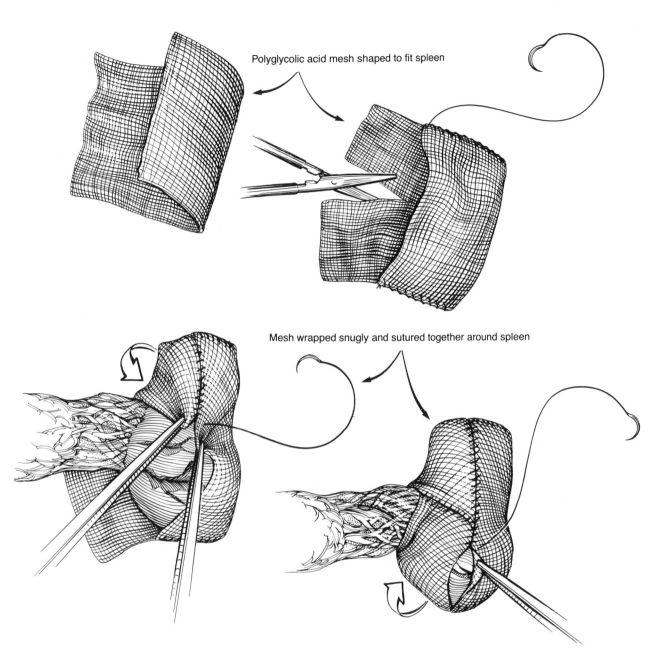

Polyglycolic acid mesh shaped to fit spleen

Mesh wrapped snugly and sutured together around spleen

FIGURES 104–16 and 104–17. We have found that fashioning a supportive mesh of absorbable polyglycolic acid is a good means of management for the spleen that seems to be otherwise not salvageable. Follow-up image studies have demonstrated the efficacy of this technique in salvaging splenic function. With good control of the segmental hilar vessels, it has been found unnecessary to use special equipment such as argon beam coagulators. Indeed, only minimal use of the Bovie electrocautery unit is required. We have found that the adjunctive use of topical hemostatic agents such as Avitene or thrombin-soaked gel foam will, when appropriately placed, provide complete and successful hemostasis should oozing continue following ligation of the appropriate segmental and intrasplenic vessels. We have also found that, if available, a patch of omentum laid about the repair site is helpful.

Whereas splenic repair is commonly employed in the patient with pediatric trauma, its use in adults is more controversial. In selected adults in whom splenic repair is considered appropriate, the preceding technical principles are also applicable.

Endocrine and Head and Neck Procedures

105

Subtotal and Total Thyroidectomy and Thyroid Lobectomy

GEORGE S. LEIGHT, JR., M.D.

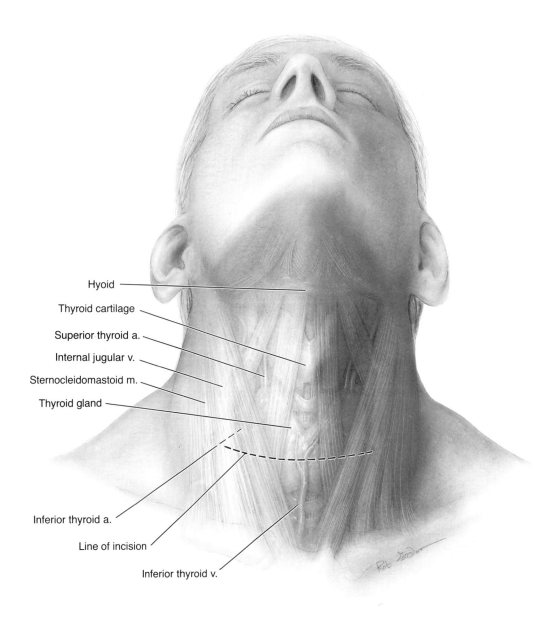

Hyoid

Thyroid cartilage

Superior thyroid a.

Internal jugular v.

Sternocleidomastoid m.

Thyroid gland

Inferior thyroid a.

Line of incision

Inferior thyroid v.

FIGURE 105–1. Proper positioning of the patient on the operating table is critical for achieving optimal exposure of the thyroid gland. Hyperextension of the neck, which moves the thyroid from under the manubrium, is accomplished by placing a rolled sheet under the patient and parallel to the spine. This allows the patient's shoulders to fall posteriorly while the head is supported on a foam rubber pad to prevent motion.

The incision must be carefully planned so that it is positioned to give optimal access to the entire thyroid gland. The optimal site is dependent on the patient's anatomy and thyroid pathology; in general, an area approximately two fingerbreadths above the clavicular heads is selected. The incision should conform to Langer's lines, and a more prominent skin fold is selected if it is properly positioned. The incision should be symmetric, extending for equal distances from the midline, and should have a gentle upward curve.

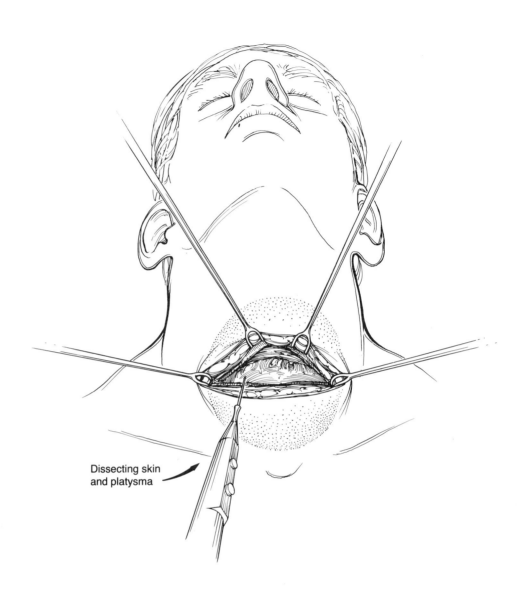

Dissecting skin
and platysma

FIGURE 105–2. The incision extends through the subcutaneous tissues, and the platysma muscle is divided with the cutting cautery. Flaps are then mobilized superiorly and inferiorly, dividing with the cautery the tissues just deep to the platysma muscle. The superior flap is taken to the level of the thyroid cartilage while the dissection is extended inferiorly to the clavicular heads and suprasternal notch.

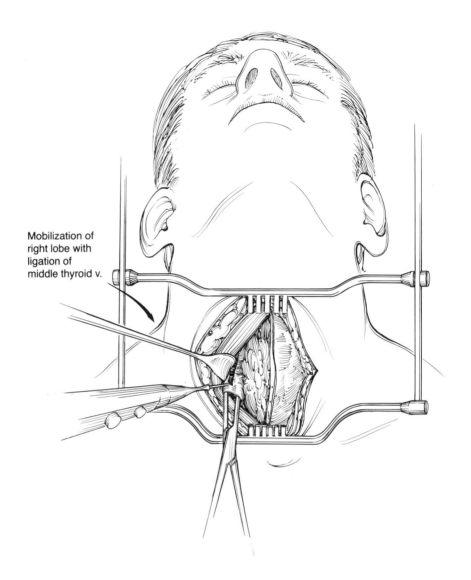

Mobilization of
right lobe with
ligation of
middle thyroid v.

FIGURE 105–3. A Mahorner retractor is inserted, and towels (not shown) are placed, so that only the incision is exposed. The strap muscles (sternohyoid and sternothyroid) are then separated by dividing the tissues in the avascular midline plane from the thyroid cartilage to the suprasternal notch. The thyroid lobe is exposed by mobilizing the strap muscles away from the lobe by means of lateral retraction on the muscles and blunt dissection with a Kuettner ("peanut") dissector. The middle vein is exposed, divided, and ligated.

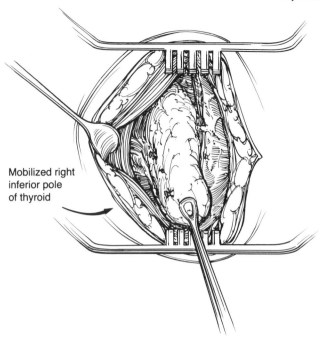

Mobilized right
inferior pole
of thyroid

FIGURE 105–4

Mobilization of thyroid near inferior thyroid a.
and recurrent laryngeal n.

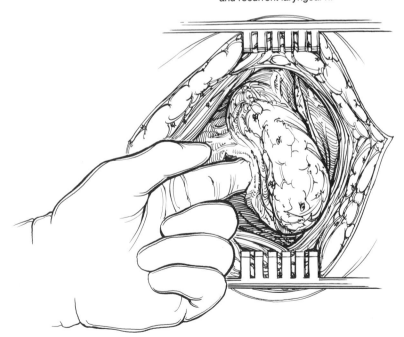

FIGURE 105–5

FIGURES 105–4 and 105–5. Babcock clamps are applied to inferior and superior (not shown) aspects of the thyroid lobe to facilitate medial retraction on the gland. This exposes the area where the parathyroid glands and recurrent laryngeal nerve are located.

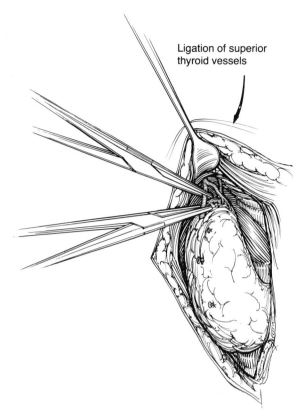

FIGURE 105–6. Downward traction on the superior Babcock clamp exposes the superior pole vessels, including the branches of the superior thyroid artery. The external laryngeal nerve courses along the cricothyroid muscle just medial to the superior pole vessels. To avoid injury to this nerve, which controls tension of the vocal cords, the superior pole vessels are divided individually as close as possible to the point where they enter the thyroid gland.

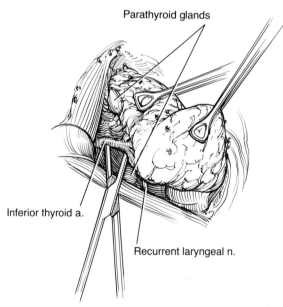

FIGURE 105–7. As the thyroid is retracted medially, gentle dissection with a Hoyt clamp is done to expose the parathyroid glands, inferior thyroid artery, and recurrent laryngeal nerve. The recurrent nerve usually passes behind the inferior thyroid artery but occasionally lies anterior to it. It is best found by careful dissection just inferior to the artery. The nerve can then be traced upward, and its position in relation to the thyroid determined. Parathyroid glands that lie on the thyroid surface can be mobilized with their vascular supply and thus preserved.

Ligation and division of distal branches of inferior thyroid a.
for **total thyroidectomy**

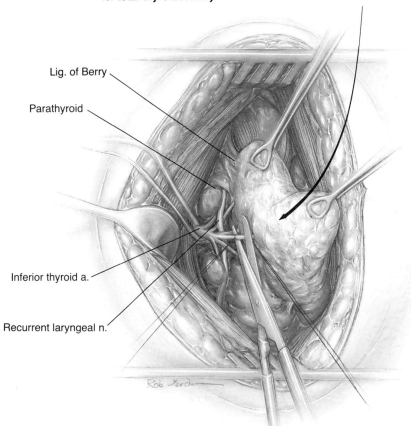

Lig. of Berry

Parathyroid

Inferior thyroid a.

Recurrent laryngeal n.

FIGURE 105–8. To perform total lobectomy, the branches of the inferior thyroid artery are divided at the surface of the thyroid gland. The inferior thyroid veins can now be ligated and divided. Superiorly, the connective tissue (ligament of Berry), which binds the thyroid to the tracheal rings, is carefully divided. There are usually several small accompanying vessels, and the recurrent nerve is closest to the thyroid and most vulnerable at this point. Division of the ligament allows the thyroid to be mobilized medially.

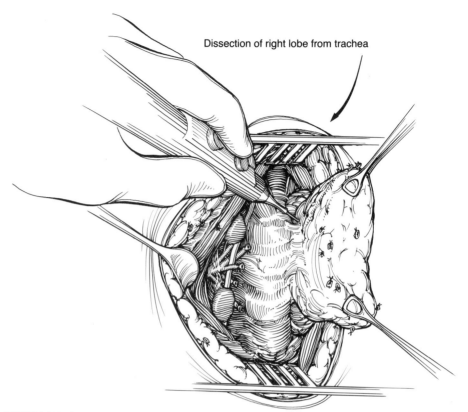

FIGURE 105–9. The dissection of the thyroid from the trachea can be performed with the cautery by division of the loose connective tissue between these structures. Dissection is extended under the isthmus, and the specimen is divided, so that the isthmus is included with the resected lobe. The pyramidal lobe also should be included if present.

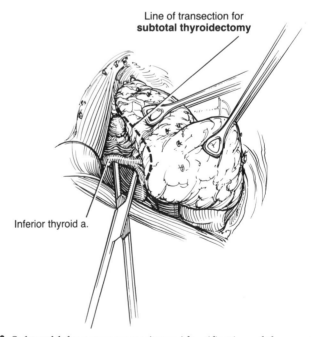

FIGURE 105–10. Subtotal lobectomy necessitates identification of the parathyroid glands, inferior thyroid artery, and recurrent laryngeal nerve, as previously described. The line of resection is selected to preserve the parathyroid glands and their blood supply and to protect the recurrent laryngeal nerve. It should be based on the inferior thyroid artery or its major branches.

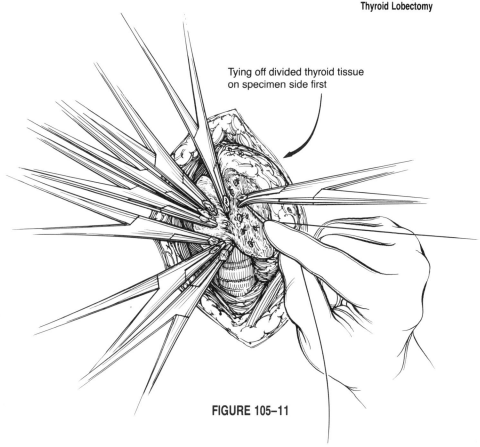

Tying off divided thyroid tissue
on specimen side first

FIGURE 105–11

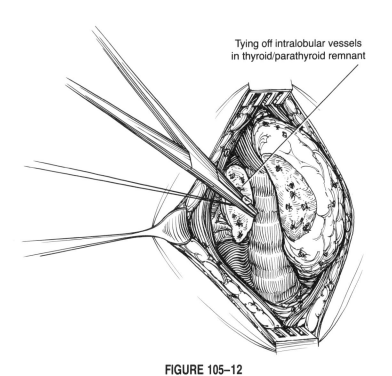

Tying off intralobular vessels
in thyroid/parathyroid remnant

FIGURE 105–12

FIGURES 105–11 and 105–12. Clamps are placed along the line of resection, and the thyroid gland is divided. The divided tissue is ligated or suture-ligated with 3-0 silk. The dissection is extended to the trachea.

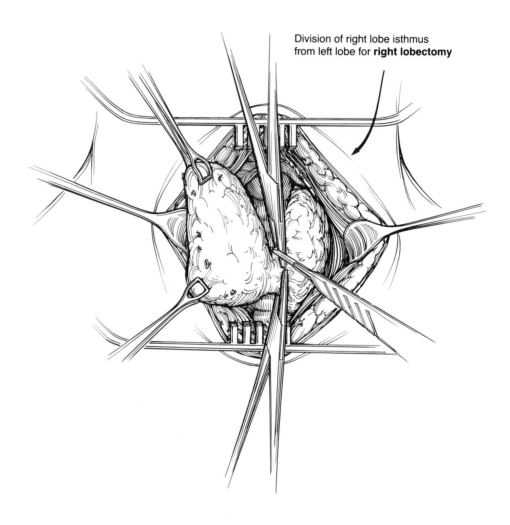

Division of right lobe isthmus
from left lobe for **right lobectomy**

FIGURE 105–13. The thyroid can now be divided so that the isthmus is included in the specimen. A running 2-0 silk suture is used to secure the line of division along the remaining thyroid lobe.

106

Radical Neck Dissection with Spinal Accessory Nerve Preservation Technique

SAMUEL R. FISHER, M.D.

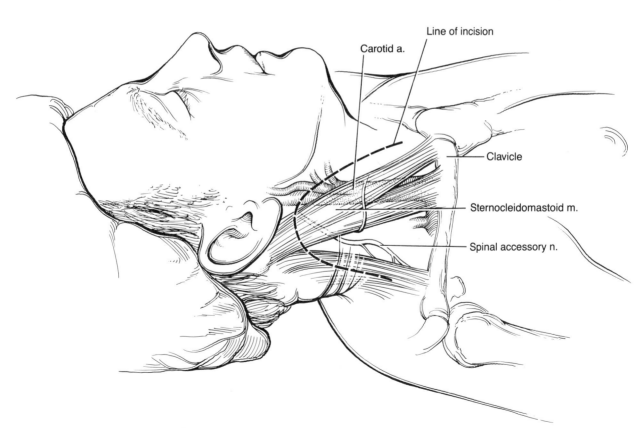

FIGURE 106–1. A curvilinear, inferiorly based U-shaped flap designed by the author is used as the neck incision. The anterior limb parallels the border of the sternocleidomastoid muscle, then gently tapers inferiorly. The posterior vertical limb parallels the edge of the trapezius muscle. The posterior limb ends 2 to 3 cm. medial to the clavicle and need not traverse it for exposure. The width-to-height ratio of this flap is adequate to maintain excellent viability and cosmesis.

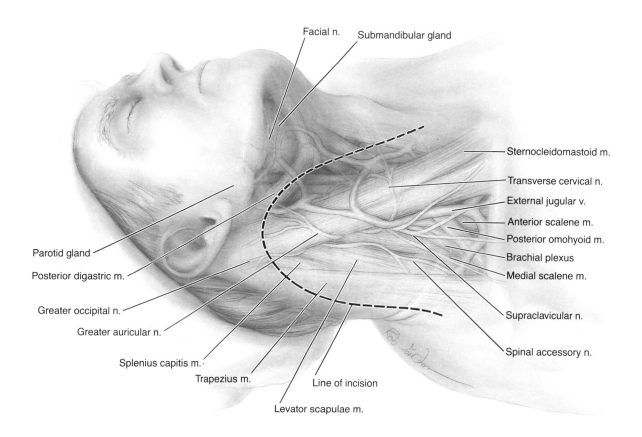

FIGURE 106–2. A close-up view of the neck incision with the underlying muscles and cutaneous nerves and vessels. Excellent exposure is achieved of the submandibular triangle contents and the posterior triangle (levels I to V). It should be noted that the inferior extent of the incision need not traverse the clavicles either medially or laterally.

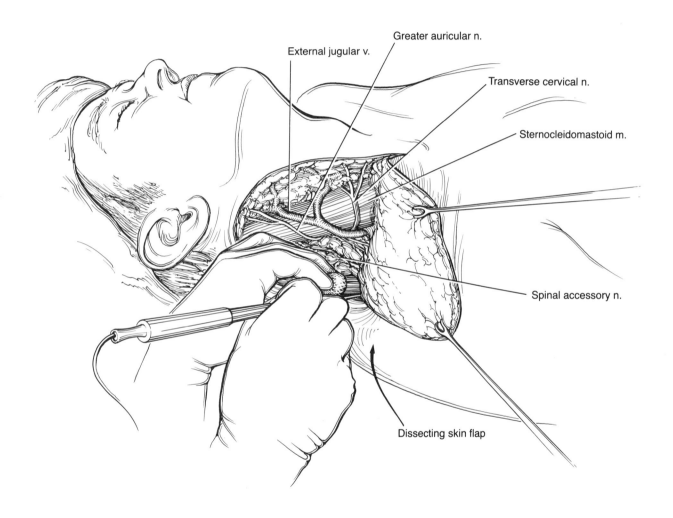

FIGURE 106–3. Elevation of the subplatysmal flap proceeds from superior to inferior lateral to the external jugular vein. Dissection proceeds posteriorly to the trapezius muscle, anteriorly to the sternocleidomastoid muscle, and inferiorly to the clavicle. Because the spinal accessory nerve lies in the superficial fascia exiting at the proximal third (Erb's point) of the sternocleidomastoid muscle, care should be taken in elevation of the flap in the posterior triangle.

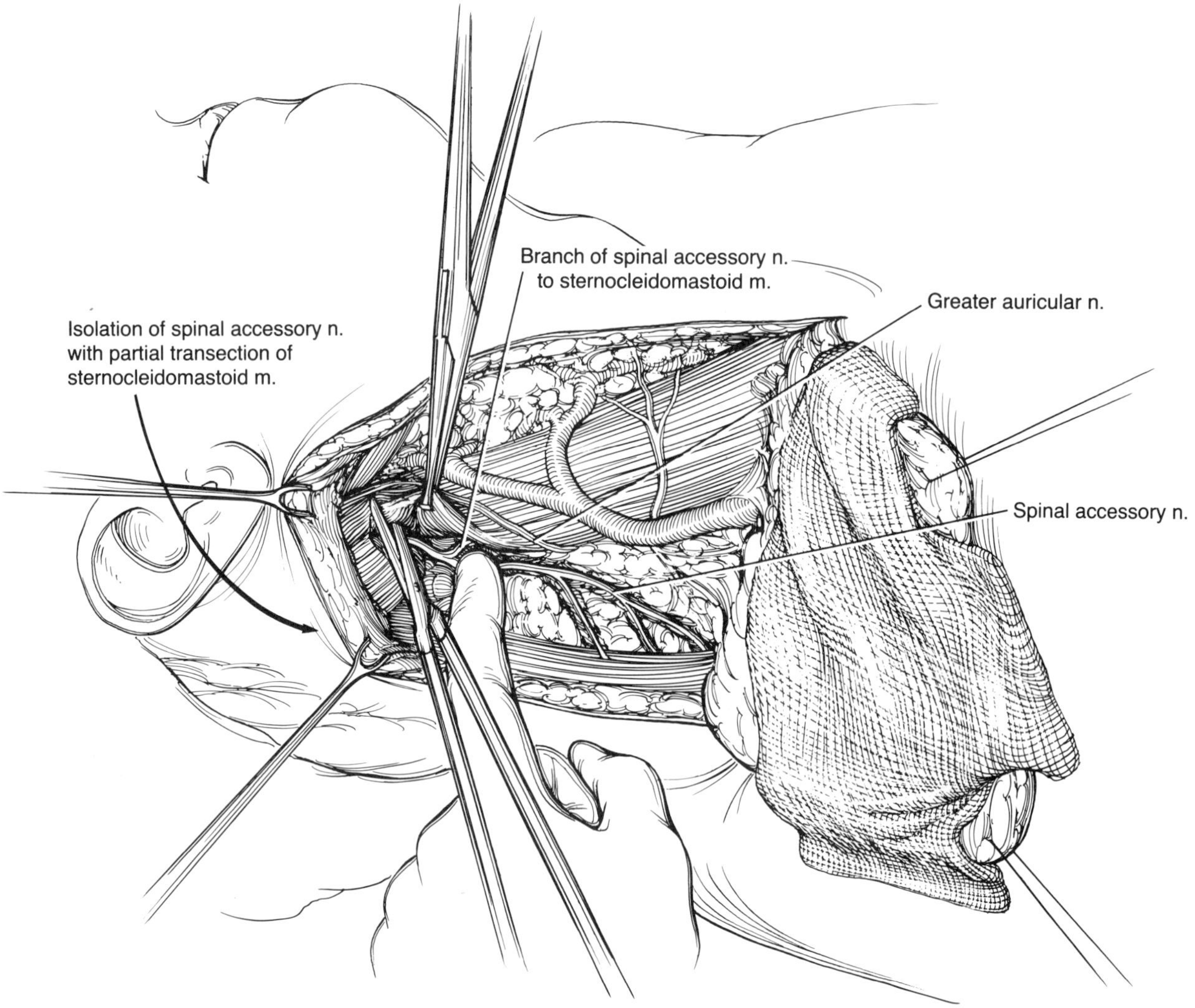

FIGURE 106–4. The neck flap is protected with a moist sponge, and the spinal accessory nerve is further identified and traced through the sternocleidomastoid muscle to the base of the skull by sharp dissection. Branches of the spinal accessory nerve to the superior and middle portion of the trapezius muscle are not uncommon and should be preserved.

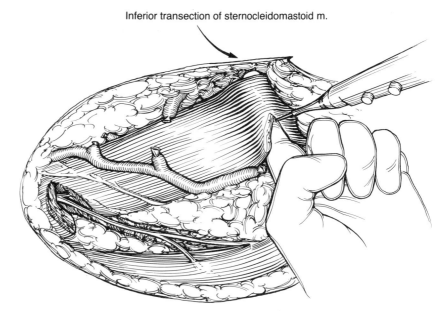

FIGURE 106–5. The external jugular veins have been ligated proximally and distally, and the clavicular head of the sternocleidomastoid muscle is transected. The surgeon should protect the carotid sheath contents during the division of the muscle.

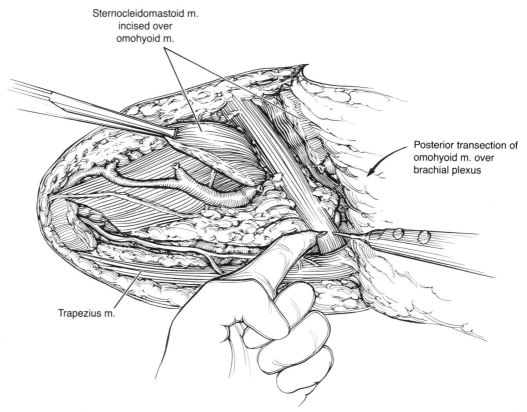

FIGURE 106–6. The omohyoid muscle is divided laterally as it courses under the clavicle, and then medially. This provides full access to the internal jugular vein and the contents of the jugular chain and is a good landmark in identifying the carotid artery, internal jugular vein, and vagus nerve.

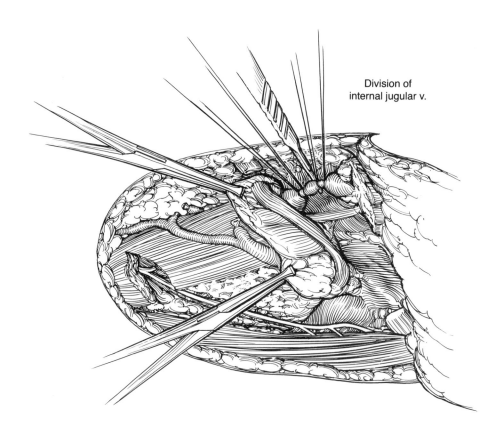

Division of internal jugular v.

FIGURE 106–7. The proximal stump of the internal jugular vein is identified and dissected free from the carotid artery and vagus nerve. The vessel is doubly ligated with 2-0 silk and transected.

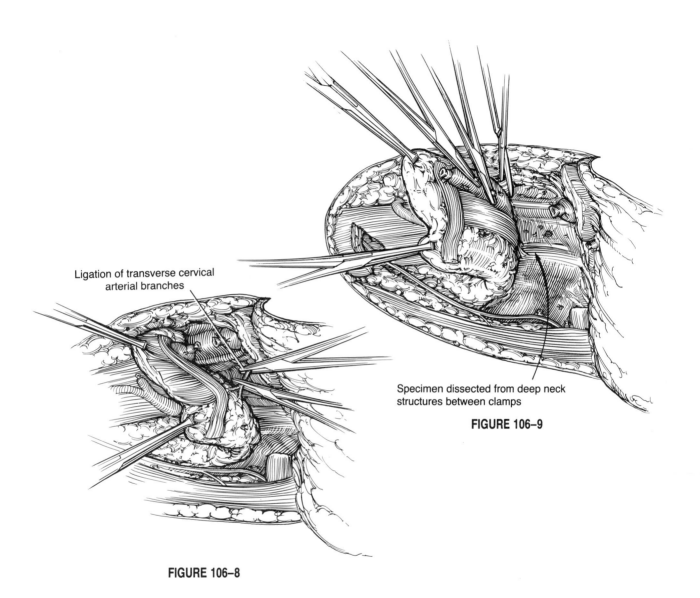

Ligation of transverse cervical
arterial branches

Specimen dissected from deep neck
structures between clamps

FIGURE 106–9

FIGURE 106–8

FIGURE 106–8. Fasciae in the supraclavicular fossa and internal chain have been incised, exposing the deep cervical fascia. The transverse cervical artery is located just lateral to the deep cervical fascia and is identified and ligated. The tissue in the supraclavicular fossa anterior and medial to the spinal accessory nerve is then elevated by sharp and blunt dissection after the vessels have been ligated laterally. The dissection then proceeds from inferior to superior with identification and ligation of branches of the internal jugular vein. The brachial plexus and phrenic nerve should be easily identified and protected during this dissection.

FIGURE 106–9. The specimen, including the sternocleidomastoid muscle, internal jugular vein, and lymph-bearing tissue, is then reflected superiorly. Identification and protection of the hypoglossal nerve can be achieved by first locating it lateral to the internal carotid artery, generally just cephalic to the carotid bifurcation.

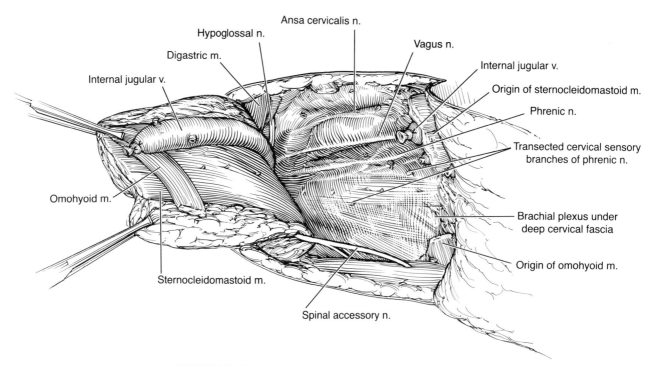

FIGURE 106–10. The contents of the posterior triangle are then modified by gentle traction on the spinal accessory nerve.

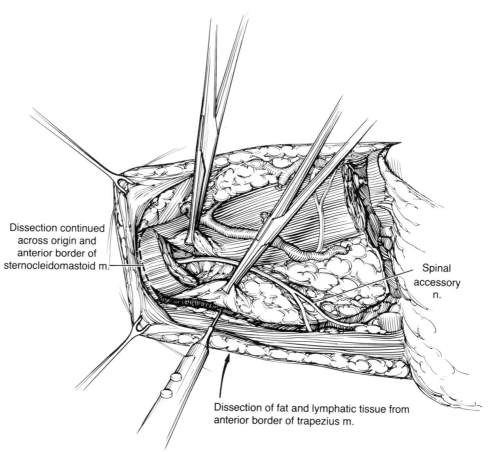

FIGURE 106–11. These contents and the resected superior aspect of the sternocleidomastoid muscle are easily passed underneath the spinal accessory nerve, which has been dissected to the base of the skull adjacent to the internal jugular vein. This maneuver should hinge all neck contents medial to the spinal accessory nerve.

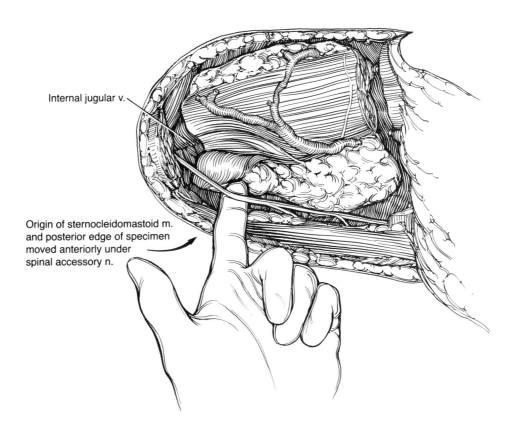

Internal jugular v.

Origin of sternocleidomastoid m.
and posterior edge of specimen
moved anteriorly under
spinal accessory n.

FIGURE 106–12. The internal jugular vein is doubly ligated at the base of the skull just medial and superior to the digastric muscle.

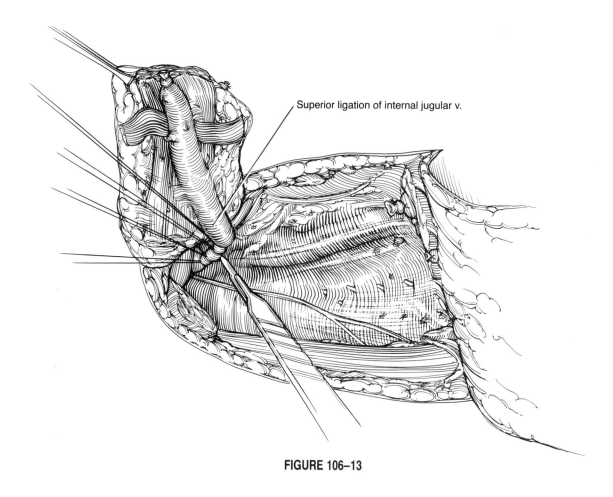

Superior ligation of internal jugular v.

FIGURE 106–13

FIGURES 106–13 and 106–14. The radical neck dissection is completed with preservation of the carotid artery, vagus nerve, phrenic nerve, spinal accessory nerve, and brachial plexus. The submandibular triangle contents (level I nodes) have not been resected at this point. These structures may be resected with the radical neck dissection when indicated and left attached to the neck dissection *en bloc*, or dissected in discontinuity.

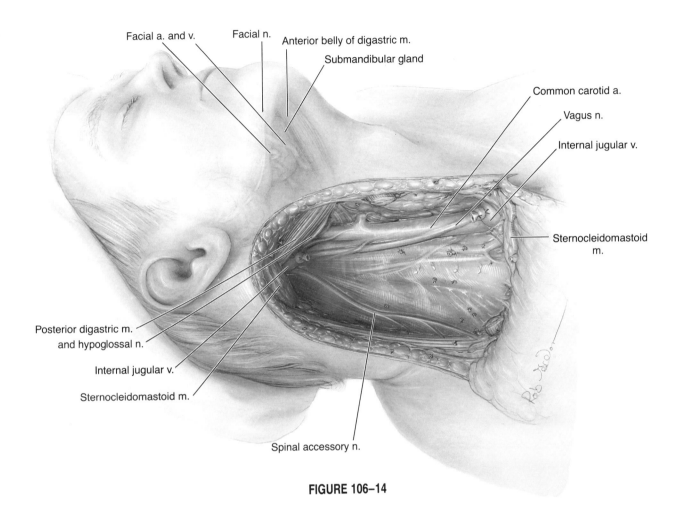

Facial a. and v.   Facial n.   Anterior belly of digastric m.

Submandibular gland

Common carotid a.

Vagus n.

Internal jugular v.

Sternocleidomastoid
m.

Posterior digastric m.
and hypoglossal n.

Internal jugular v.

Sternocleidomastoid m.

Spinal accessory n.

FIGURE 106–14

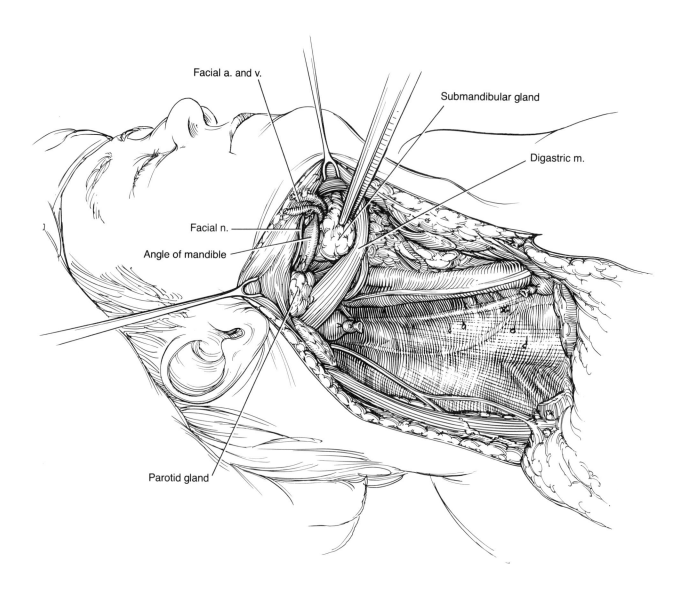

Facial a. and v.

Submandibular gland

Digastric m.

Facial n.

Angle of mandible

Parotid gland

FIGURE 106–15. The contents of the submandibular triangle are resected, preserving the ramus mandibularis branch of the facial nerve. This can be accomplished by dissecting beneath the anterior facial vein, which has been ligated and reflected superiorly. The submandibular gland and surrounding lymph nodes are then resected after the excito-gustatory fibers of the lingual nerve have been transected medially.

107

Parathyroidectomy for Hyperplasia and Adenoma

GEORGE S. LEIGHT, JR., M.D.

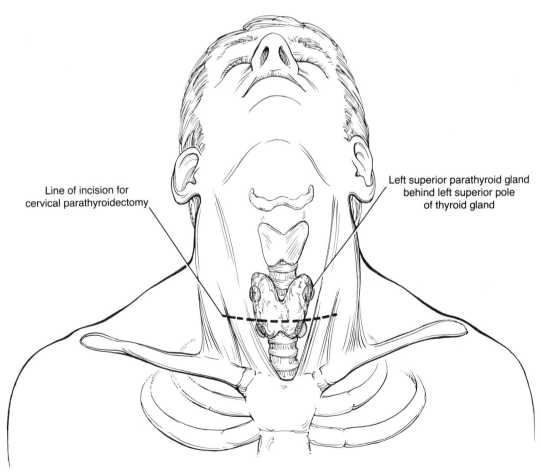

Line of incision for
cervical parathyroidectomy

Left superior parathyroid gland
behind left superior pole
of thyroid gland

FIGURE 107–1. The patient is positioned as described for thyroidectomy, and the incision is similar, although extending farther laterally to provide optimal exposure. The primary areas where parathyroid glands are most frequently found are indicated by the stippled areas.

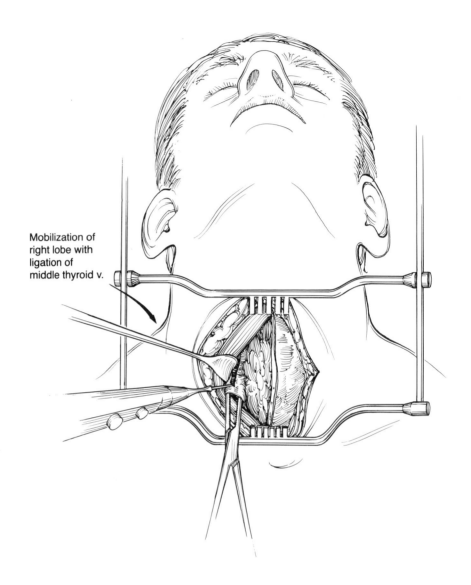

Mobilization of
right lobe with
ligation of
middle thyroid v.

FIGURE 107–2. The plane between the strap muscles is divided, and they are retracted laterally, exposing the thyroid lobe. The middle thyroid vein is divided and ligated, allowing medial mobilization of the thyroid gland.

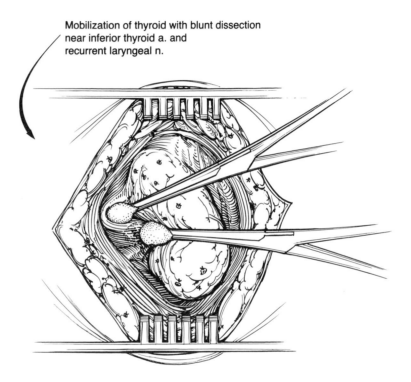

Mobilization of thyroid with blunt dissection
near inferior thyroid a. and
recurrent laryngeal n.

FIGURE 107–3. The mobilization of the right thyroid lobe is carefully performed with a combination of sharp and blunt dissection. Absolute hemostasis must be maintained during this and subsequent portions of the procedure because blood-stained tissue makes parathyroid identification much more difficult. Meticulous surgical technique produces the best results in parathyroid surgery.

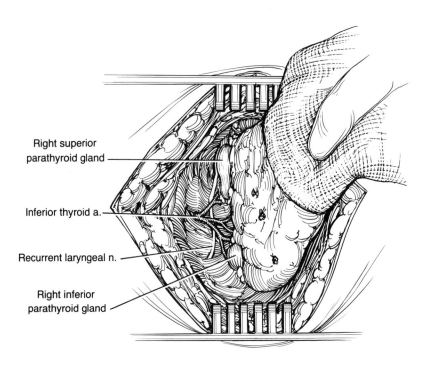

Right superior
parathyroid gland

Inferior thyroid a.

Recurrent laryngeal n.

Right inferior
parathyroid gland

FIGURE 107–4. After mobilization is complete, Babcock clamps are applied to the thyroid lobe, which is retracted medially. The inferior thyroid artery and the recurrent laryngeal nerve are identified and carefully protected. The recurrent nerve usually passes posterior to the inferior thyroid artery, although it may be anterior to the artery or may interdigitate with the artery's branches. The surgeon should also be aware of the existence of a nonrecurrent laryngeal nerve, although this is a rare finding. The parathyroid glands should be sought in their primary locations. The upper gland is more constant in location and is most frequently found in fatty tissue above the inferior thyroid artery just lateral to the thyroid gland. The characteristic tan color of normal parathyroid glands is very important in differentiating them from fat, lymph nodes, thyroid tissue, and other structures. A normal right inferior gland and an enlarged right superior gland are shown.

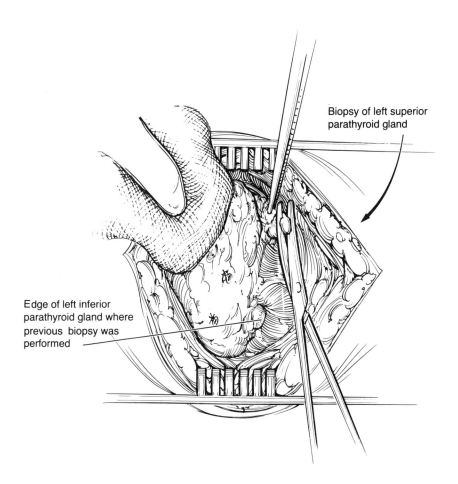

Biopsy of left superior
parathyroid gland

Edge of left inferior
parathyroid gland where
previous biopsy was
performed

FIGURE 107–5. The left side is explored in a similar manner. When the lower gland cannot be identified, the tissues between the lower thyroid pole and the thymus, as well as the thymus itself, should be carefully searched. When an upper gland cannot be identified, it will most likely be found posteriorly behind the inferior thyroid artery or its branches. Two glands of normal size, color, and consistency are depicted, with small slivers from the part of the gland opposite the blood supply being taken for histologic confirmation to be certain that it is parathyroid tissue.

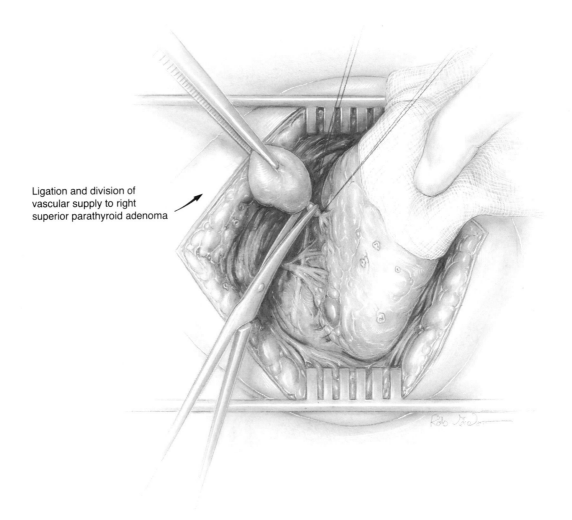

Ligation and division of
vascular supply to right
superior parathyroid adenoma

FIGURE 107–6. Attention is returned to the right side, where the right upper parathyroid adenoma is carefully dissected from the surrounding tissues with a fine Hoyt clamp. The adenoma is submitted to the pathologist for weight and histologic examination. A biopsy of the normal right lower gland also is obtained. All remaining normal glands are always marked with a suture.

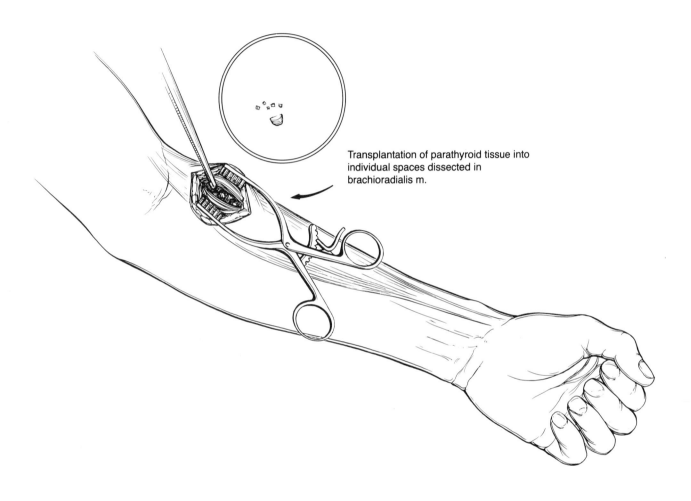

Transplantation of parathyroid tissue into
individual spaces dissected in
brachioradialis m.

FIGURE 107–7. If two or three parathyroid glands are abnormal, they are removed; a biopsy of the normal gland(s) is performed, and they are marked with a suture and left in place. If all four parathyroid glands are abnormal, the surgeon must decide whether to perform subtotal (3.5 glands) parathyroidectomy or total parathyroidectomy with autotransplantation. If the latter is chosen, 15 to 20 slivers of parathyroid tissue are implanted into individual pockets in the brachioradialis muscle of the nondominant forearm. Each pocket is closed with a single nonabsorbable suture to secure the tissue in place and mark its position.

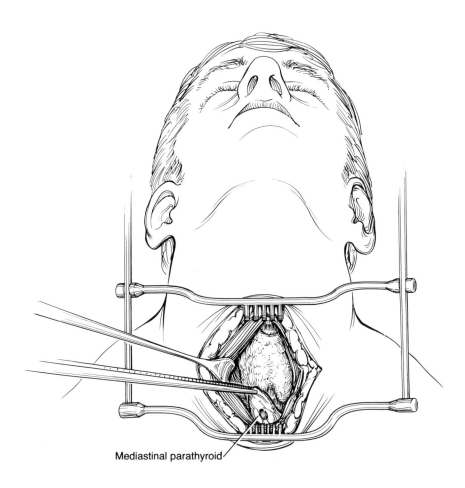

Mediastinal parathyroid

FIGURE 107–8. Parathyroid adenomas are frequently found in the thymus. Even when these intrathymic adenomas are in the superior mediastinum, they can usually be mobilized through a cervical incision and brought to the neck for removal.

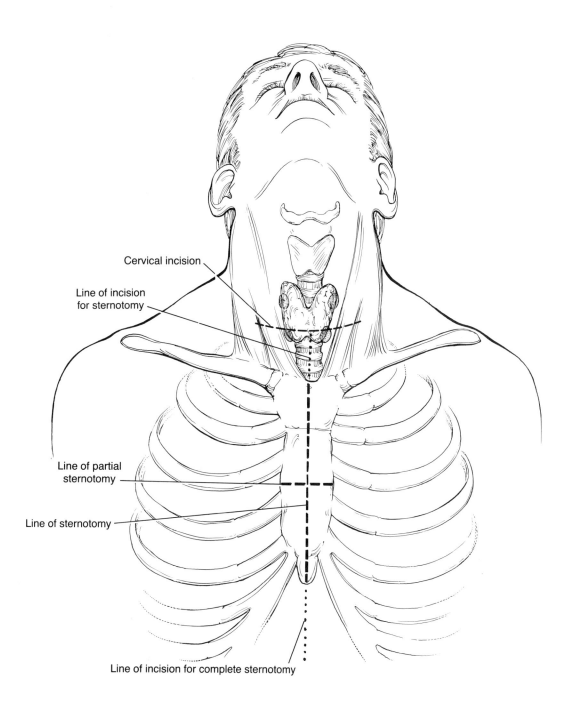

Cervical incision

Line of incision
for sternotomy

Line of partial
sternotomy

Line of sternotomy

Line of incision for complete sternotomy

FIGURE 107–9. A median sternotomy is sometimes necessary for mediastinal parathyroid adenomas that cannot be reached through a cervical incision. Partial sternotomy to the level of the third intercostal space may provide adequate exposure of the superior mediastinum. For exploration of the entire mediastinum, a complete sternotomy is needed.

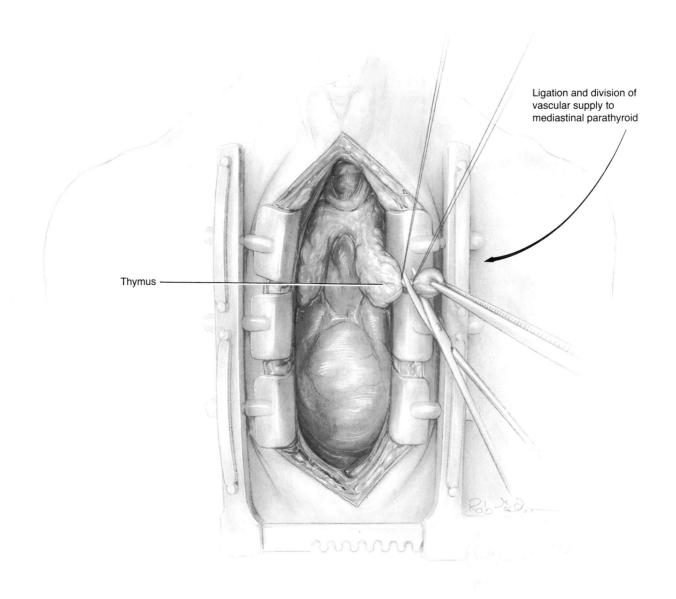

Thymus

Ligation and division of
vascular supply to
mediastinal parathyroid

FIGURE 107–10. The divided sternum is retracted laterally, allowing exposure of the thymus and other mediastinal structures. The recurrent and phrenic nerves should be identified and protected. A careful search can then be conducted, and the mediastinal parathyroid adenoma resected.

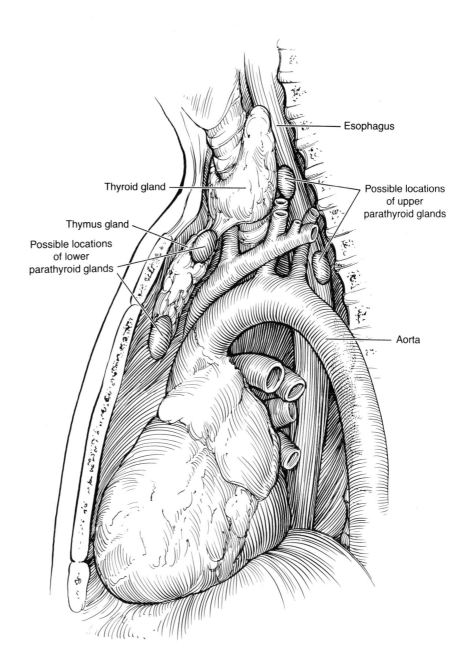

Esophagus

Thyroid gland

Possible locations
of upper
parathyroid glands

Thymus gland

Possible locations
of lower
parathyroid glands

Aorta

FIGURE 107–11. The most common ectopic locations of parathyroid adenomas are depicted. When a lower parathyroid gland is absent, it can usually be located in the thymus or surrounding perithymic tissues. When an upper gland is absent, it is usually situated within the posterior mediastinum. (Drawn after L. Schlossberg.)

108

Excision of Benign Adrenal Neoplasm
(POSTERIOR ADRENALECTOMY, RIGHT)

GEORGE S. LEIGHT, JR., M.D.

Posterior adrenalectomy is the preferred approach for the management of small functioning and nonfunctioning adrenal tumors. Pheochromocytomas, because of the possibility of multiple or extra-adrenal tumors, and large adrenal tumors, when malignancy is suspected, should be resected by a transabdominal approach to permit wide exposure and complete resection. The posterior approach avoids potential injury to the intra-abdominal organs, and postoperative ileus is usually minimal. The procedure is better accepted by patients because they experience less pain and can be discharged from the hospital more quickly than those who undergo transabdominal procedures.

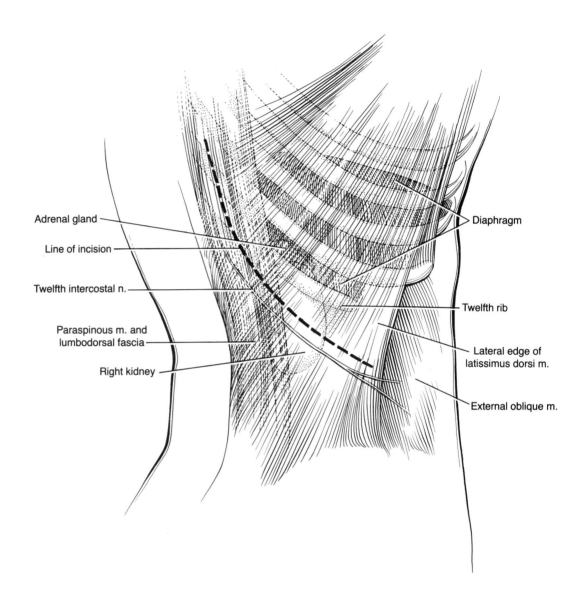

Adrenal gland

Line of incision

Twelfth intercostal n.

Paraspinous m. and
lumbodorsal fascia

Right kidney

Diaphragm

Twelfth rib

Lateral edge of
latissimus dorsi m.

External oblique m.

FIGURE 108–1. The patient is anesthetized and placed in the prone position, with rolled pillows placed beneath the chest and pelvis. The incision is started over the eleventh rib two to three fingerbreadths lateral to the midline and is extended in a curvilinear manner to a point below the tip of the twelfth rib.

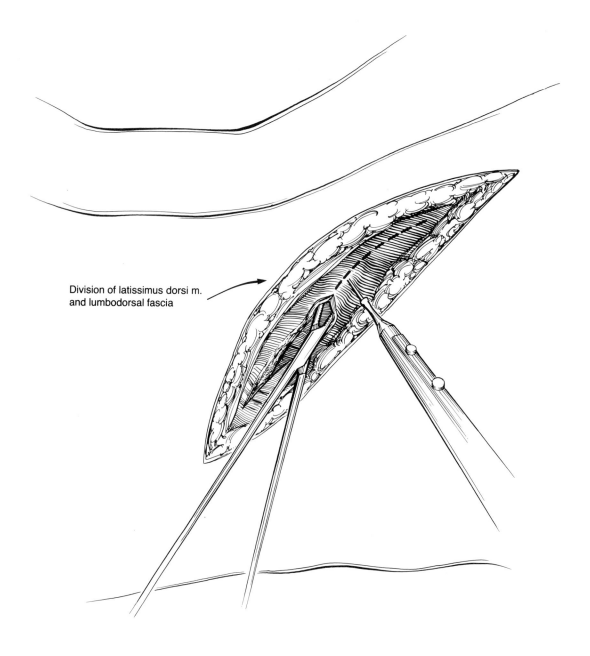

Division of latissimus dorsi m.
and lumbodorsal fascia

FIGURE 108–2. The incision is extended through the posterior lamella of the lumbodorsal fascia and the fibers of the latissimus dorsi muscle. The paraspinal (erector spinae) muscles can then be retracted medially, exposing the twelfth rib.

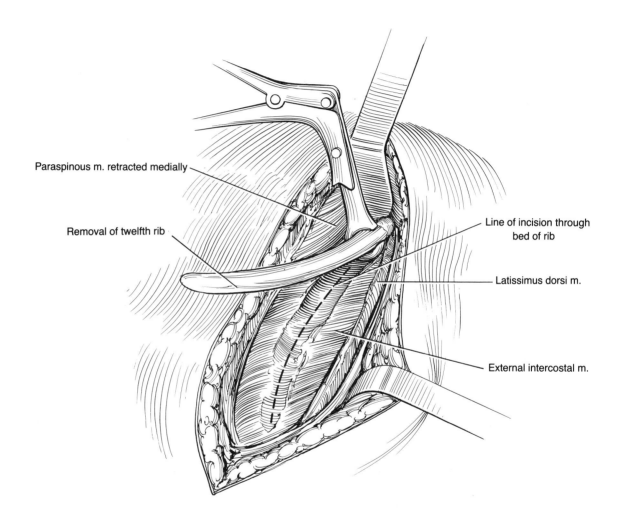

Paraspinous m. retracted medially

Removal of twelfth rib

Line of incision through
bed of rib

Latissimus dorsi m.

External intercostal m.

FIGURE 108–3. The twelfth rib is mobilized as far medially as possible and is resected. The inferior extent of the pleura can be determined by having the anesthesiologist inflate the lung, which slides down to the inferior margin of the pleura. The lumbodorsal fascia and Gerota's fascia are then divided, with care being taken to remain approximately 1 cm. below the pleura. The intercostal nerve, which lies inferior to the bed of the rib, should be protected.

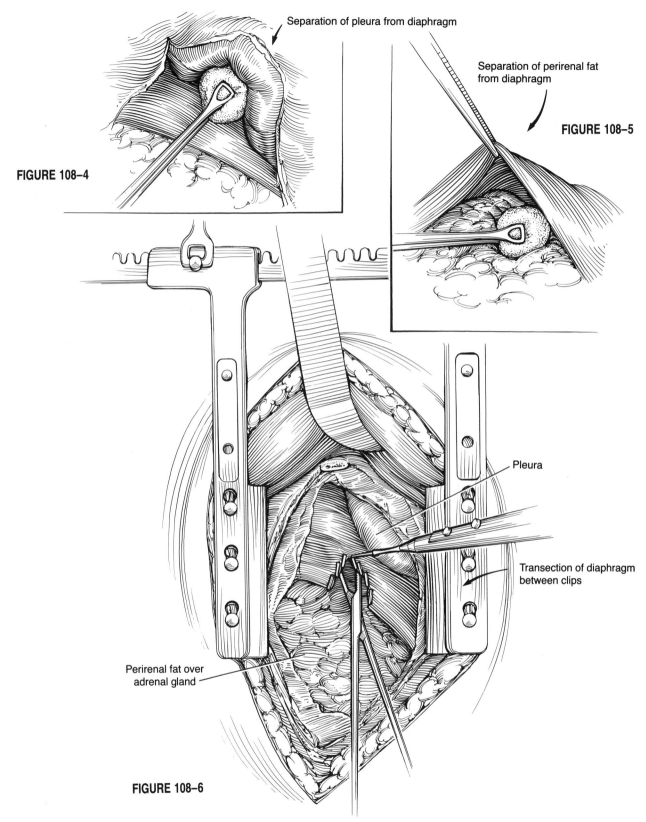

Separation of pleura from diaphragm

FIGURE 108–4

Separation of perirenal fat
from diaphragm

FIGURE 108–5

Pleura

Transection of diaphragm
between clips

Perirenal fat over
adrenal gland

FIGURE 108–6

FIGURES 108–4 to 108–6. The posterior fibers of the diaphragm, which insert into the periosteum of the twelfth rib, are separated from the pleura. This muscular insertion of the diaphragm is divided between clips, allowing the pleura to be retracted upward. A small tear in the pleura can be closed with sutures.

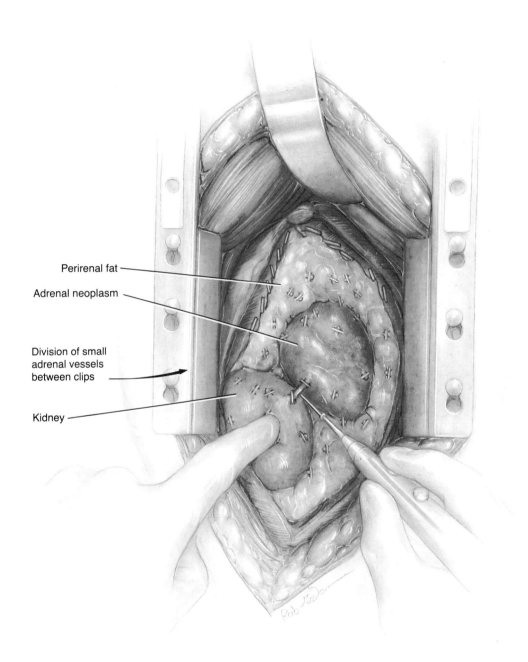

Perirenal fat

Adrenal neoplasm

Division of small
adrenal vessels
between clips

Kidney

FIGURE 108–7. The kidney is retracted inferiorly and laterally. Gentle blunt dissection is used to expose the adrenal tumor. Beginning laterally, one should mobilize the small vessels entering the adrenal tumor with a fine right-angle clamp, clip them on the parietal side, and divide them with the electrocautery. Larger vessels are clipped on both sides. The dissection is extended around the superior and inferior aspects of the tumor. The anterior surface can usually be mobilized with gentle blunt dissection.

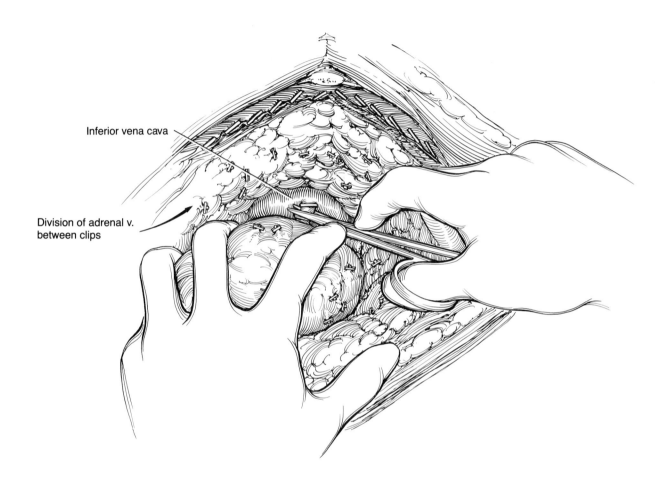

Inferior vena cava

Division of adrenal v.
between clips

FIGURE 108–8. The tumor can now be retracted laterally to expose the small vessels and the adrenal vein, which, on the right side, enters directly into the vena cava. After all the other small vessels have been divided, the adrenal vein can be divided between clips or ligatures if it is of sufficient length.

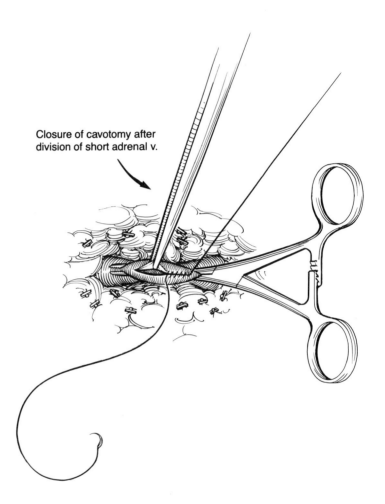

Closure of cavotomy after
division of short adrenal v.

FIGURE 108–9. If the adrenal vein is very short, a vascular clamp is applied to occlude the vena cava partially; the adrenal vein is divided, and the vena cava is closed with 3-0 or 4-0 Prolene sutures.

The lumbodorsal fascia is closed to the lateral aspect of the paraspinal muscles with absorbable sutures. The latissimus dorsi and posterior lumbodorsal fasciae are closed with nonabsorbable sutures, and the skin is closed with surgical clips. A chest x-ray film is obtained postoperatively to check for pneumothorax.

109

Total Adrenalectomy (ANTERIOR)

GEORGE S. LEIGHT, JR., M.D.

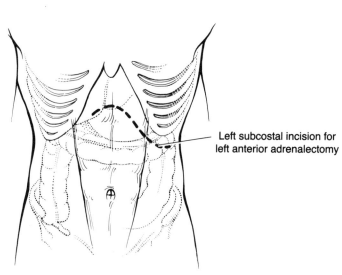

FIGURE 109–1. The anterior approach to the left adrenal is performed via a left subcostal incision, which can be extended across the midline for additional exposure.

Left subcostal incision for left anterior adrenalectomy

FIGURE 109–3

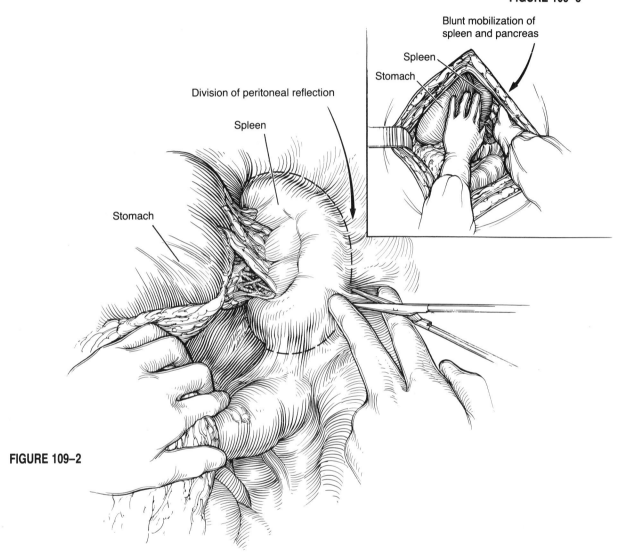

Blunt mobilization of
spleen and pancreas

Spleen

Stomach

Division of peritoneal reflection

Spleen

Stomach

FIGURE 109–2

FIGURES 109–2 and 109–3. The left adrenal gland can be approached by entering the lesser sac and mobilizing the pancreas superiorly or by mobilizing the spleen and tail of the pancreas medially. The latter method involves a higher risk of splenic injury but provides wider exposure of the left adrenal gland and is of particular importance when the tumor is large. The stomach is decompressed with a nasogastric tube, and the splenic flexure is mobilized inferiorly. The peritoneum at the posterolateral aspect of the spleen is divided with scissors, and small vessels are electrocoagulated. The spleen is carefully mobilized medially by a combination of sharp and blunt dissection. The tail of the pancreas is carefully retracted medially with the spleen.

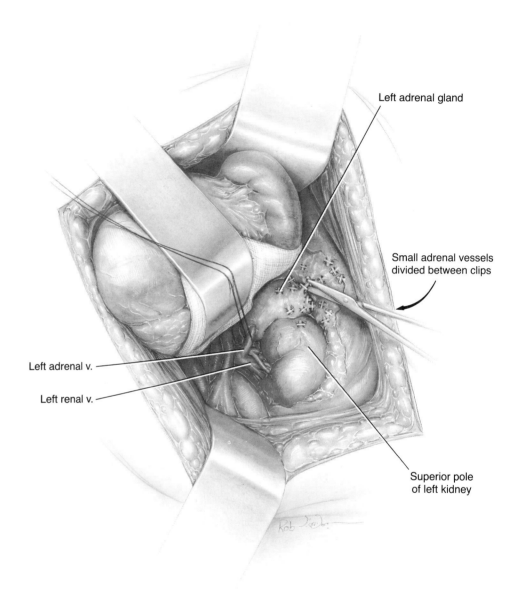

Left adrenal gland

Small adrenal vessels
divided between clips

Left adrenal v.

Left renal v.

Superior pole
of left kidney

FIGURE 109–4. The spleen is covered with a moist gauze pad and retracted medially. The kidney and left adrenal are exposed. For a large adrenal tumor, dissection is begun laterally and continued around the superior and inferior aspects of the mass. Small veins are clipped on the parietal side and coagulated on the adrenal side. Large veins or arteries necessitate clips on both sides. The tumor can then be retracted laterally to expose the multiple small arteries and the adrenal vein for ligation and division. When the operation is being performed for pheochromocytoma, the adrenal vein is identified and ligated as the first step to diminish catecholamine efflux into the systemic circulation.

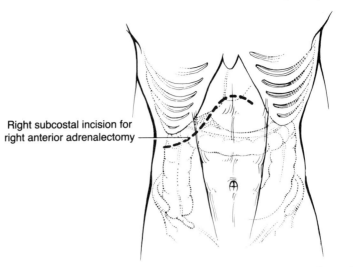

Right subcostal incision for
right anterior adrenalectomy

FIGURE 109–5. The right adrenal gland is approached through a right subcostal incision, which is extended across the midline for additional exposure.

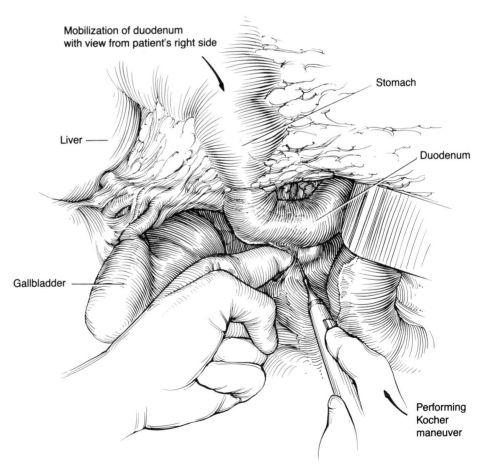

Mobilization of duodenum
with view from patient's right side

Stomach

Liver

Duodenum

Gallbladder

Performing
Kocher
maneuver

FIGURE 109–6. The duodenum is mobilized by dividing the peritoneum just lateral to its lateral margin. The attachments of the liver to the posterior peritoneal surface are sharply divided, and the liver is then retracted superiorly.

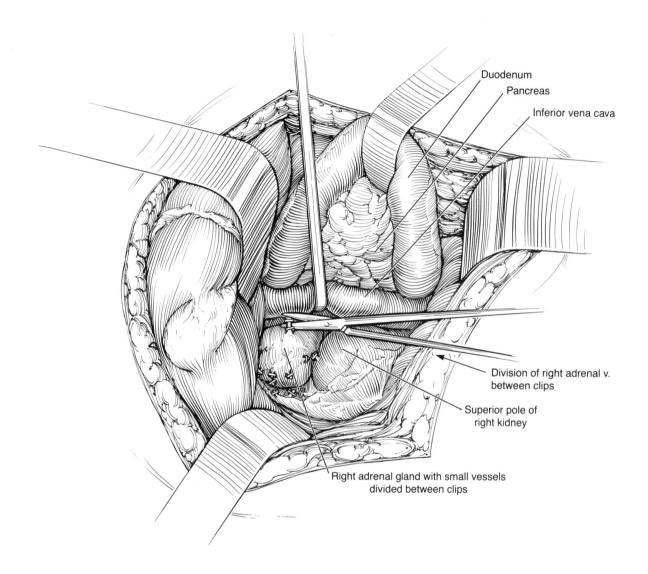

Duodenum

Pancreas

Inferior vena cava

Division of right adrenal v.
between clips

Superior pole of
right kidney

Right adrenal gland with small vessels
divided between clips

FIGURE 109–7. The right kidney, vena cava, and right adrenal vein can now be visualized. The peritoneum overlying the adrenal is sharply divided. The lateral, inferior, and superior aspects of the tumor are mobilized as described for the left adrenal. The adrenal vein is quite short on the right side, and lateral retraction of the tumor and medial retraction of the vena cava provide the best exposure. If the adrenal vein is of sufficient length, it can be doubly clipped or ligated. If the adrenal vein is very short, a curved vascular clamp should be applied to the vena cava before division of the vein. The divided end of the adrenal vein is oversewn with 4-0 Prolene at the site where it enters the vena cava. Drains are not ordinarily used unless the tumor is quite large or unless extensive dissection of lymphatics has been necessary.

110

Parotidectomy

SAMUEL R. FISHER, M.D.

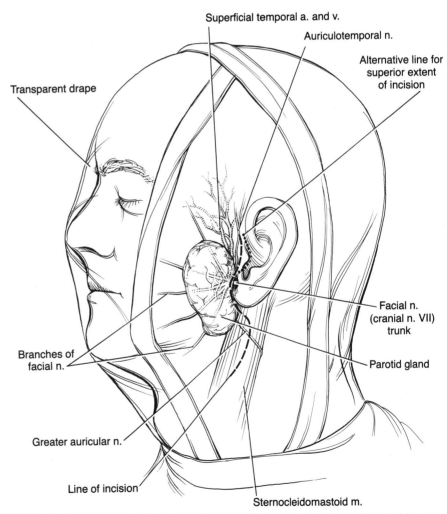

FIGURE 110–1. The standard incision for parotidectomy is in the relaxed skin tension crease in the preauricular sulcus. The incision courses under the lobule, sweeping gently posteriorly and then paralleling the midportion of the sternocleidomastoid muscle. An alternative incision would be hidden along the border of the tragus and extended under the lobule and over the sternocleidomastoid muscle.

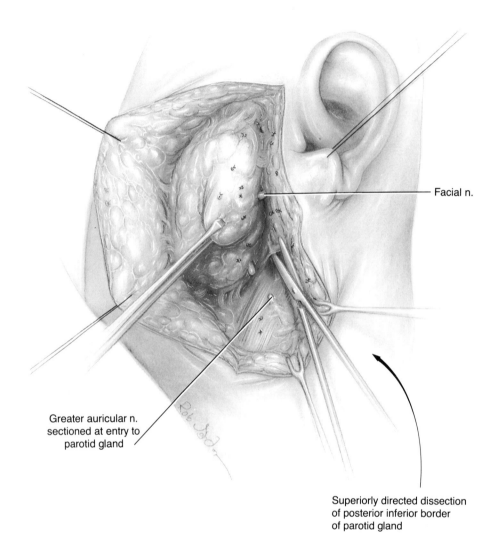

Facial n.

Greater auricular n.
sectioned at entry to
parotid gland

Superiorly directed dissection
of posterior inferior border
of parotid gland

FIGURE 110–2. An anterior skin flap is elevated in the subcuticular plane to the midface level, and a posterior flap is lifted to the superior border of the sternocleidomastoid muscle. Care should be taken not to dissect the skin flap too thin, especially in males because damage to the hair follicles may follow, causing alopecia. If the flap is too thick, the capsule of the parotid gland can be penetrated. The greater auricular nerve is identified along the anterior border of the sternocleidomastoid muscle and sectioned as it enters the gland on its inferior surface.

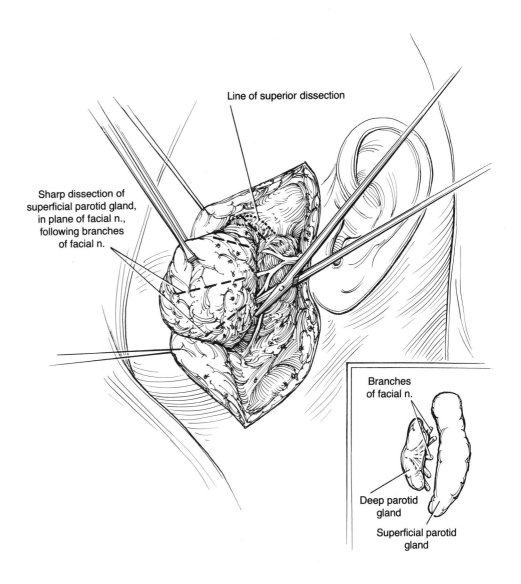

Line of superior dissection

Sharp dissection of
superficial parotid gland,
in plane of facial n.,
following branches
of facial n.

Branches
of facial n.

Deep parotid
gland

Superficial parotid
gland

FIGURE 110–3. The trunk of the facial nerve is identified as it exits the base of the skull at the stylomastoid foramen. This is adjacent to the styloid process and inferomedial to the stylomastoid structures. A common method of locating the nerve trunk involves tracing the anterior cartilaginous border of the ear inferiorly with the ''pointer'' cartilage as a guide. This method can be cumbersome but is facilitated if the tail and inferior body of the parotid gland are first separated from the sternocleidomastoid muscle. This greatly widens the field and provides exposure of the facial nerve trunk. The greater auricular nerve is divided, and the tail and inferior aspect of the parotid gland are dissected free from the border of the sternocleidomastoid muscle.

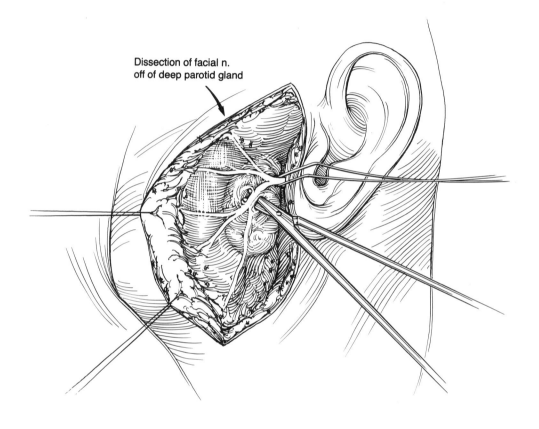

Dissection of facial n.
off of deep parotid gland

FIGURE 110–4. Once the trunk of the facial nerve has been identified and/or confirmed with a facial nerve stimulator, the superficial lobe is removed lateral to each facial nerve branch. This is done by tracing each branch distally, which allows transection of the parotid tissue between each branch without risk to the nerves. Once all facial nerve branches have been identified and traced distally into the face, the superficial lobe is removed. It should be noted that, especially in the frontozygomatic and orbital branches, the nerve is oftentimes tortuous and relatively superficial. Great care must be taken in dissecting these branches to prevent accidental transection. The nerve is most superficial just adjacent to the zygomatic arch. The entire gland should be removed peripherally in order to prevent parotid tissue from remaining laterally.

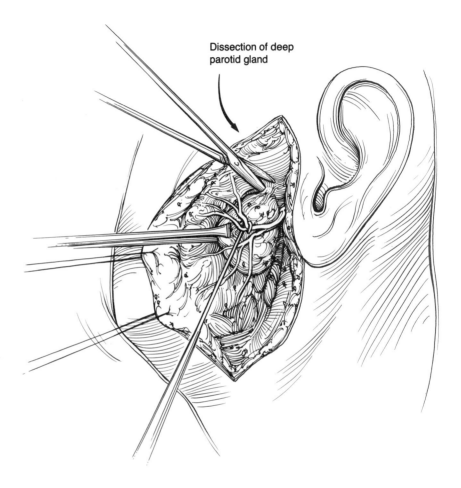

Dissection of deep
parotid gland

FIGURE 110–5. The deep lobe of the parotid gland is resected by mobilizing the entire
facial nerve branches and resecting the medial remaining parotid tissue. Gentle traction
of the facial nerve with a blunt nerve hook or blunt retractors assists in removing the
deep tissue. Meticulous care should be taken in the traction on the facial nerves during
the dissection to prevent iatrogenic trauma and neuropraxia. Although sacrifice of
individual branches should be at the discretion of the surgeon, it is generally required
only with neural invasion by malignant tumor. The optimal time for facial nerve grafting
is at the time of the initial operation.

Gynecology

111

Abdominal Hysterectomy

DANIEL CLARKE-PEARSON, M.D.

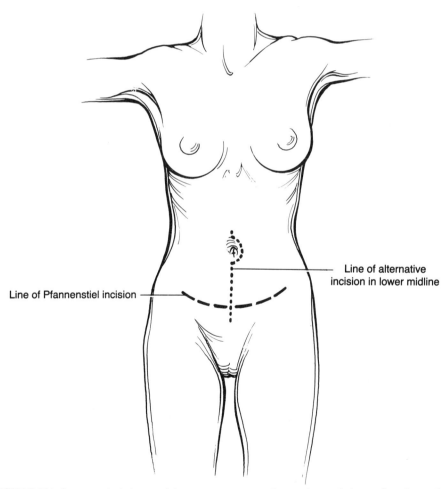

FIGURE 111–1. A total abdominal hysterectomy may be performed through either a low midline incision or a transverse Pfannenstiel incision. The selection of the surgical incision depends on several factors, including the patient's habitus and the extent of exposure required to perform the hysterectomy and associated procedures such as pelvic and para-aortic lymphadenectomy.

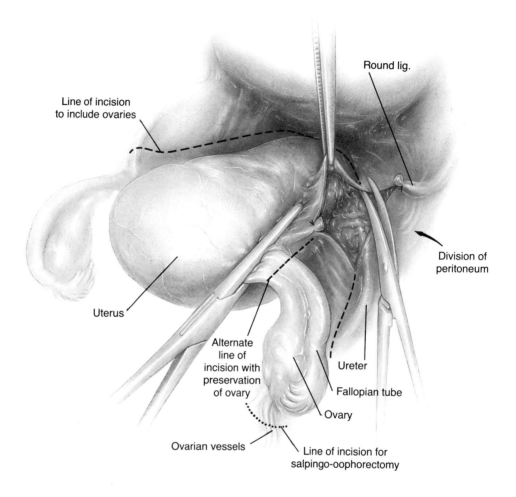

Round lig.

Line of incision
to include ovaries

Division of
peritoneum

Uterus

Alternate
line of
incision with
preservation
of ovary

Ureter

Fallopian tube

Ovary

Ovarian vessels

Line of incision for
salpingo-oophorectomy

FIGURE 111–2. The abdomen and pelvis should be explored, and, after adequate exposure is obtained by packing the small intestine out of the pelvis, the uterus is grasped across the round ligament and fallopian tube, near the uterine cornu, to elevate the uterus and manipulate it during the surgical procedure. The round ligament is ligated and divided. The peritoneum of the broad ligament is incised toward the cervix, dividing the peritoneum at the juncture between the bladder and the cervix. The peritoneum is also incised caudad parallel to the external iliac artery. If the fallopian tube and ovary are to be removed along with the uterus, the ovarian vessels proximal to the ovary should be isolated, clamped, divided, and ligated. Care must be taken to identify the ureter so that it is not incorporated in this clamp. Once the ovarian vessels have been ligated, the posterior leaf of the broad ligament may be incised beneath the fallopian tube, extending this incision toward the uterus.

If the fallopian tube and ovary are to be retained, the proximal fallopian tube and the utero-ovarian vessels should be clamped, divided, and suture-ligated. The bladder is mobilized from its loose attachments to the cervix and upper vagina by a process of blunt and sharp dissection.

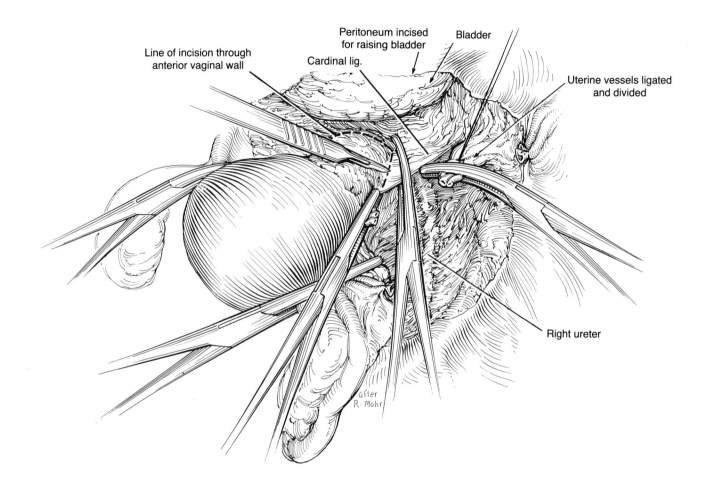

Line of incision through
anterior vaginal wall

Peritoneum incised
for raising bladder

Cardinal lig.

Bladder

Uterine vessels ligated
and divided

Right ureter

after
R. Mohr

FIGURE 111–3. The uterine vessels are clamped adjacent to the upper cervix, divided, and suture-ligated. The author prefers 2-0 Vicryl for all sutures and ligatures. All clamps should be placed immediately adjacent to the uterus to avoid injury to the ureter, which courses in the paracervical tissue approximately 1 to 2 cm. lateral to the cervix and upper vagina. The cardinal ligament is likewise clamped next to the cervix, divided, and suture-ligated. The bladder must be continually advanced off the lower cervix and upper vagina until the cervicovaginal junction is encountered. The lateral vaginal "angle" should be clamped and the vagina incised at its junction with the cervix. The uterus and cervix may then be handed off the operating field.

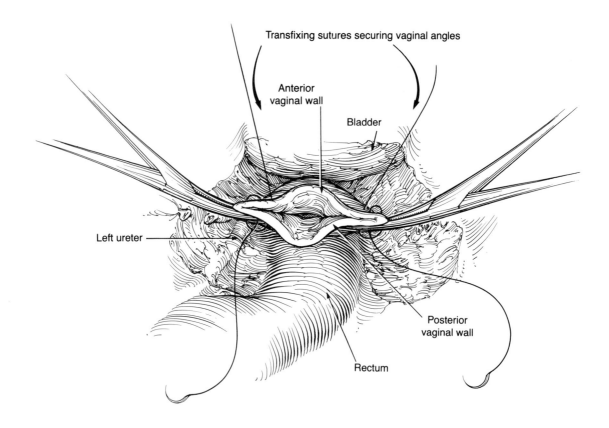

FIGURE 111–4. The vaginal angles are secured with transfixing sutures using a 2-0 or 1-0 Vicryl suture. The remainder of the vaginal cuff may be closed with figure-of-eight sutures or, where drainage of the deep pelvis is required because of infection, the vaginal margins may be secured with a continuous figure-of-eight suture, leaving the central vaginal cuff open for drainage. The peritoneum of the bladder flap is reapproximated with the vaginal cuff and the peritoneum adjacent to the posterior vaginal cuff and rectum. Unless infection is present, closed suction drainage of the vaginal cuff or pelvis is not required.

112

Salpingectomy-Oophorectomy

DANIEL CLARKE-PEARSON, M.D.

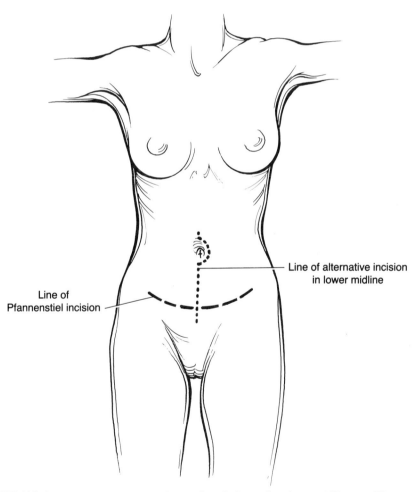

FIGURE 112–1. The abdomen may be explored through a low midline or Pfannenstiel incision. Selection of incisions depends on the patient's habitus and the expected disease. When ovarian carcinoma is suspected, the low midline incision is most appropriate because it allows extension of the incision into the upper abdomen to perform an omentectomy, a para-aortic lymphadenectomy, and tumor debulking from the upper abdomen.

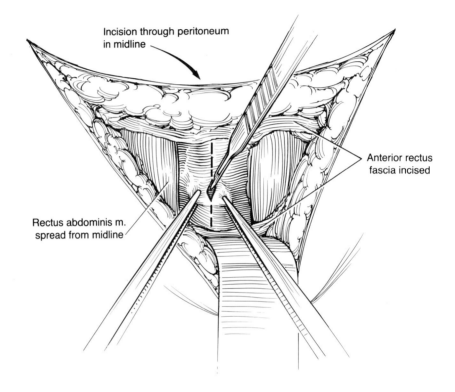

Incision through peritoneum
in midline

Anterior rectus
fascia incised

Rectus abdominis m.
spread from midline

FIGURE 112–2. The Pfannenstiel incision is most appropriate for premenopausal women who are slender or of average habitus and are suspected of having a benign adnexal mass. The incision is made approximately 3 cm. above the pubic ramus and extends laterally, with a gentle curve cephalad extending toward the anterior iliac crest. The length of the incision depends on the required exposure. The rectus fascia is incised transversely and mobilized cephalad and caudad from its attachments to the rectus muscle. The peritoneum is incised between the two rectus bellies, with care being taken to avoid injury to the bladder in the lower part of the incision.

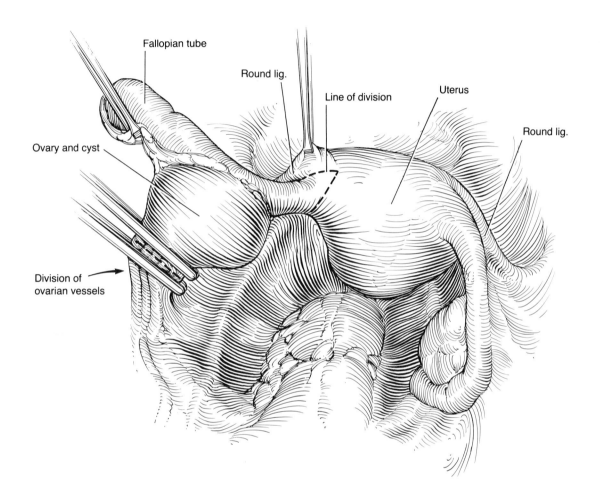

Fallopian tube

Round lig.

Line of division

Uterus

Round lig.

Ovary and cyst

Division of
ovarian vessels

FIGURE 112–3. The abdomen and pelvis should be explored, and the adnexal process identified. If there is suspicion of ovarian malignancy, peritoneal washings should be obtained from the pelvis and upper abdomen and submitted for cytopathologic evaluation. A salpingo-oophorectomy may be performed in conjunction with a total abdominal hysterectomy (see Chapter 111). When the tube and ovary are to be removed and the uterus and contralateral tube and ovary remain, the ovarian vessels proximal to the ovary should be clamped, divided, and doubly ligated using a 2-0 synthetic absorbable suture. Care should be taken to avoid the ureter, which is located medial and inferior to the ovarian vessels. Once the ovarian vessels are secured, the peritoneum of the anterior and posterior leaves of the broad ligament is incised toward the uterine cornu. The junction of the fallopian tube and uterine cornu is then clamped, and the fallopian tube and utero-ovarian vascular anastomosis is divided and ligated with figure-of-eight sutures of 1-0 Vicryl.

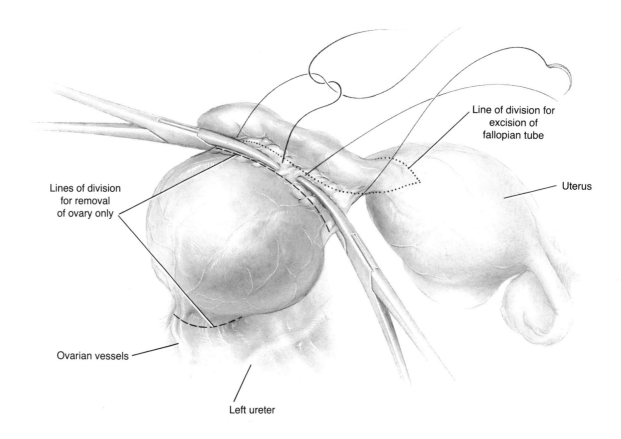

Line of division for
excision of
fallopian tube

Uterus

Lines of division
for removal
of ovary only

Ovarian vessels

Left ureter

FIGURE 112–4. When a benign ovarian cyst necessitates oophorectomy, the ipsilateral fallopian tube may be preserved to improve future fertility. In performing an oophorectomy, the ovarian vessels are divided and ligated. The mesosalpinx and utero-ovarian vascular supply is divided adjacent to the fallopian tube, and the pedicles are suture-ligated. Conversely, disease processes in the fallopian tube (such as a large, ruptured ectopic pregnancy) may be treated by salpingectomy with preservation of the ipsilateral ovary. In this figure, clamps are placed along the mesosalpinx, dividing the fallopian tube from the ovary, and the mesosalpinx is suture-ligated for hemostasis. The attachment of the fallopian tube to the uterus is transected, and figure-of-eight suture ligatures are used to secure hemostasis.

Transplantation of Organs

113

Kidney Transplantation

JOHN L. WEINERTH, M.D.

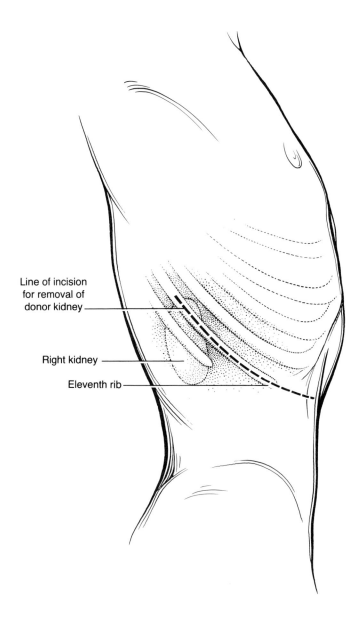

Line of incision
for removal of
donor kidney

Right kidney

Eleventh rib

FIGURE 113–1. Positioning of the patient for living donor nephrectomy is 30 degrees posterior to the true flank, allowing anterior and posterior access to the kidney. An incision is made over the tenth or eleventh rib, beginning at the anterior axillary line and directed horizontally from the tip of the rib to the rectus fascia. The external and internal oblique muscles are divided with the cautery. The transversalis muscles are separated in the line of their fibers after the anterior portion of the rib is resected subperiosteally, and the peritoneum is bluntly dissected away from the undersurface of the transversalis muscles.

Gerota's fascia is entered posteriorly in a vertical line, and all perinephric tissue is dissected from the anterior, posterior, and inferior surfaces of the kidney, exposing the hilum.

An alternative approach is a subcostal incision from the xiphoid to the tip of the twelfth rib and subsequent extraperitoneal dissection with the patient in the supine position.

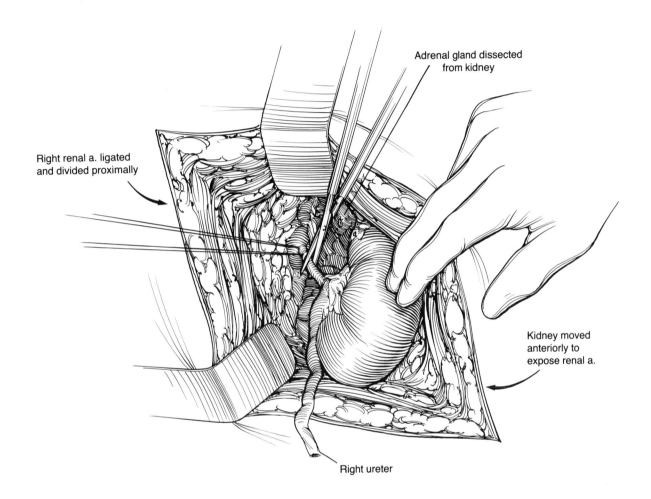

Adrenal gland dissected
from kidney

Right renal a. ligated
and divided proximally

Kidney moved
anteriorly to
expose renal a.

Right ureter

FIGURE 113–2. The adrenal gland is separated from the upper pole of the kidney. The ureter is dissected with a band of adventitia (to preserve the ureteral blood supply) to the level of the common iliac artery. The distal portion of the ureter is secured with a surgical clip or suture, and the ureter is divided.

After dissection of the renal artery and veins, including the anterior and posterior surfaces of the vena cava, the kidney is placed in a diuretic state with mannitol or furosemide and is ready to be removed.

The kidney is rotated anteriorly, and the renal artery is doubly ligated with 1-0 silk (a smaller suture, especially monofilament, may cut through the artery) and divided without clamps for maximal length.

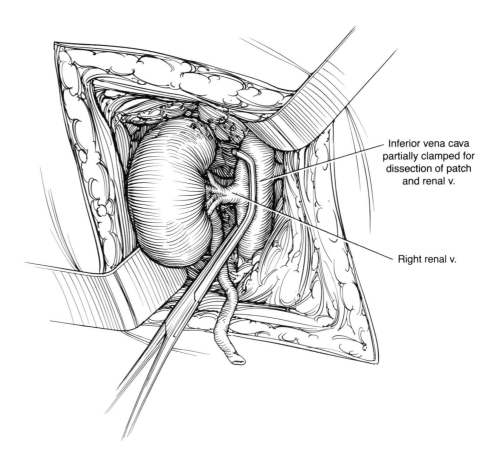

Inferior vena cava
partially clamped for
dissection of patch
and renal v.

Right renal v.

FIGURE 113–3. The kidney is rotated posteriorly (original position). A partially occluding Satinsky clamp is applied to the vena cava to permit a cuff of vena cava to be harvested with the renal vein, which is often thin and short. A back-up Satinsky clamp behind the first clamp is recommended. The cuff is divided, and the kidney is removed to another table for perfusion with cold preservative solution.

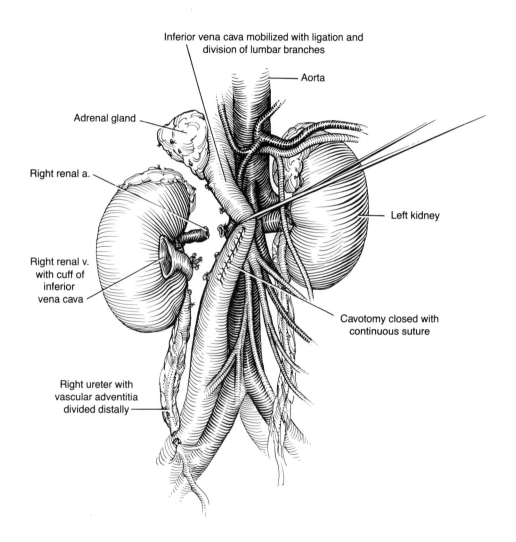

Inferior vena cava mobilized with ligation and division of lumbar branches

Aorta

Adrenal gland

Right renal a.

Right renal v. with cuff of inferior vena cava

Left kidney

Cavotomy closed with continuous suture

Right ureter with vascular adventitia divided distally

FIGURE 113–4. The opening in the vena cava is closed with a running 4-0 monofilament suture. Lumbar veins that impede the dissection should be doubly ligated with fine silk and divided to avoid avulsion during renal manipulation.

LINES OF DISSECTION FOR LEFT KIDNEY
FROM LIVING DONOR

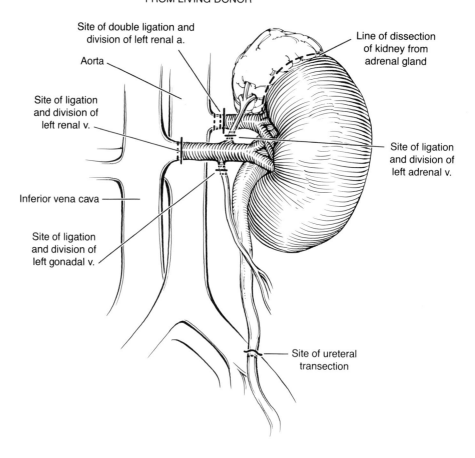

Site of double ligation and
division of left renal a.

Aorta

Site of ligation
and division of
left renal v.

Line of dissection
of kidney from
adrenal gland

Site of ligation
and division of
left adrenal v.

Inferior vena cava

Site of ligation
and division of
left gonadal v.

Site of ureteral
transection

FIGURE 113–5. The approach to the left kidney of the living donor is identical. The differences involve the dissection of the vein, which is much longer. Both the adrenal and the gonadal veins should be doubly ligated and divided for mobility and length of the renal vein.

It is very important to inspect the posterior aspect of the left renal vein for lumbar veins, which can be numerous and treacherous. They should be ligated and divided before full mobilization of the renal vein. The renal artery is doubly ligated and divided close to the aorta. By double ligation and division, a 5- to 6-cm. segment of left renal vein is provided.

CADAVERIC DONOR DISSECTION

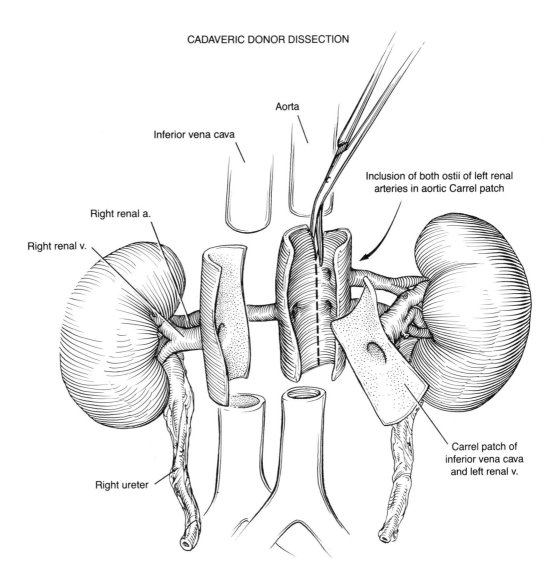

Aorta

Inferior vena cava

Inclusion of both ostii of left renal
arteries in aortic Carrel patch

Right renal a.

Right renal v.

Carrel patch of
inferior vena cava
and left renal v.

Right ureter

FIGURE 113–6. Cadaver donor kidneys are dissected *en bloc*, including the aorta, vena cava, and ureters with ample adventitia. However, because preoperative arteriograms are generally not obtained, the aorta and vena cava should be split anteriorly and posteriorly, producing large Carrel patches that may include secondary or tertiary arteries and veins.

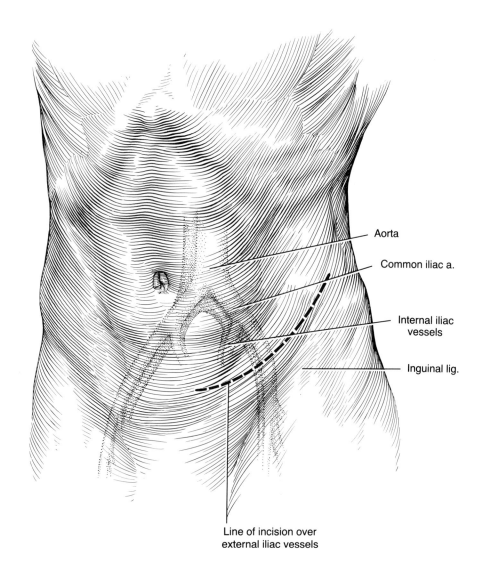

Aorta

Common iliac a.

Internal iliac
vessels

Inguinal lig.

Line of incision over
external iliac vessels

FIGURE 113–7. The recipient incision is made opposite to the side of the kidney harvested
so that the kidney can be turned front to back, thus shortening the distance needed for
the venous anastomosis. The incision is curvilinear, following the line of the inguinal
ligament but two to three fingerbreadths medial to it, extending from the midportion
of the rectus fascia to a point cephalad to the anterior superior iliac spine. All muscle
layers are divided, and the peritoneum is reflected medially, exposing the iliac vessels
and the anterior and lateral aspect of the bladder.

The round ligament can be ligated and divided. The spermatic cord, if it does not
seriously impede the operation, should be freed superiorly and inferiorly and retracted
laterally. At closure, the spermatic cord should be anterior to the kidney and ureter to
avoid ureteral obstruction. Preservation of the cord may have an impact on fertility and
possibly reduce the occurrence of a postoperative hydrocele.

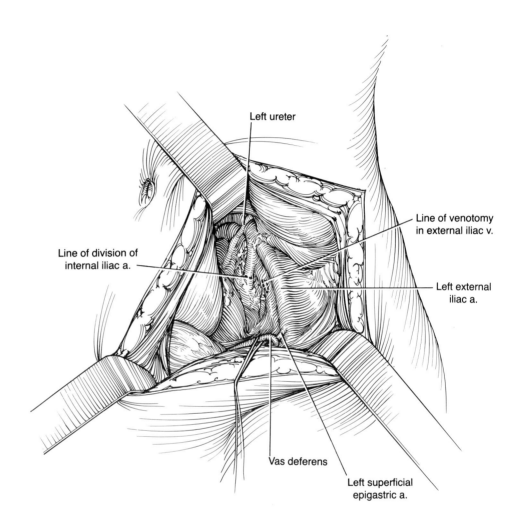

Left ureter

Line of venotomy
in external iliac v.

Line of division of
internal iliac a.

Left external
iliac a.

Vas deferens

Left superficial
epigastric a.

FIGURE 113–8. The pelvic vessels are mobilized, and any visible lymphatics are ligated with fine sutures to reduce the postoperative complication of lymphocele. The iliac vein should be adequately exposed and mobilized to select the proper position for anastomosis of the renal vein.

The internal iliac artery, as well as the bifurcation of the common iliac artery, should be fully dissected to allow some external rotation, avoiding kinking of the iliac artery at its origin. The distal dissection of the internal iliac artery is to the point where it divides into its several vesical arteries. The distal segment is secured with both a silk tie and a suture ligature.

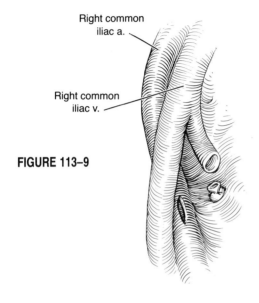

Right common
iliac a.

Right common
iliac v.

FIGURE 113-9

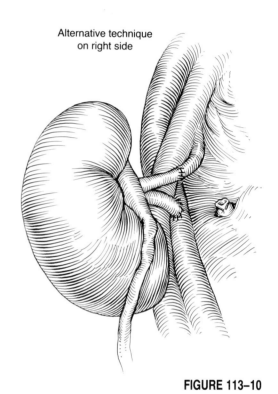

Alternative technique
on right side

FIGURE 113-10

FIGURE 113-9. Prior to division of the internal iliac artery, vascular clamps should be placed both proximally and distally on the iliac vein, proximally on the common iliac artery, and distally on the external iliac artery. If a sufficient length of internal iliac artery is present, a single clamp can be placed at the bifurcation of the common iliac artery.

FIGURE 113-10. The final position of the transplanted kidney is such that the posterior surface of the kidney, the ureter, and the renal pelvis is now anterior, the venous anastomosis is directed posterior from the renal hilum, and the renal artery crosses over the iliac vein to the internal iliac artery.

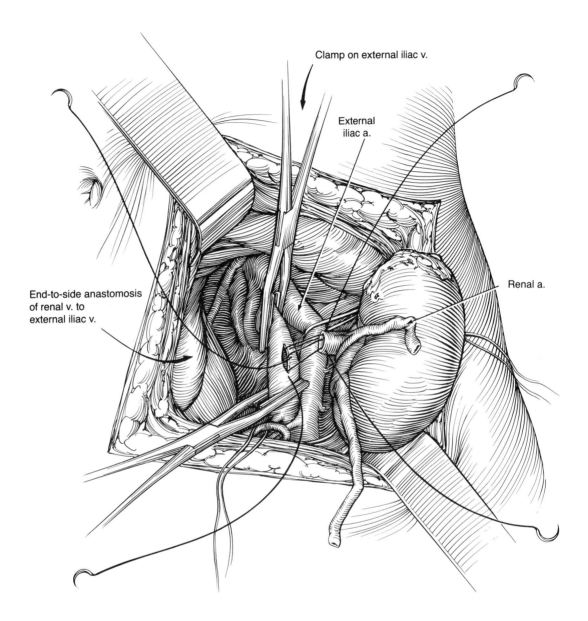

Clamp on external iliac v.

External
iliac a.

End-to-side anastomosis
of renal v. to
external iliac v.

Renal a.

FIGURE 113–11. The venous anastomosis is done first, and an adequate venotomy, most often in the form of an ellipse, is performed. The anastomosis begins on the posterior portion, followed by an anterior continuous suture.

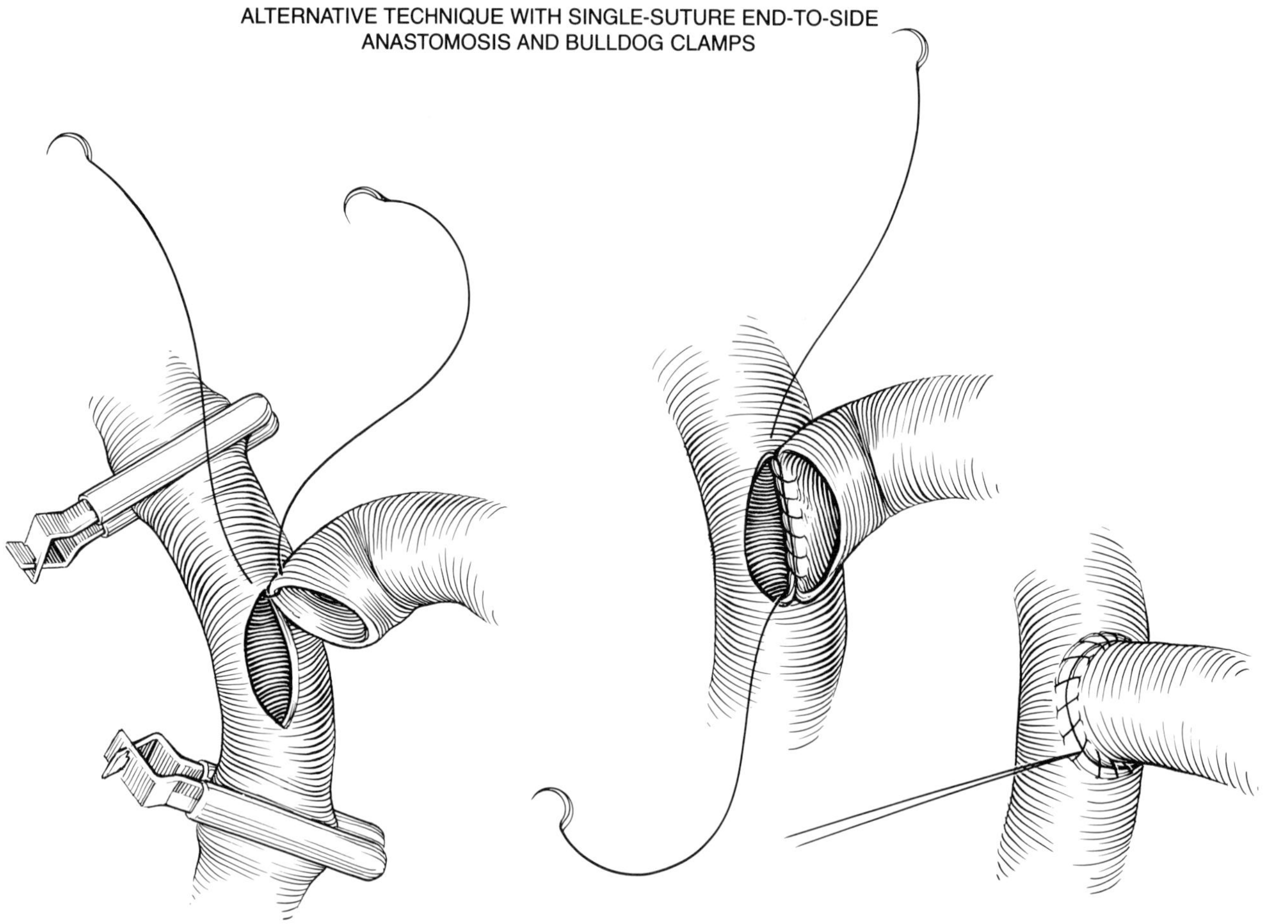

ALTERNATIVE TECHNIQUE WITH SINGLE-SUTURE END-TO-SIDE
ANASTOMOSIS AND BULLDOG CLAMPS

FIGURES 113–12 to 113–14. Variations include starting two sutures in the middle posteriorly and joining them anteriorly or using a single double-ended monofilament suture.

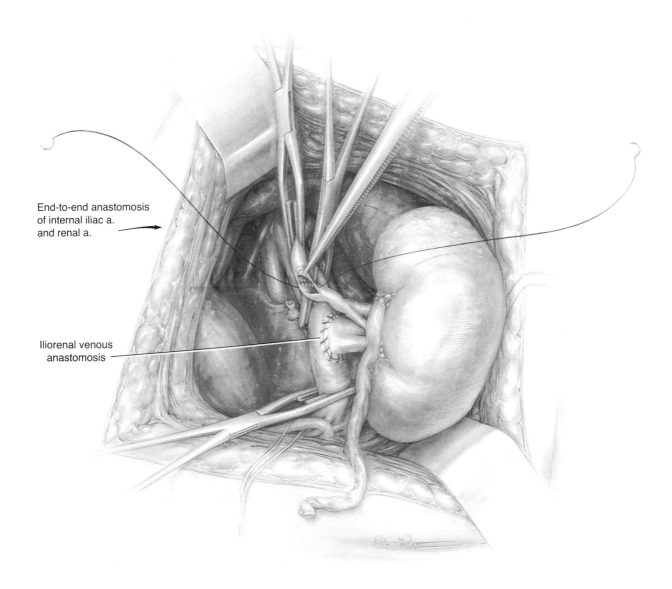

End-to-end anastomosis
of internal iliac a.
and renal a.

Iliorenal venous
anastomosis

FIGURE 113–15. The arterial anastomosis is performed next with a continuous monofilament suture, starting from the back and finishing and tying in front, or with two
sutures at the superior and inferior points, completing the back row first, joining the
second suture, and then completing the front row. When positioning the kidney, one
should take care that there is no angulation at the point of anastomosis.

ALTERNATIVE TECHNIQUE WITH END-TO-SIDE ANASTOMOSIS
OF RENAL A. AND EXTERNAL ILIAC A.

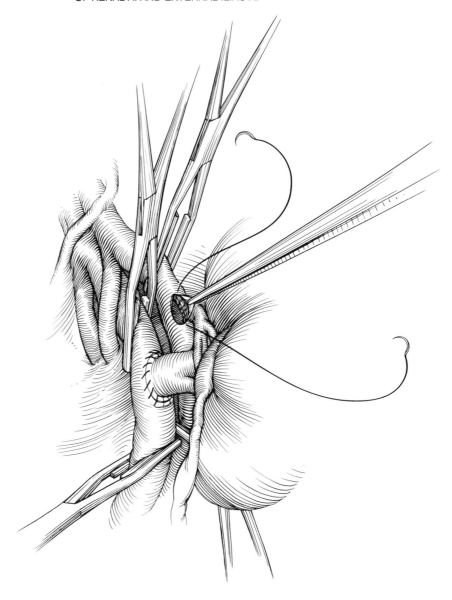

FIGURE 113–16. If the internal iliac artery or its origin from the common iliac artery is
diseased or the internal iliac artery is too short, an alternative arterial anastomosis can
be end-to-side with the external iliac artery.

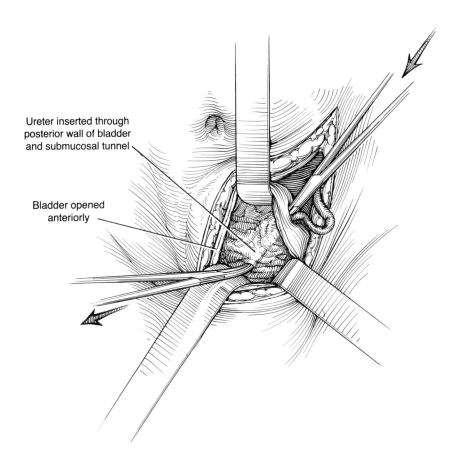

Ureter inserted through
posterior wall of bladder
and submucosal tunnel

Bladder opened
anteriorly

FIGURE 113–17. The ureter is anastomosed to the bladder by opening the bladder with an anterior, slightly lateral incision, exposing the *bas-fond*. An incision is made in the bladder mucosa medial to the native ipsilateral ureteral orifice, and, with a curved clamp, a 2.5-cm. submucosal tunnel is developed. The clamp is then exited obliquely through the bladder musculature to the paravesical space. The ureter is grasped and brought into the bladder without torsion, tension, or kinks.

A slight redundancy of the ureter is left outside the bladder to allow movement or positioning of the kidney. The ureter is sutured to the bladder at the point of mucosal entry with interrupted 4-0 chromic catgut through-and-through sutures. Ureteral stents are optional. The bladder is closed with mucosal, muscular, and serosal running chromic catgut sutures. If the spermatic cord is preserved, the ureter must run beneath it to avoid obstruction.

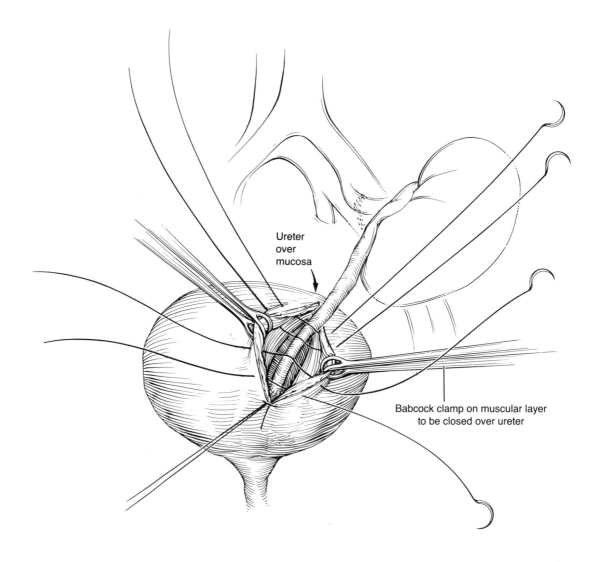

Ureter
over
mucosa

Babcock clamp on muscular layer
to be closed over ureter

FIGURE 113–18. An alternative technique is the extravesical approach. The bladder is
distended with saline via a Foley catheter placed in a sterile manner. The anterolateral
bladder serosa is opened in a straight line with the ureter. With sharp and blunt
dissection, the bladder musculature is separated to create a wide trough, the base of
which is the bulging bladder mucosa. An incision is made in the bladder mucosa in the
most distal aspect, and the ureter is sutured to the opening with interrupted chromic
catgut sutures. The ureter is placed in the trough, and the muscles are closed over the
ureters, starting distally. Care is taken not to compress the ureter excessively. To prevent
this occurrence, a small clamp can be inserted over the ureter as each suture is tied.

114

Liver Transplantation

WILLIAM C. MEYERS, M.D.

When the first liver transplants were performed, the operation was fraught with complications. With knowledge gained through experience, the operation has become a straightforward surgical procedure. The major reasons for this improvement are better patient selection, standardization of the procedure, and better control of bleeding. Better liver preservation also has led to improved liver transplants, and the operation can usually be done during the regular schedule. A smooth operation requires excellent teamwork by experienced nurses, skilled anesthesiologists, and perfusion teams.

There are essentially five determinants for an acceptable liver replacement: selection of the donor, the harvest procedure, warm or cold ischemia time, intraoperative anesthetic management, and the technical process of removal of the native liver and replacement with the transplant.

PERFUSION AND HARVEST OF DONOR LIVER

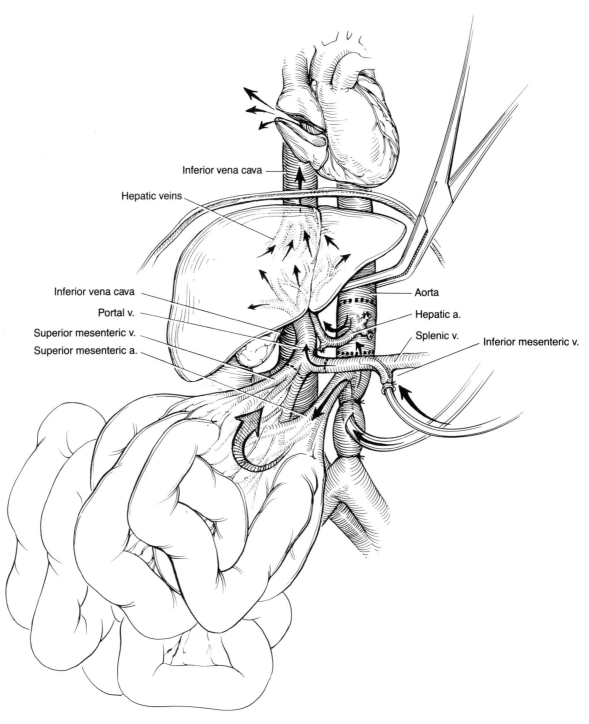

Inferior vena cava

Hepatic veins

Inferior vena cava

Portal v.

Superior mesenteric v.

Superior mesenteric a.

Aorta

Hepatic a.

Splenic v.

Inferior mesenteric v.

FIGURE 114–1 *See legend on opposite page*

FIGURE 114–1. Donor selection involves a number of considerations, including the size of the liver and ABO blood group compatibility. For both the *fast* and *slow* methods of harvest, a long midline incision with transverse extensions is used for exposure. The fast method refers to performing most of the dissection after perfusion of the cold preservation solution. The transverse incisions only extend several inches to maintain the cold solution within the abdominal cavity. The abdominal incision is extended as a median sternotomy whether or not the heart or lungs are harvested.

The liver is mobilized, and the aberrant ("replaced") right or left hepatic arteries are identified to prevent injury. A replaced right artery traverses posterior to the portal vein, and a replaced left artery arises from the left gastric artery and enters the left lobe of the liver beneath the left lateral segment. Later, the arteries are removed *en bloc* with a patch of aorta. The common bile duct is divided and either ligated or allowed to drain freely. At some point, the gallbladder is opened and the biliary system is irrigated with Belzer's solution. On a back table, the common duct is later perfused retrograde with the same solution.

The gastroduodenal, splenic, and gastric arteries are ligated and divided in a manner to provide a patch of aorta with the hepatic artery. If a replaced artery is present, the patch should include all of the aortic orifices necessary. The proximal aorta is encircled with an umbilical tape below the diaphragm, and the aorta is cannulated at or above the bifurcation with the iliac artery. The irrigant solution is vented through either the intra-abdominal vena cava, the atrium, or the inferior vena cava above the diaphragm. The latter is preferred unless the lungs are to be harvested. After the liver is mobilized, the portal vein is exposed to include the confluence of the splenic and superior mesenteric veins. The right renal vein is identified, and a cannula is placed into the portal system through the inferior mesenteric vein, which can easily be identified as it courses along the colonic mesentery near the ligament of Treitz.

As soon as the aorta is crossclamped in the chest (if the heart is to be taken) or below the diaphragm, both the arterial and the portal perfusions are begun. An incision is made in the inferior hepatic vena cava or right atrium for venting. Five liters of Belzer's solution are infused—3 liters into the aorta and 2 liters into the portal vein— and the liver is removed with long cuffs of the suprahepatic and infrahepatic vena cavae, the confluence of the portal vein, and the aortic patch. The common duct is divided with sufficient length for easy implantation but above the pancreas to preserve the hepatic arterial blood supply. The gallbladder is removed prior to implantation.

There are several other important points concerning the harvest. The abdominal cavity is filled with cold saline solution as soon as the aorta is crossclamped, and perfusion is begun. Continuous perfusion is important, as is monitoring, to be certain that proper venting and appropriate change in the color of the liver have occurred. In the event of a concomitant harvest of the heart, the liver is retracted inferiorly when the supradiaphragmatic vena cava is divided to ensure a reasonable cuff for the implantation. For a donor heart, the atrium is removed prior to cardiac transplantation. Some of the diaphragm is excised with the vena cava, and the liver is excised to prevent injury to the cava.

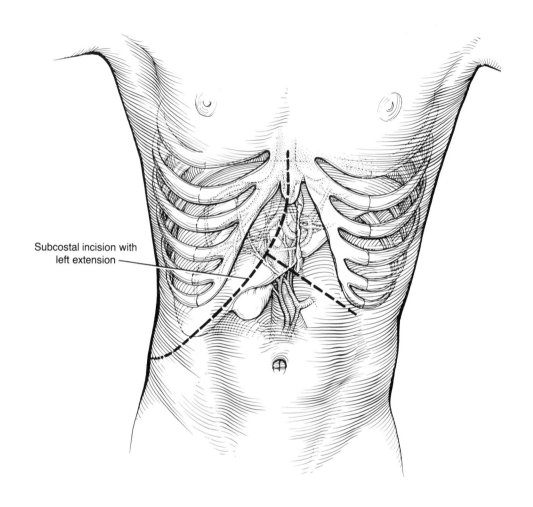

Subcostal incision with left extension

FIGURE 114–2. A liver transplant is performed through a generous right subcostal incision, extending approximately an inch above the xiphoid process and including the right gutter. A left subcostal extension completes the incision.

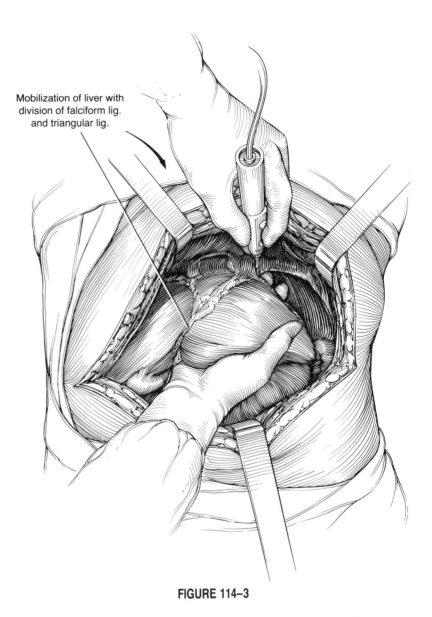

Mobilization of liver with
division of falciform lig.
and triangular lig.

FIGURE 114–3

FIGURE 114–3. The liver is completely mobilized as is done for an extensive hepatic resection.

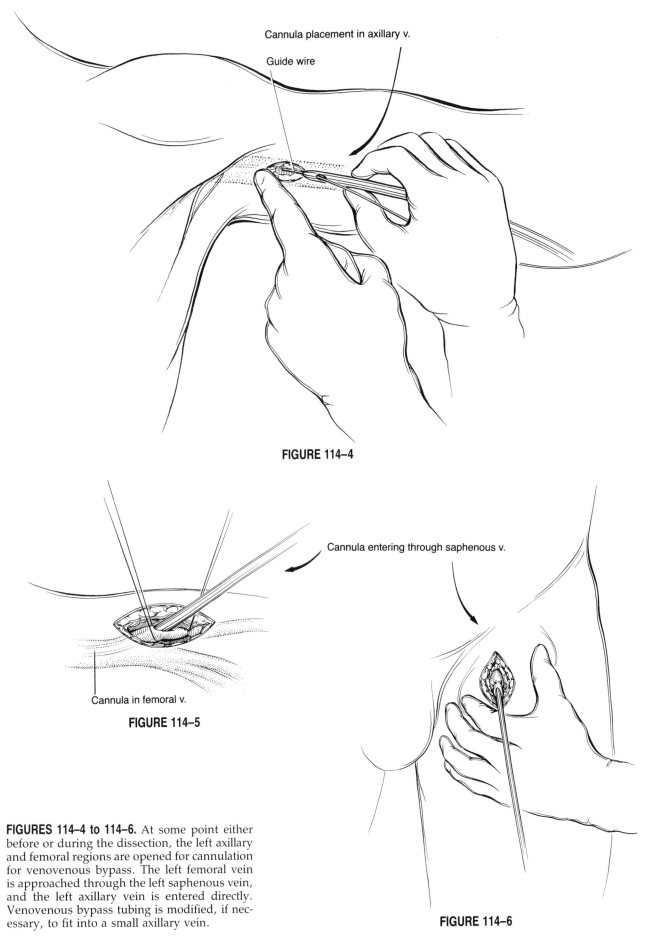

Cannula placement in axillary v.

Guide wire

FIGURE 114–4

Cannula entering through saphenous v.

Cannula in femoral v.

FIGURE 114–5

FIGURES 114–4 to 114–6. At some point either before or during the dissection, the left axillary and femoral regions are opened for cannulation for venovenous bypass. The left femoral vein is approached through the left saphenous vein, and the left axillary vein is entered directly. Venovenous bypass tubing is modified, if necessary, to fit into a small axillary vein.

FIGURE 114–6

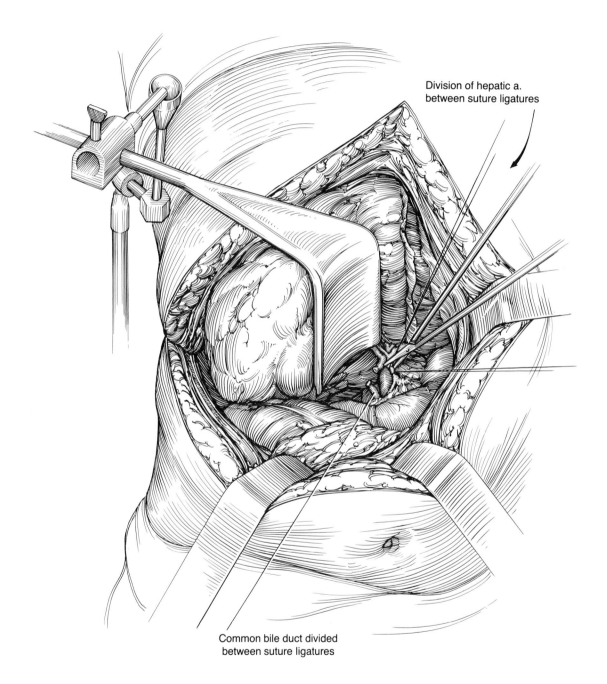

Division of hepatic a.
between suture ligatures

Common bile duct divided
between suture ligatures

FIGURE 114–7. Essentials of the portal dissection include *en bloc* ligation of the portal varices after identification of the key vessels, extensive use of cautery for the small varices, division of the common duct with an approximately 1-inch long stump, and ligation and division of the hepatic artery near the bifurcation, which is later trimmed. The hepatic arterial anastomosis is generally performed at the junction of the gastro-duodenal and hepatic arteries or to the aorta.

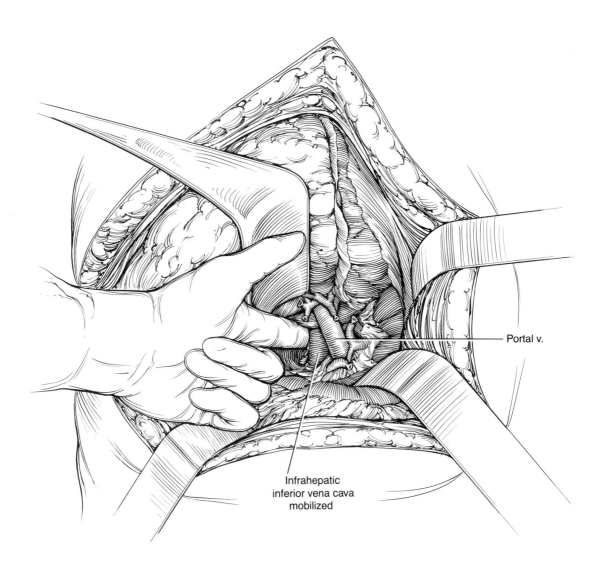

Portal v.

Infrahepatic
inferior vena cava
mobilized

FIGURE 114–8. Following division of the bile duct and hepatic artery, one can easily identify the portal vein. Adjacent lymphatic, neural, and other tissues are divided, and a generous length of portal vein is dissected.

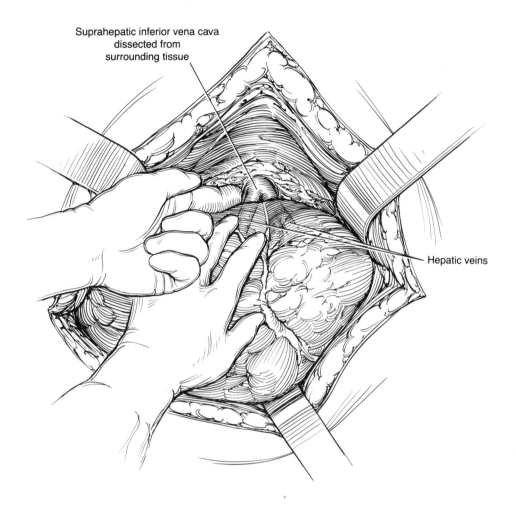

Suprahepatic inferior vena cava
dissected from
surrounding tissue

Hepatic veins

FIGURE 114–9. The key parts of the suprahepatic and infrahepatic vena caval dissections are usually reserved until after the portal dissection. A portion of diaphragm is usually left with the suprahepatic vena cava.

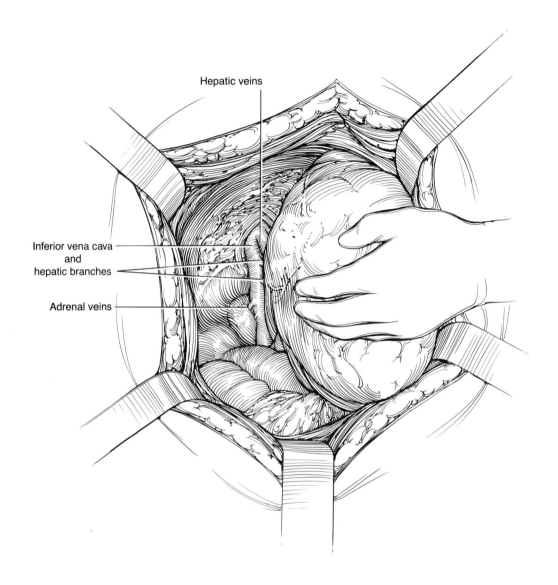

FIGURE 114–10. The infrahepatic vena cava is dissected between the adrenal and the
renal veins.

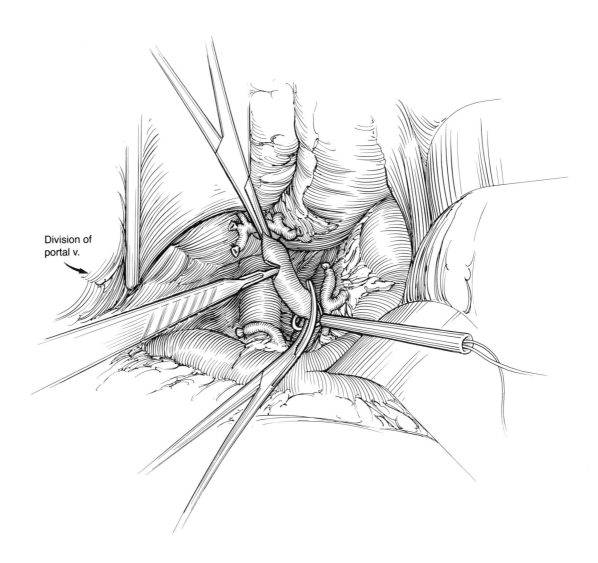

Division of
portal v.

FIGURE 114–11. After the dissections of the portal vein and inferior vena cava are completed, the portal vein is ready for cannulation. A long-angled DeBakey clamp is placed on the portal vein anterior to a Rumel tourniquet. The portal vein is clamped, divided, and ligated near its bifurcation to the hilum of the liver to leave a long stump.

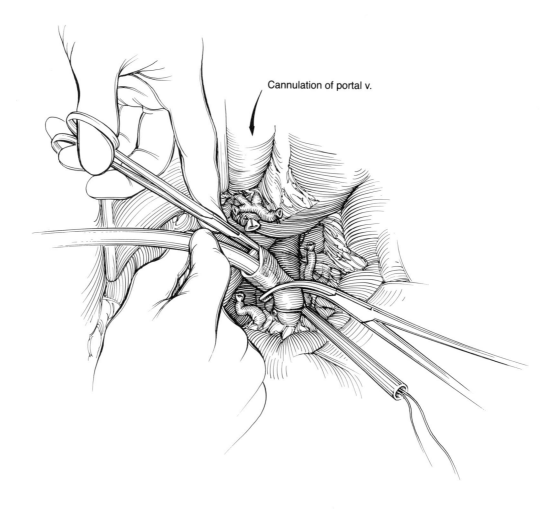

Cannulation of portal v.

FIGURE 114–12. The cannulation of the portal vein, an important part of the operation, is performed next. A small tonsil-type clamp is placed on the medial aspect of the portal vein for control. With traction on this clamp, and with both hands, the surgeon places the cannula into the portal vein. In *one* step to minimize bleeding, the vascular clamp is removed and the Rumel tourniquet is secured above the opening for the cannula. With the same exposure, the assistant retracts the portal vein cannula while a Crafoord clamp is applied on the infrahepatic vena cava.

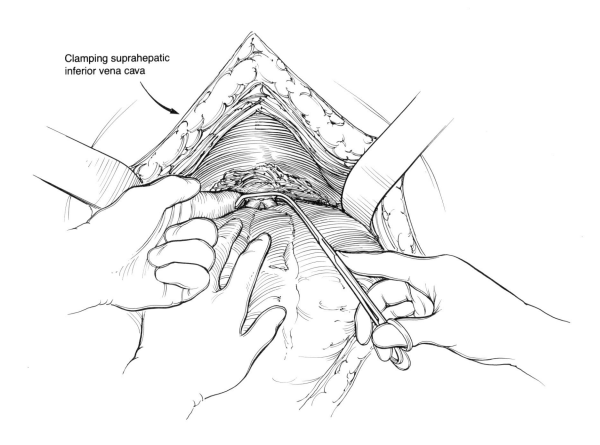

Clamping suprahepatic
inferior vena cava

FIGURE 114–13. The suprahepatic vena cava is then clamped. It is essential to incorporate
a portion of the diaphragm in the clamp to prevent slippage.

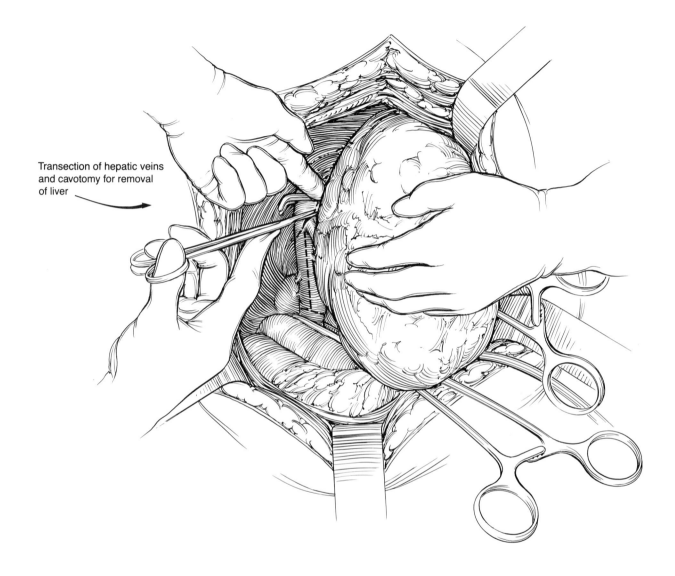

Transection of hepatic veins
and cavotomy for removal
of liver

FIGURE 114–14. All that remains in order to remove the liver is excision of the intrahepatic portion of the inferior vena cava. The suprahepatic vena cava is divided to include the junction of the hepatic veins and is later trimmed. Preserving an inch or more of infrahepatic vena caval cuff is preferable but not always achievable.

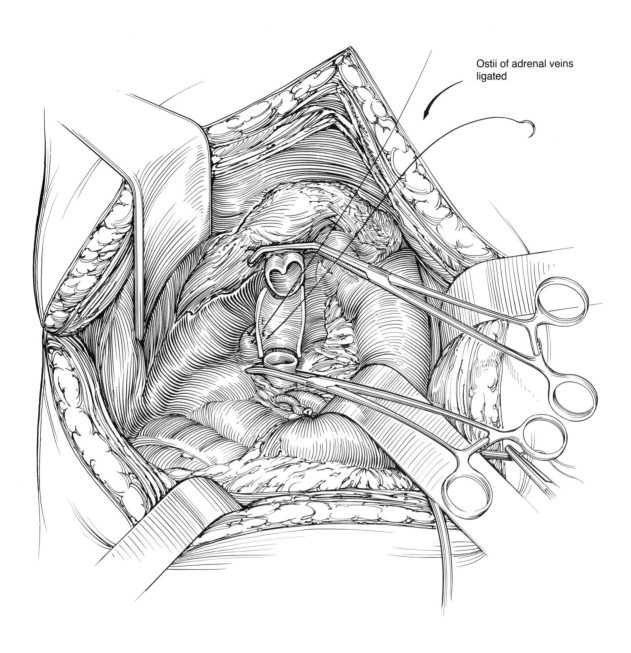

Ostii of adrenal veins
ligated

FIGURE 114–15. It is not necessary to dissect the adrenal veins separately; rather, the back wall of the infrahepatic vena cava is left intact but oversewn with 3-0 Prolene suture after the liver is removed.

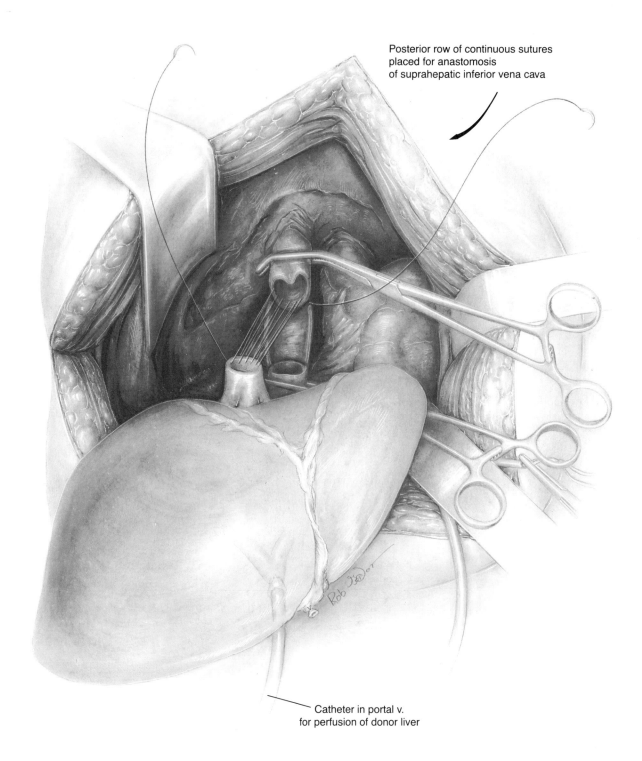

Posterior row of continuous sutures
placed for anastomosis
of suprahepatic inferior vena cava

Catheter in portal v.
for perfusion of donor liver

FIGURE 114–16. The anastomosis of the new liver is straightforward. The liver, which has been prepared at a back table, is placed into the recipient's abdomen with cold slush packing.

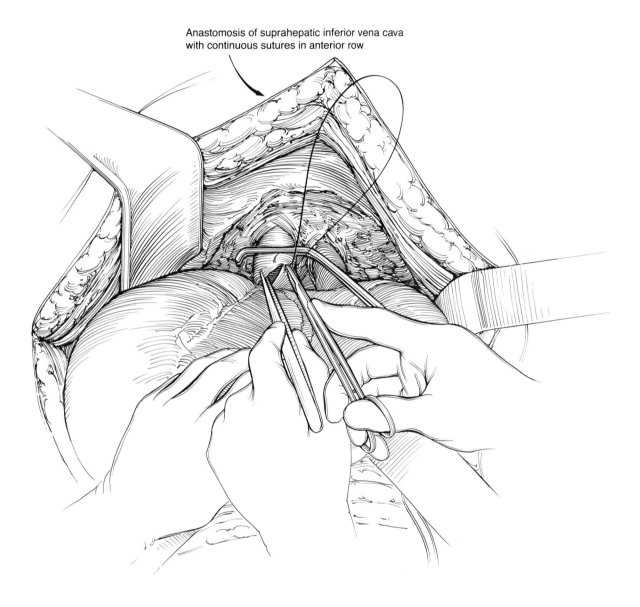

Anastomosis of suprahepatic inferior vena cava
with continuous sutures in anterior row

FIGURE 114–17. A long 3-0 Prolene suture is used for the suprahepatic vena caval anastomosis, with most of the posterior wall of the vena cava sewn with the liver lifted superiorly. The anterior anastomosis is completed after the liver has been placed into the subdiaphragmatic location. El-med retractors are very helpful and preclude the need for an additional assistant. After the suprahepatic vena caval anastomosis is completed, a *deep* Deaver retractor is placed into one El-med retractor to retract the liver while the infrahepatic vena cava anastomosis is performed.

Anastomosis of infrahepatic
inferior vena cava
with continuous sutures

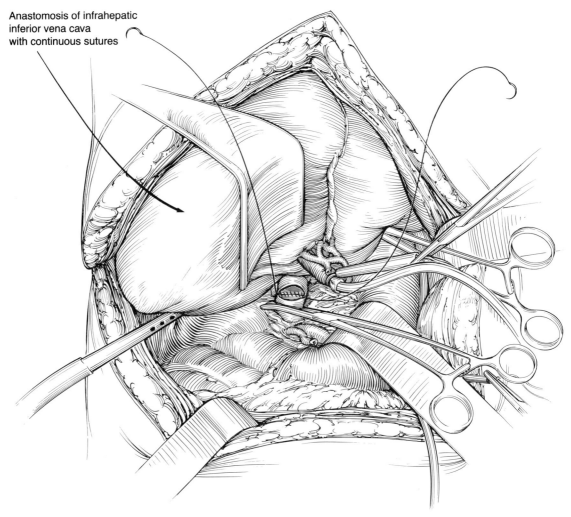

FIGURE 114–18. The inferior vena caval anastomosis (with 3-0 Prolene suture) is not completed until near the end of the procedure.

FIGURE 114–19. Most of the portal vein anastomosis is performed with 5-0 Prolene suture with the patient on portal-venous bypass.

FIGURE 114–20. The arterial anastomosis is performed with 6-0 Prolene suture. The portal vein is then flushed with 5 per cent albumin solution in Ringer's solution to remove the high potassium, and the portal vein anastomosis is then completed. The infrahepatic anastomosis is secured, and the anesthesia team prepares for release of the clamps. The clamps are released, and stability is achieved with cessation of mechanical bleeding. The anastomosis of the bile duct is performed in a dry field.

FIGURE 114–21. The anastomosis of the bile duct is usually performed by direct choledochocholedochostomy.

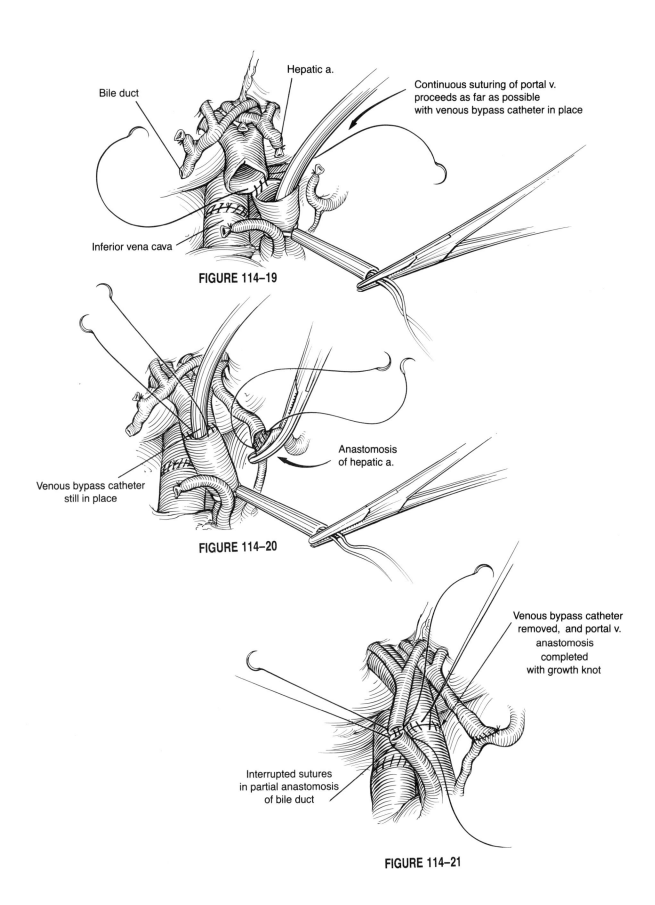

Bile duct

Hepatic a.

Continuous suturing of portal v. proceeds as far as possible with venous bypass catheter in place

Inferior vena cava

FIGURE 114–19

Venous bypass catheter still in place

Anastomosis of hepatic a.

FIGURE 114–20

Venous bypass catheter removed, and portal v. anastomosis completed with growth knot

Interrupted sutures in partial anastomosis of bile duct

FIGURE 114–21

Anastomosis of bile duct
completed with hepatoduodenal stent

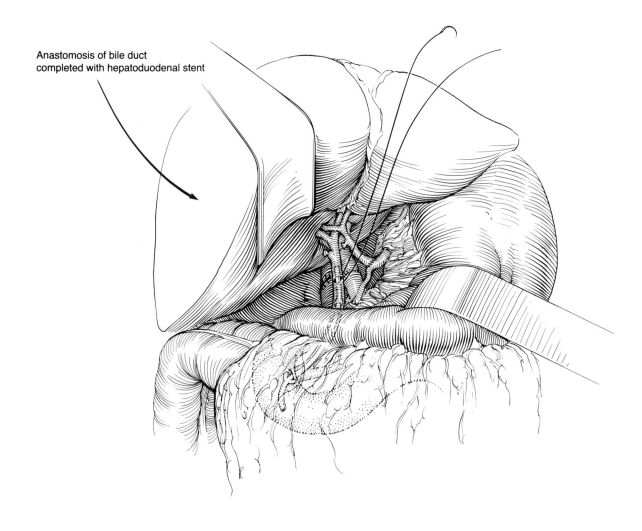

FIGURE 114–22. The anastomosis is accomplished directly with interrupted 4-0 Prolene sutures and placement of an intraluminal stent similar to that used by endoscopists.

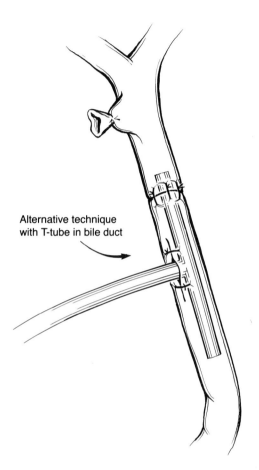

Alternative technique
with T-tube in bile duct

FIGURE 114–23. Alternative methods of biliary reconstruction include use of a T-tube via the recipient duct, with the proximal end stenting the anastomosis, or performance of a Roux-en-Y hepaticojejunostomy with 18 inches of Roux segment.

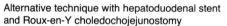

Alternative technique with hepatoduodenal stent
and Roux-en-Y choledochojejunostomy

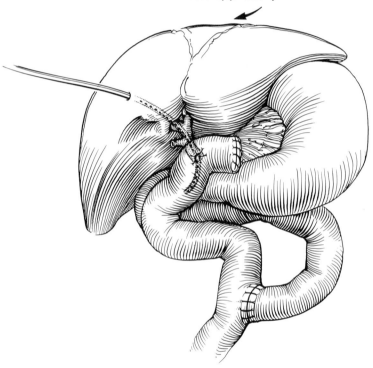

FIGURE 114–24. For the Roux-en-Y biliary reconstruction, the duct is either not stented, stented with a transhepatic tube, or stented with an intraluminal Silastic stent that later passes spontaneously.

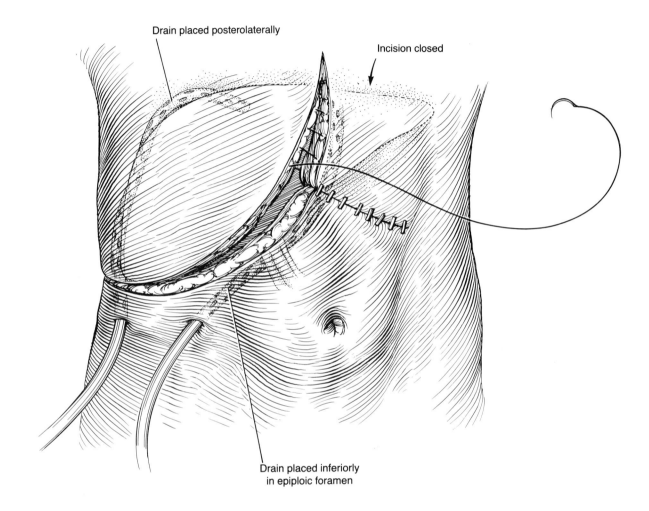

Drain placed posterolaterally

Incision closed

Drain placed inferiorly
in epiploic foramen

FIGURE 114–25. After hemostasis is achieved, the transplant incision is closed with a continuous heavy nylon suture. Two Silastic (Blake type) drains are placed: one along the left of the liver inferiorly, which also drains the biliary anastomosis area, and the other along the right gutter. The axillary and femoral incisions are closed with absorbable sutures. The left axillary vein is repaired with 6-0 Prolene suture, and the saphenous vein is ligated. Three loads of staples are usually necessary for closure of the abdominal skin.

115

Pancreas Transplantation

WALTER B. VERNON, M.D.

Pancreatic transplantation is performed most commonly in conjunction with cadaver renal transplantation for end-stage renal disease secondary to insulin-dependent diabetes mellitus. However, it can be performed singly or subsequent to kidney transplantation. Current preservation techniques allow for 24 hours of hypothermic storage. After graft procurement, the recipient is prepared for the procedure while a cross-match is performed. Preparation includes enemas, dialysis if indicated, intravenous hydration, intravenous insulin therapy to control blood glucose, and initial doses of immunosuppressive medications. Oral azathioprine, intravenous cyclosporine, and an intravenous bolus of methylprednisolone are administered preoperatively.

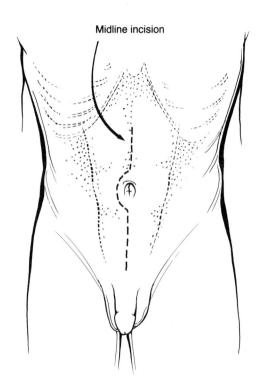

Midline incision

FIGURE 115–1. The patient is placed in the supine position, and attention is given to cushioning the patient's heels and other pressure points. Because of the viscid properties of pancreatic juice, a large-bore (22 to 24 French) Foley catheter is placed in the bladder, and the bladder is irrigated with a solution containing bacitracin and neomycin. After complete evacuation of the bladder, 200 ml. of this irrigant is instilled and the catheter is clamped.

The abdomen is prepared from the xiphoid to the thighs and draped into the sterile field. A midline abdominal incision is made from halfway between the xiphoid and the umbilicus to the pubis. On entering the peritoneal cavity, one should pay attention to entering exactly between the lateral umbilical folds or between the right lateral umbilical fold and the urachus. The right and left umbilical folds are taken down from the anterior abdominal wall with the electrocautery and preserved for subsequent use as "bladder ears" (see Figs. 115–14 and 115–15).

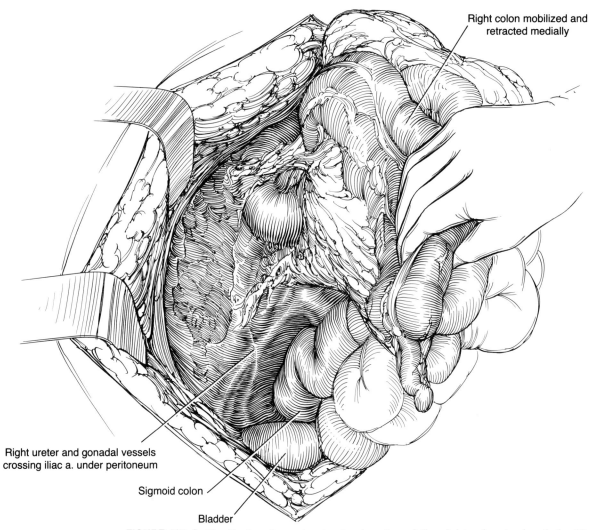

Right colon mobilized and
retracted medially

Right ureter and gonadal vessels
crossing iliac a. under peritoneum

Sigmoid colon

Bladder

FIGURE 115–2. The Buchwalter retractor is placed, and the right colon is elevated with ligation of the vascular tributaries at the hepatic flexure.

FIGURE 115–3. The gonadal vessels are ligated proximally and distally, and the midportion is excised.

FIGURE 115–4. The right ureter is elevated with care in order to maintain an adequate pedicle of periureteral tissue to prevent ischemia of the ureter. This mobilization is taken well up into the retroperitoneum and into the pelvis to allow easy mobilization of the ureter and retraction during the anastomoses.

FIGURE 115–5. The right common iliac artery is exposed from its origin, and the external iliac artery is exposed to the inguinal ligament. The artery is carefully dissected free of its surrounding areolar tissue over this length, and the internal iliac artery is dissected from its areolar tissue sufficiently to allow easy application of a vascular clamp.

   The iliac vein is now exposed from the inferior vena cava to the inguinal ligament. It is carefully dissected free of its surrounding areolar tissue. All the posterior branches are divided between ligatures of fine silk. This permits ready mobilization of the vein from the pelvis, which renders the venous anastomosis easier to perform and, after final placement of the graft, allows the anastomosed portal and iliac veins to lie in a position to eliminate obstruction.

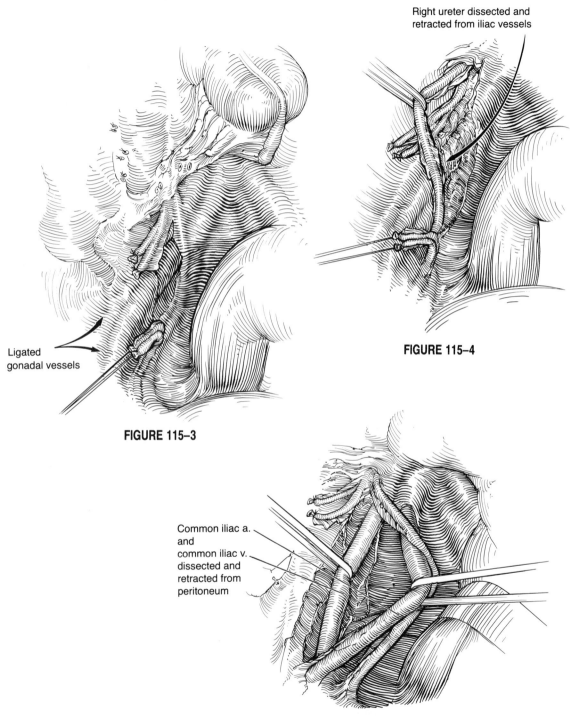

Right ureter dissected and
retracted from iliac vessels

FIGURE 115–4

Ligated
gonadal vessels

FIGURE 115–3

Common iliac a.
and
common iliac v.
dissected and
retracted from
peritoneum

FIGURE 115–5

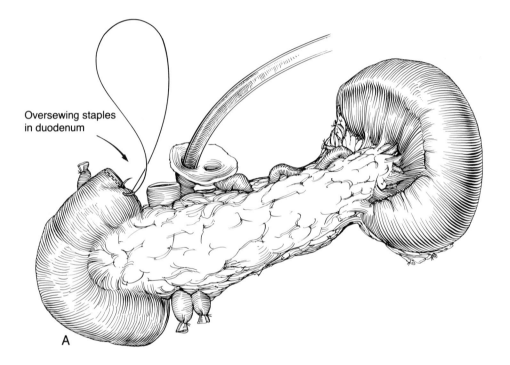

Oversewing staples
in duodenum

A

FIGURE 115–6. *A,* Prior to or during the initial dissection at the operating table, the graft
is prepared in preservation solution on ice at a back table. Key elements of this dissection
include (1) secure closure of the common bile duct; (2) dissection of the portal vein free
of surrounding areolar tissue to provide sufficient length for the anastomosis and
performance of a venous extension graft of donor iliac vein, if absolutely necessary; (3)
double and secure ligation of the superior mesenteric artery and vein with care in order
to preserve the inferior pancreaticoduodenal vessels; and (4) dissection of the duodenum
proximally and distally to the point where it is intimately associated with the head of
the pancreas. The duodenum is divided with a stapling device, and the ends are
inverted with multiple 3-0 silk Lembert sutures; the arterial inflow is prepared by
dissecting a Carrel patch of aorta containing both the celiac axis and the superior
mesenteric artery from their surrounding nervous and areolar tissue. In this dissection,
care must be paid to secure closure of the orifices of the hepatic and left gastric arteries.

ALTERNATIVE METHODS

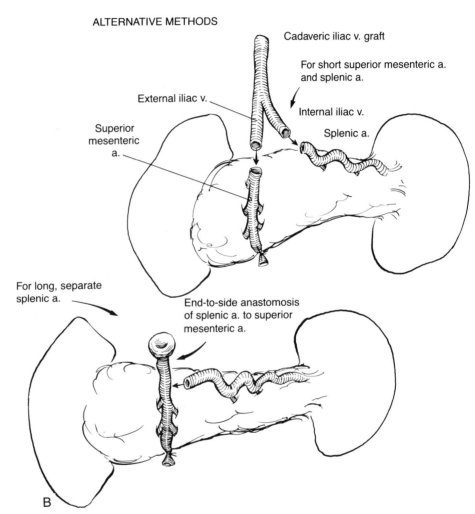

FIGURE 115–6 *Continued B,* Alternative methods for arterial reconstruction for a graft in which the celiac axis has been harvested with the liver.

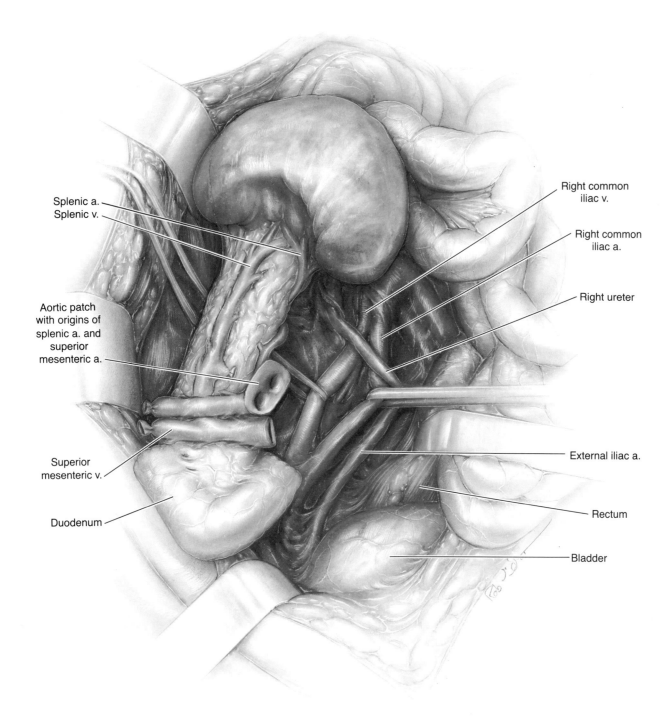

Splenic a.
Splenic v.

Aortic patch
with origins of
splenic a. and
superior
mesenteric a.

Superior
mesenteric v.

Duodenum

Right common
iliac v.

Right common
iliac a.

Right ureter

External iliac a.

Rectum

Bladder

FIGURE 115–7. An appropriate position is chosen for the graft. As the assistant holds
the graft, the surgeon chooses a convenient site for the venous anastomosis. In
determining this site, it is important to judge correctly the distance from the venous
anastomosis to the duodenocystostomy.

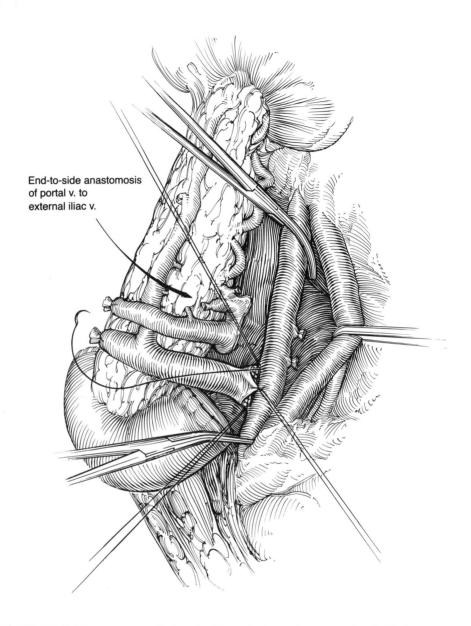

End-to-side anastomosis
of portal v. to
external iliac v.

FIGURE 115–8. Clamps are applied to the iliac vein (note the ties on the divided posterior pelvic branches), and a venotomy is made by excising a small ellipse of iliac vein. Four stay sutures of 5-0 Prolene are placed, and a running anastomosis is sewn with knots proximally and distally.

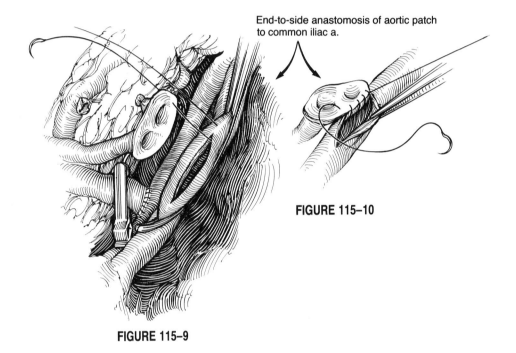

End-to-side anastomosis of aortic patch
to common iliac a.

FIGURE 115–10

FIGURE 115–9

FIGURES 115–9 and 115–10. After completion of the venous anastomosis, clamps are applied to the common, external, and internal iliac arteries. The frequent occurrence of relatively advanced atherosclerotic plaques in these vessels usually mandates the use of Fogarty arterial clamps and careful selection of a site for the arterial anastomosis. The arterial anastomosis of a Carrel patch of aorta end-to-side to the common iliac artery is demonstrated. This is performed with running 5-0 Prolene suture.

During the suturing of the arterial anastomosis, the final prereperfusion immunosuppressant medication is administered intravenously with mannitol to limit reperfusion injury from superoxide radicals.

At the conclusion of the vascular anastomosis, the arterial anastomosis is tested by temporarily occluding the superior mesenteric and celiac tributaries and releasing the external iliac clamp. If hemostasis is satisfactory, the venous clamps are removed, followed by the arterial clamps.

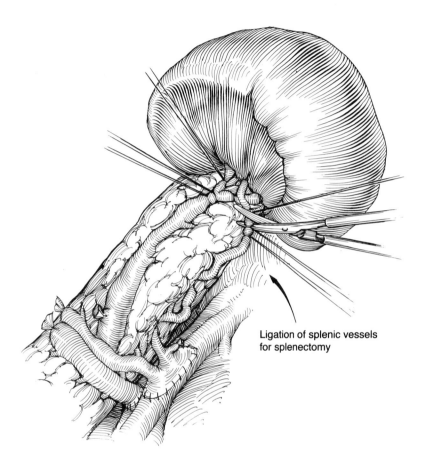

Ligation of splenic vessels
for splenectomy

FIGURE 115–11. Release of the vascular clamps may be attended by some hemorrhage, and it is wise to advise the anesthesiology team of this prior to reperfusion. The spleen has been left attached by its vascular pedicle to the pancreas, and now the turgor of the spleen and the pressure within the easily palpated splenic vein can be compared with the pressure in the iliac vein to assess and relieve any stenosis in venous drainage. Once its turgor is thought to be acceptable, the spleen is removed, taking care to doubly ligate the vascular tributaries on the pancreatic side. The splenic cells may be frozen and used in the future as a source of donor tissue in the immunologic management of the recipient. The graft is now carefully inspected a second time, and all bleeding points are controlled. Frequently, fine sutures of 5-0 and 6-0 polypropylene produce better control of small bleeders in the pancreatic parenchyma than does electrocautery.

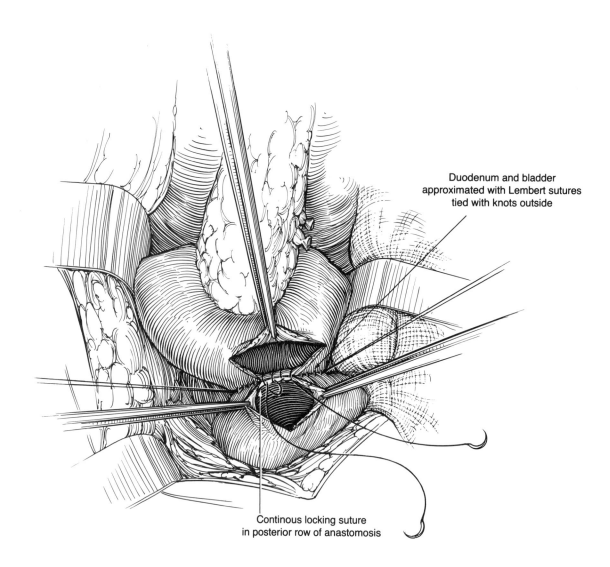

Duodenum and bladder
approximated with Lembert sutures
tied with knots outside

Continous locking suture
in posterior row of anastomosis

FIGURE 115–12. After acceptable vascular anastomoses and hemostasis are accomplished, the dome of the bladder is identified, and, on its posterior portion in a right parasagittal plane, an incision is made in the bladder with the electrocautery. The duodenum is opened longitudinally, and a transplant duodenocystostomy is performed in two layers. A posterior row of inverting 3-0 braided polyester Lembert sutures is placed, with attention given to keeping the knots outside. An inner row of running 3-0 polydioxanone is placed in lock stitch fashion and turned when convenient on the anterior row to a Connell suture and securely tied.

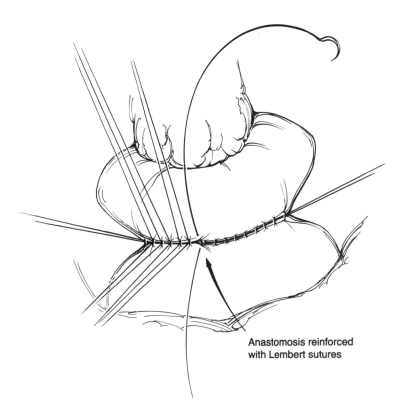

Anastomosis reinforced
with Lembert sutures

FIGURE 115–13. An anterior row of inverting 3-0 braided polyester Lembert sutures is placed. Extreme care should be taken in placing these sutures both posteriorly and anteriorly to be certain that none penetrate the mucosa of the bladder.

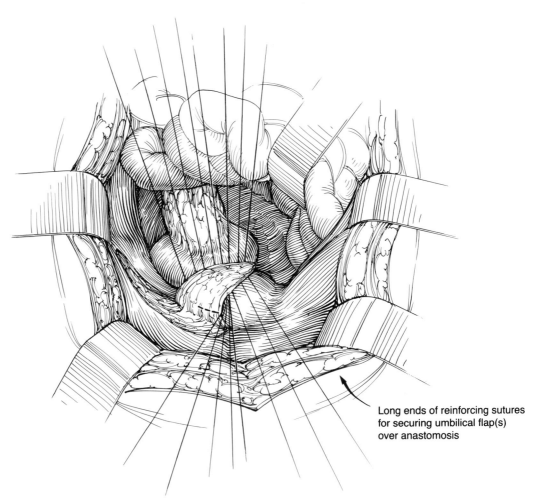

Long ends of reinforcing sutures
for securing umbilical flap(s)
over anastomosis

FIGURE 115–14. *See legend on opposite page*

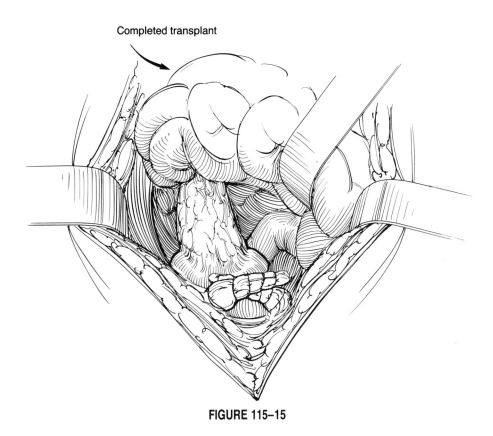

Completed transplant

FIGURE 115–15

FIGURES 115–14 and 115–15. The tails of every other Lembert suture on the anterior wall are left long, and now the right lateral umbilical fold is placed over the anterior suture line and tied in place. The same procedure is repeated for the urachus or left lateral umbilical fold.

The graft is inspected a third time as meticulous hemostasis is obtained, with careful attention to the ligated splenic vessels in the tail of the pancreas and the frequently annoying small vessels in the bed of the celiac and superior mesenteric arteries. The pancreas is placed in the right gutter; a Jackson-Pratt drain is placed medially along the pancreas through the right abdominal wall, and another is placed laterally, both with the tips in the pelvis. The abdomen is copiously irrigated with saline, and the right colon is replaced over the pancreatic transplant. Care is taken to replace the small bowel in an orderly manner. To assist in the differential diagnosis of subsequent graft pancreatitis, an inversion appendectomy is often performed. The omentum is replaced, and the linea alba is reapproximated with multiple interrupted figure-of-eight sutures of No. 1 polydioxanone. The drains are sutured in place, and the skin is reapproximated with a stapling device. The wound is washed, dried, and dressed.

Amputations

116

Below-Knee Amputation

RICHARD L. McCANN, M.D.

Below-knee amputation is usually feasible in patients with gangrene limited to the foot. Eighty-five per cent of below-knee amputations heal sufficiently to allow attempts at fitting a prosthesis. Modern below-knee prostheses use total contact sockets, with weight-bearing primarily on the patellar tendon. Adequate knee motion occurs if 4 or 5 cm. of tibia is preserved below the tibial tubercle. Skin flaps are designed to cover the bone ends with an adequate cushion and without tension. Because weight-bearing is on the tibial tubercle and not on the end of the stump, the position of the suture line in the skin is less important. Either a long posterior flap or symmetric anterior and posterior skin flaps are acceptable designs. Both designs provide adequate muscle coverage of the bone ends, and the choice may depend on assessment of the local integrity of the skin.

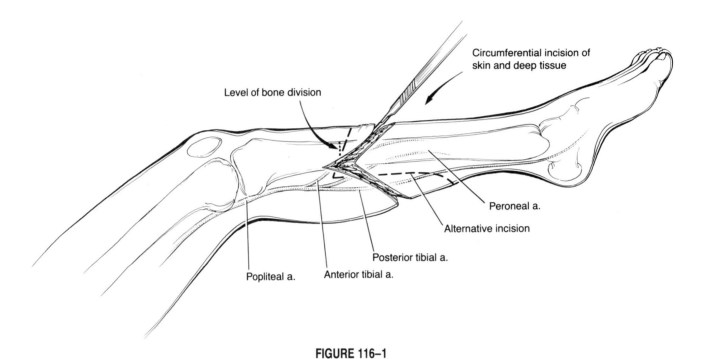

FIGURE 116–1

FIGURES 116–1 and 116–2. The skin, subcutaneous tissue, and superficial fascia are incised sharply in the chosen configuration. The muscle bellies are divided sharply or with the electrocautery. Each neurovascular bundle is doubly clamped, divided, and ligated as encountered. It is important not to place excessive traction on the nerves before severing them to avoid a nerve stretch injury and a troublesome pain syndrome postoperatively.

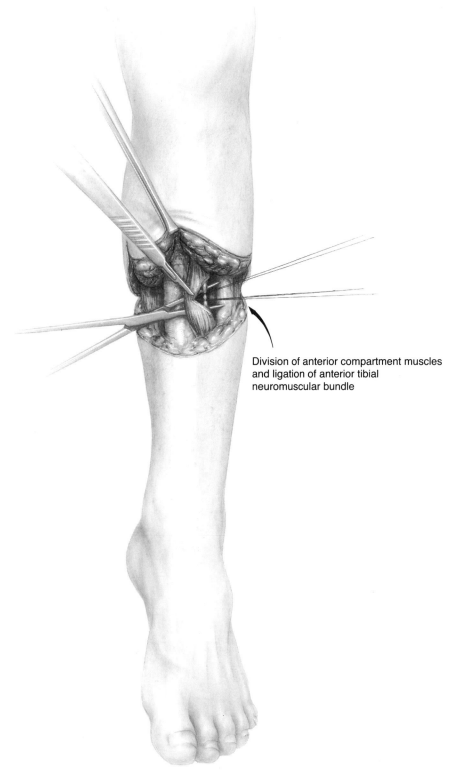

Division of anterior compartment muscles
and ligation of anterior tibial
neuromuscular bundle

FIGURE 116–2

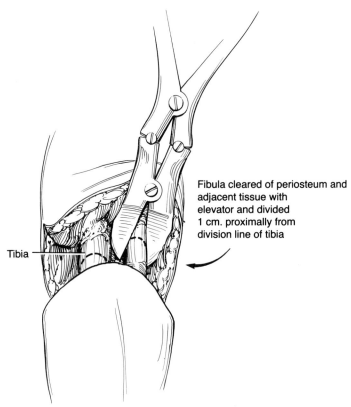

Tibia

Fibula cleared of periosteum and adjacent tissue with elevator and divided 1 cm. proximally from division line of tibia

FIGURE 116–3. The fibula is divided 1 cm. proximal to the intended line of division of the tibia to form a conical shape to the stump.

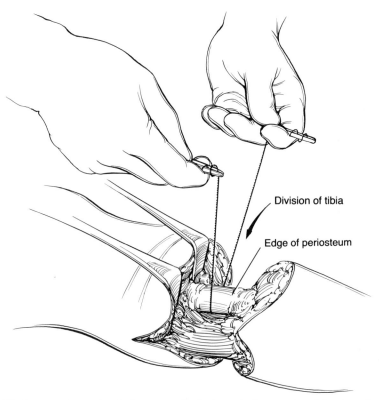

Division of tibia

Edge of periosteum

FIGURE 116–4. The tibia is divided perpendicularly to its long axis with a hand or power bone saw.

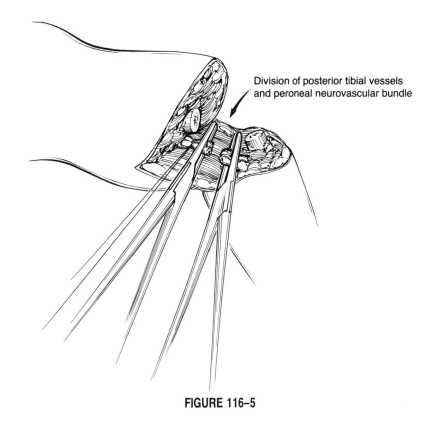

Division of posterior tibial vessels
and peroneal neurovascular bundle

FIGURE 116–5

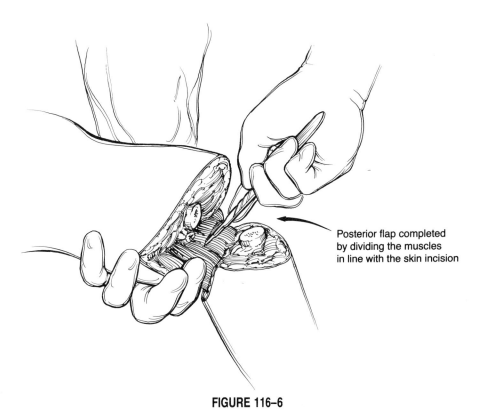

Posterior flap completed
by dividing the muscles
in line with the skin incision

FIGURE 116–6

FIGURES 116–5 and 116–6. The posterior flap is made, with care taken to control the posterior tibial and peroneal vessels.

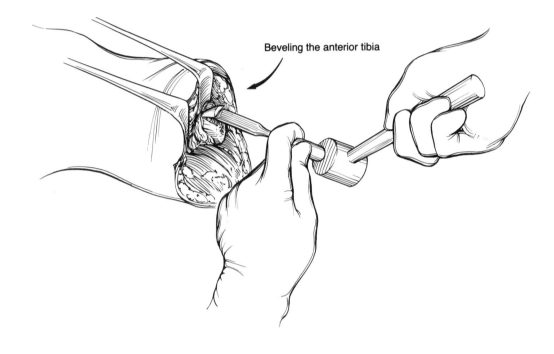

Beveling the anterior tibia

FIGURE 116–7. The anterior aspect of the tibia is rounded and beveled with a power saw or hand osteotome in order to avoid a bony prominence in the stump. The wound is irrigated with antibiotic solution, and the muscles are assessed for viability.

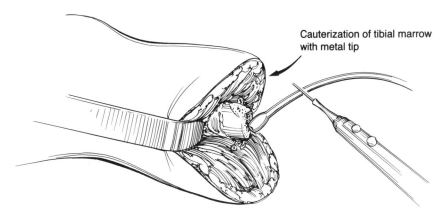

Cauterization of tibial marrow
with metal tip

FIGURE 116–8. Careful hemostasis is obtained to avoid a hematoma. Drainage is not used and, in patients amputated for peripheral vascular disease, a tourniquet is contraindicated.

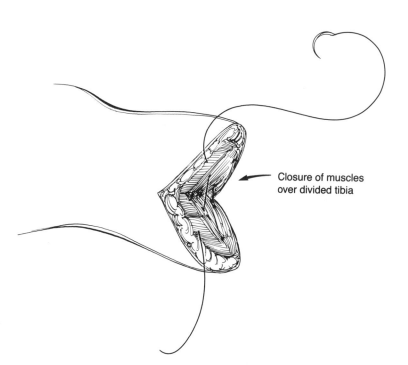

Closure of muscles
over divided tibia

FIGURE 116–9. Simple myodesis approximates the calf muscles over the bone ends, and the superficial fascia is sutured with interrupted absorbable sutures.

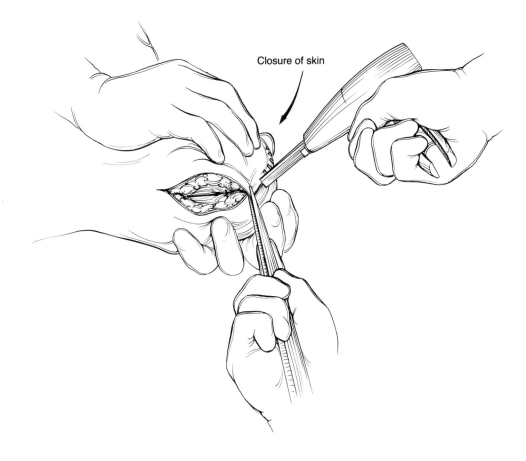

Closure of skin

FIGURE 116–10. The skin is approximated carefully with stainless steel staples, and any dog ears are carefully tailored.

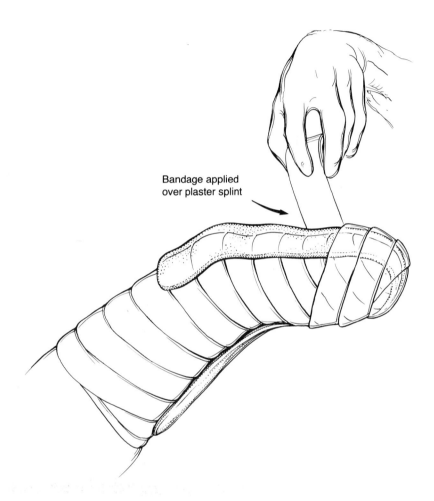

Bandage applied
over plaster splint

FIGURE 116–11. Appropriate dressing is important to minimize postoperative swelling and pain. Appropriate immobilization also improves the chance of successful healing and minimizes the time of rehabilitation. The suture line is covered with sterile gauze, and the area from the stump to the upper thigh is wrapped with cast padding. A plaster splint is used to immobilize the knee in a position of minimal flexion, is firmly secured with a wrap, and is covered with a tubular stockinette.

Because of the tenuous vascular supply, healing is promoted by immobilization, and immediate fitting of the prosthesis is seldom appropriate in the elderly. The dressing is removed at 5 days, and active flexion exercises are encouraged. At 3 to 4 weeks, the skin sutures are removed and stump wrapping is begun. Fitting of the prosthesis may be considered at 6 to 8 weeks following operation if healing is complete.

117

Supracondylar Amputation

RICHARD L. McCANN, M.D.

Supracondylar amputation is indicated for the nonambulatory patient or when a below-knee amputation is unfeasible or fails to heal. General or regional anesthesia is satisfactory, and, in occasional circumstances, femoral-sciatic nerve block supplemented with local anesthesia may be necessary. The length of the stump is dependent on the extent of the gangrenous process. The stump should be made as long as possible consistent with wound healing because a longer stump provides a better fulcrum for a prosthesis or transfers for the amputee. The flaps may be anterior and posterior or sagittal.

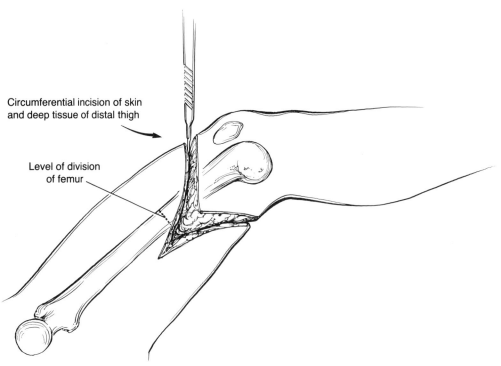

Circumferential incision of skin and deep tissue of distal thigh

Level of division of femur

FIGURE 117–1. The skin and subcutaneous tissues are incised sharply, and a tourniquet is not used in amputations performed for vascular disease.

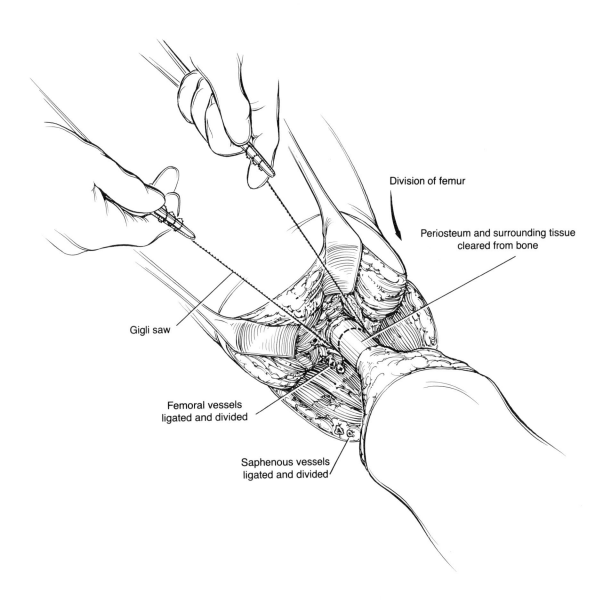

Division of femur

Periosteum and surrounding tissue
cleared from bone

Gigli saw

Femoral vessels
ligated and divided

Saphenous vessels
ligated and divided

FIGURE 117-2. The femoral vessels are doubly clamped, divided, and ligated or suture-ligated. The femoral nerve is transected and allowed to retract. Care is taken to avoid excessive traction on the femoral and sciatic nerves to avoid stretch injury and subsequent troublesome pain syndrome. The femur is divided with a hand or power bone saw at a level to allow flap approximation without tension over the end of the bone. Meticulous hemostasis is important, and drainage is not used.

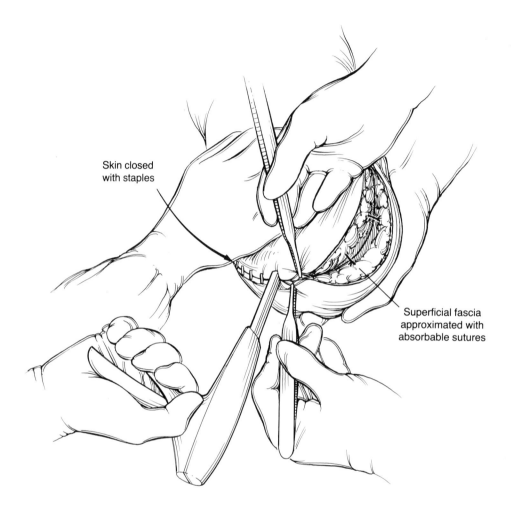

Skin closed
with staples

Superficial fascia
approximated with
absorbable sutures

FIGURE 117–3. The flaps are approximated by suturing the superficial fascia with interrupted absorbable sutures. The skin is meticulously coapted with stainless steel staples or monofilament sutures. A soft dressing rather than plaster is used. Attention is directed posteriorly to avoid a hip flexion contracture, with judicious use of physical therapy postoperatively.

118

Transmetatarsal Amputation

RICHARD L. McCANN, M.D.

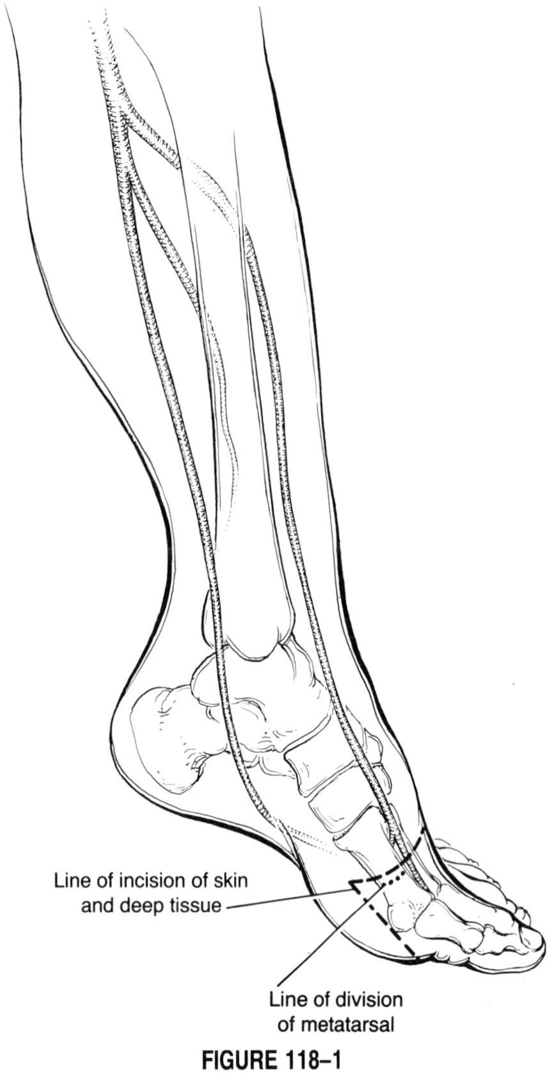

Line of incision of skin
and deep tissue

Line of division
of metatarsal

FIGURE 118–1

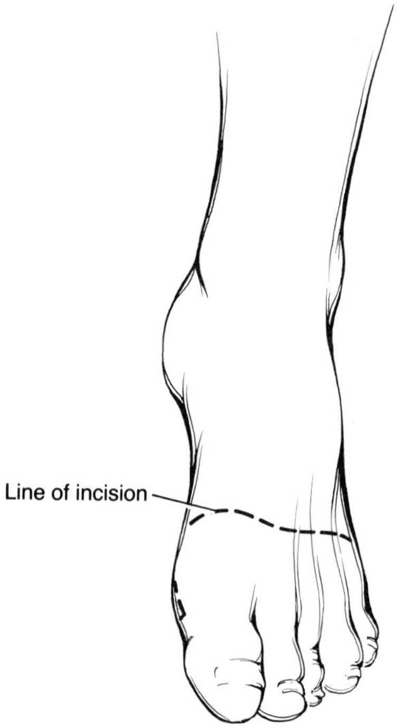

Line of incision

FIGURE 118–2

FIGURES 118–1 to 118–3. Transmetatarsal amputation is performed with a long plantar flap. The dorsal incision is made at the midtarsal level and extended sharply to the bones. The corners are curved back slightly to avoid a lateral redundancy. The plantar flap is kept as long and thick as practicable.

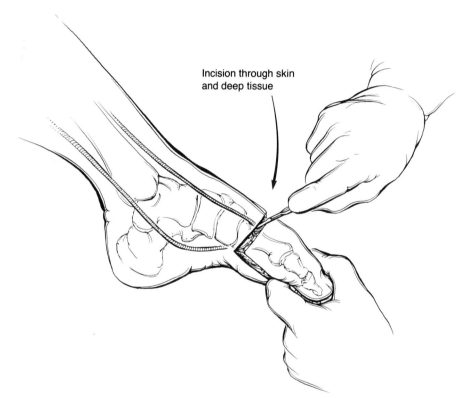

Incision through skin
and deep tissue

FIGURE 118–3

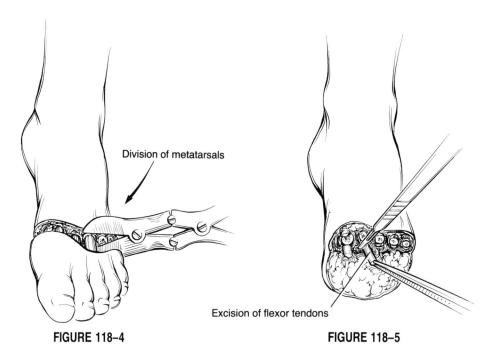

Division of metatarsals

Excision of flexor tendons

FIGURE 118–4　　　　　　**FIGURE 118–5**

FIGURES 118–4 and 118–5. The metatarsals are divided serially, and the flexor tendons are severed and allowed to retract. The flap is rotated anteriorly and tailored to achieve accurate skin coaptation.

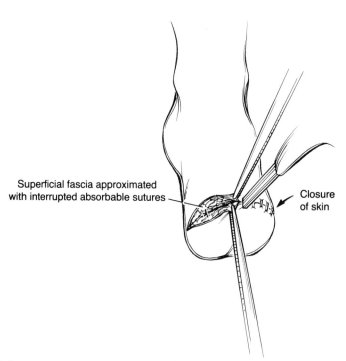

Superficial fascia approximated
with interrupted absorbable sutures

Closure
of skin

FIGURE 118–6. The deeper tissues are approximated with interrupted absorbable sutures, and the skin is closed with stainless steel staples. A rigid dressing is applied to minimize edema and to immobilize the ankle. Touch-down weight-bearing is allowed after the first dressing change at 5 days. A formal prosthesis is not required, but good shoeing is required to minimize the risk of breakdown.

Miscellaneous Procedures

119

Excision of Pilonidal Cysts and Sinuses

ONYE E. AKWARI, M.D.

Hodges introduced the term *pilonidal (pilus, hair; nidus, nest)* in 1880 and proposed a theory of congenital origin. It is now apparent that the problem that most commonly occurs in the sacrococcygeal area and has been reported in the umbilicus, the axilla, the clitoris, the interdigital web of the foot, the sole of the foot, and the anal canal is, in fact, acquired. Distorted hair follicles secondarily ingest hair, become filled with keratin and other debris, and, when infected, present as acute pilonidal abscesses.

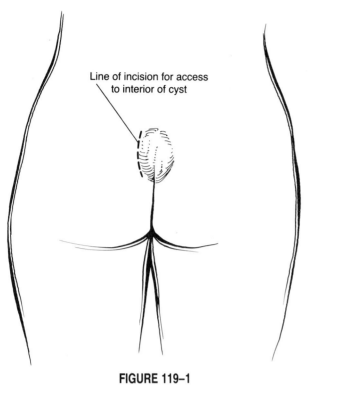

Line of incision for access
to interior of cyst

FIGURE 119–1

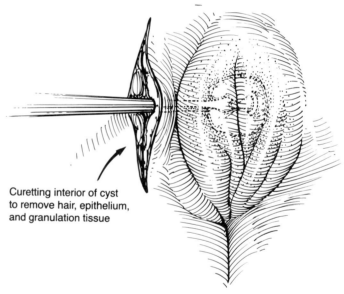

Curetting interior of cyst
to remove hair, epithelium,
and granulation tissue

FIGURE 119–2

FIGURES 119–1 and 119–2. *Acute pilonidal abscess:* Through an incision avoiding the midline pits, the abscess is incised and drained. Evacuation of the pus and hair and curetting of the granulation tissue are favored.

Chronic pilonidal disease: Eighty per cent of patients with pilonidal disease present with a chronic abscess and no history of a prior clinically apparent acute stage. Initial treatment must include medication for pain and an antibiotic regimen particularly directed against *Staphylococcus* and *Bacteroides* species. After a local or regional anesthetic is administered, the chronic abscess is opened, avoiding the midline *ditch* of pits and sinuses. The abscess cavity is scrubbed free of hair and debris. All visible small holes from the midline skin are excised with minimal skin loss. The lateral incision is left widely open to permit drainage.

Epithelial inclusion cyst: In the rare patient with very long-standing disease, the abscess wall is covered with surface epithelium that has grown into the cavity. At this stage, it is no longer a chronic abscess but an epithelial inclusion cyst and should be excised. Occasionally, multiple cavities may appear under insignificant-appearing follicles, and, again, the amount of excised tissue is kept to a minimum but with removal of all the epithelial tracts.

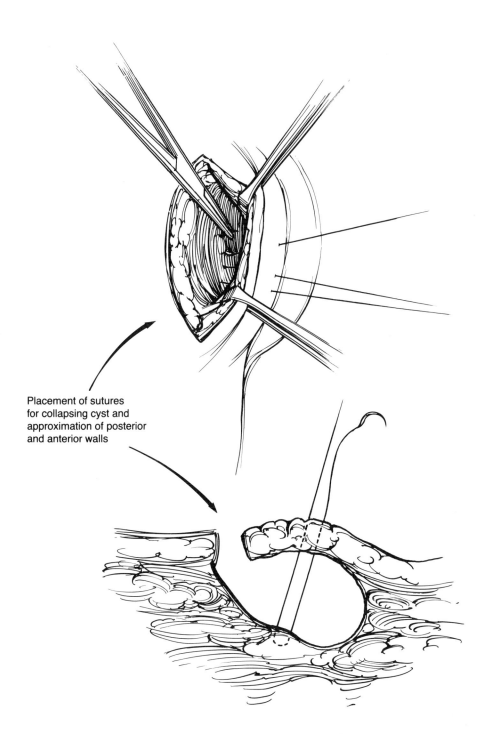

Placement of sutures
for collapsing cyst and
approximation of posterior
and anterior walls

FIGURES 119–3 and 119–4. Primary healing is aided by collapsing a portion of the far wall of the cavity against the underside of the closure.

EXCISIONAL TREATMENT OF PILONIDAL CYST (Buie, 1939)

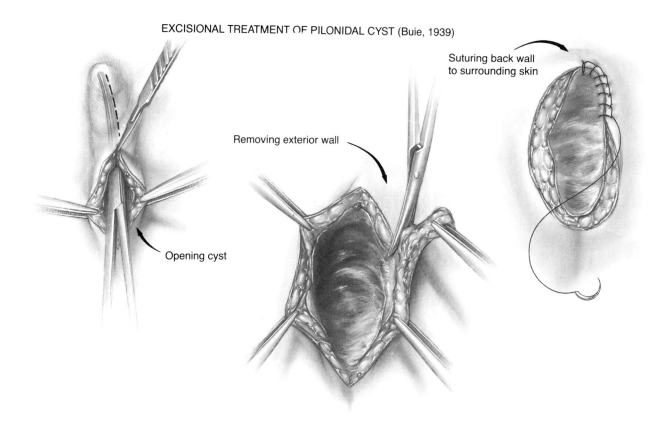

Opening cyst

Removing exterior wall

Suturing back wall
to surrounding skin

FIGURES 119–5 to 119–7. It is instructive to reflect on the thought that Buie, who popularized the marsupilization operation, must have encountered a significant number of such advanced chronic cases and had excellent results from the more radical unroofing of these cysts. There is growing consensus that management of pilonidal disease should involve conservative approaches with less loss of tissue, especially because these approaches have yielded satisfactory results and lower recurrence rates and can be undertaken in an outpatient setting.

120

Axillary Node Dissection

HILLIARD F. SEIGLER, M.D.

Solid human malignancies are associated with both hematogenous and lymphogenous metastases. Adenocarcinomas are most frequently associated with lymphogenous metastases, whereas sarcomas more frequently spread through the blood stream. Neuroectodermal tumors can involve either lymphatics or hematogenous channels. The most commonly involved lymph node basins detectable by external examination include the cervical area, ilioinguinal chain, and axilla. Infrequently involved are lymph nodes in the popliteal fossa and antecubital fossa. The surgeon is commonly involved in standard axillary dissection and groin dissection.

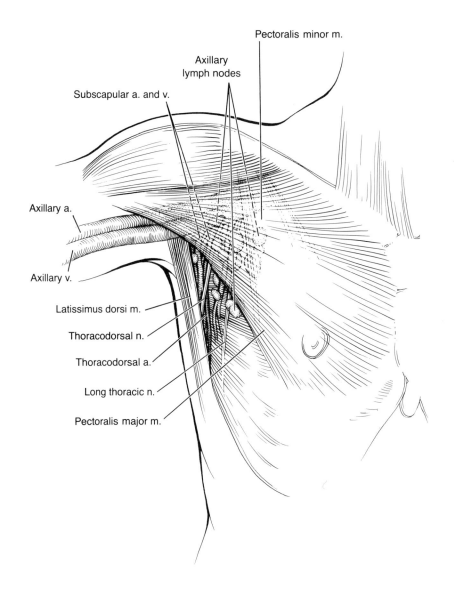

Pectoralis minor m.

Axillary
lymph nodes

Subscapular a. and v.

Axillary a.

Axillary v.

Latissimus dorsi m.

Thoracodorsal n.

Thoracodorsal a.

Long thoracic n.

Pectoralis major m.

FIGURE 120–1. Axillary lymph nodes are usually associated with adenocarcinomas or melanoma involving the ipsilateral trunk below the clavicle and above Sappey's line, which rests at the level of the umbilicus. Additionally, ipsilateral upper extremity primary lesions are frequently associated with axillary lymph node involvement.

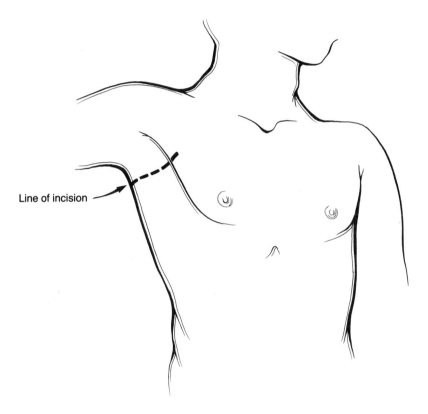

Line of incision

FIGURE 120–2. The incision for axillary dissection should be made from the border of the pectoralis major to the border of the latissimus dorsi muscle following the naturally occurring skin lines.

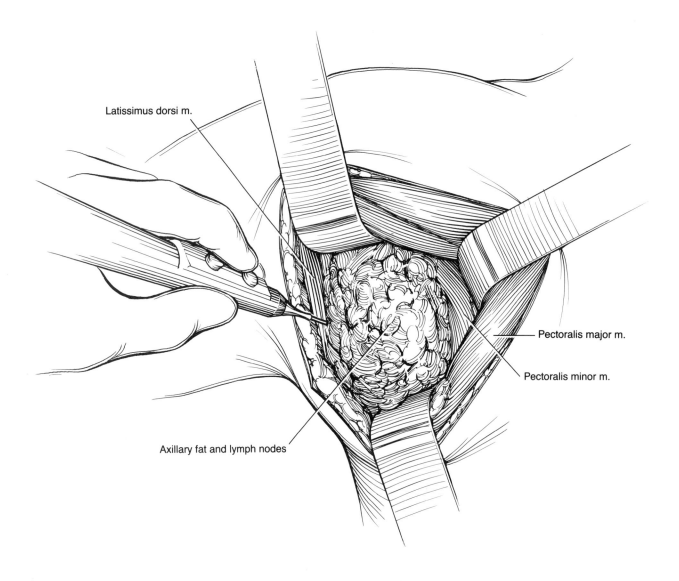

Latissimus dorsi m.

Pectoralis major m.

Pectoralis minor m.

Axillary fat and lymph nodes

FIGURE 120–3. Superior and inferior flaps are dissected with the cautery. As the adipose tissue containing the lymph nodes is mobilized, care should be taken not to interrupt the neural innervation of the pectoralis muscles. The interpectoral nodes should be included with the specimen. Access to the true axilla is gained by following the border of the pectoralis minor muscle. The axillary vein is sharply exposed by entering the vascular sheath. The small tributary vessels from the inferior surface of the axillary vein should be carefully dissected, clamped, and securely ligated. This permits dissection of the node-bearing tissue at the apex of the axilla. At this point, the vascular and lymphatic vessels should be carefully doubly clamped and ligated.

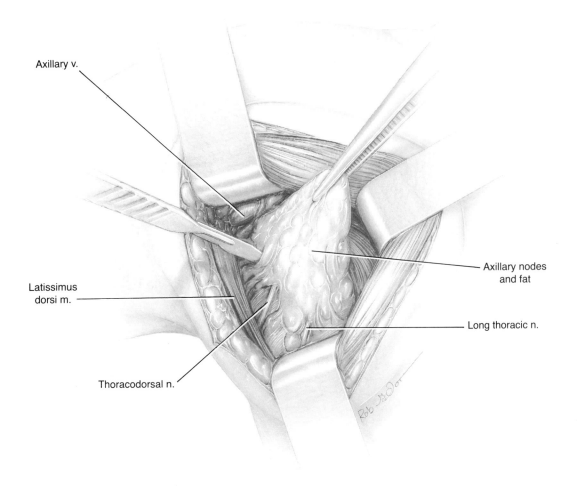

Axillary v.

Latissimus
dorsi m.

Thoracodorsal n.

Axillary nodes
and fat

Long thoracic n.

FIGURE 120–4. As the dissection progresses along the anterior serratus muscle, care is taken to identify the long thoracic nerve and to preserve its integrity. The neurovascular bundle comprising the subscapular vessels and the thoracodorsal vessels and nerves is easily identified and can be dissected away from the axillary contents and allowed to remain intact adjacent to the latissimus dorsi muscle. The entire adipose tissue with the axillary lymph nodes can be removed *en bloc*.

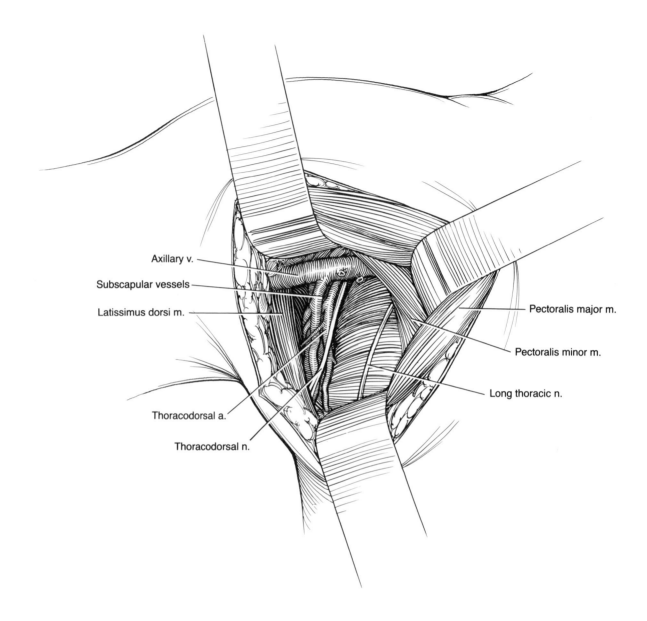

Axillary v.

Subscapular vessels

Latissimus dorsi m.

Pectoralis major m.

Pectoralis minor m.

Long thoracic n.

Thoracodorsal a.

Thoracodorsal n.

FIGURE 120–5. The superior border of the dissection is defined by the axillary vein, and medially the carefully dissected pectoralis major and minor muscles are free from adipose tissue containing lymph nodes. The lateral border of the dissection is the latissimus dorsi muscle. In the base of the wound rests the intact long thoracic nerve and thoracodorsal nerve.

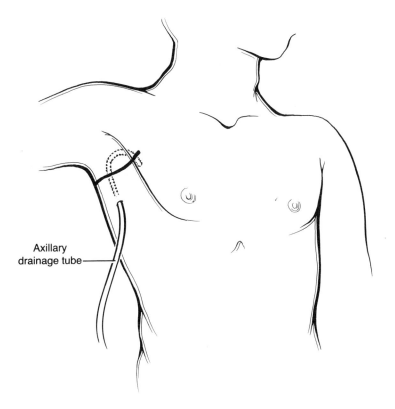

Axillary
drainage tube

FIGURE 120–6. A closed drainage tube is passed through the skin by a separate stab wound. The drain is anchored into place at the level of the skin. The fenestrated portion of the drainage catheter is placed in the depths of the axilla, with the tip resting under the pectoralis muscles, maintaining it in the correct position. Meticulous hemostasis and lymphostasis are secured with ties and electrocoagulation. The flaps are closed by approximating the subcutaneous tissue with an absorbable suture, and the skin is closed in a standard manner.

121

Inguinal Node Dissection

HILLIARD F. SEIGLER, M.D.

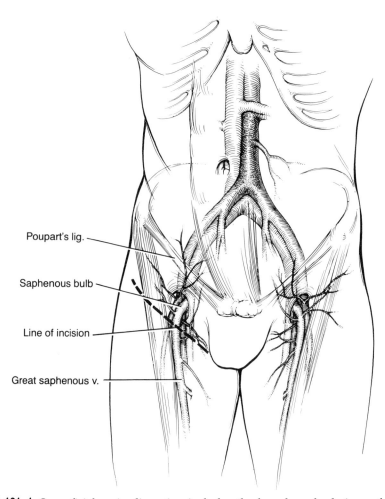

FIGURE 121–1. Superficial groin dissection includes the lymph node drainage from the ipsilateral lower extremity and ipsilateral axial sites below Sappey's line. Operations including the deep iliac and obturator nodes are of questionable value. The incision for superficial groin dissection is placed parallel to Poupart's ligament. Superior and inferior flaps are dissected with the cautery.

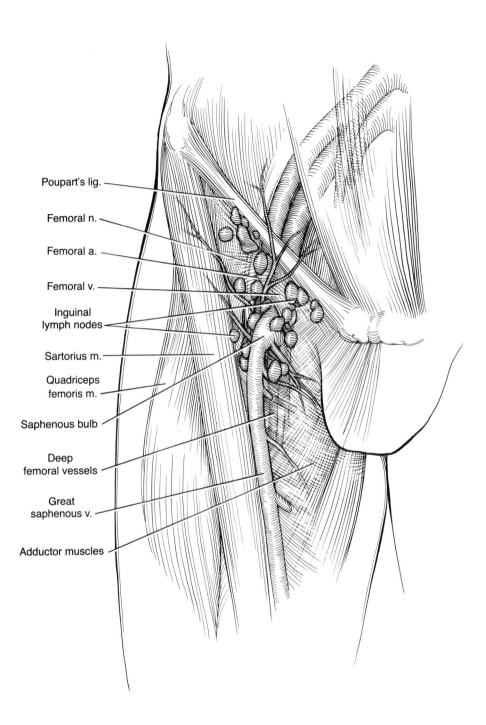

Poupart's lig.

Femoral n.

Femoral a.

Femoral v.

Inguinal
lymph nodes

Sartorius m.

Quadriceps
femoris m.

Saphenous bulb

Deep
femoral vessels

Great
saphenous v.

Adductor muscles

FIGURE 121–2. The adipose tissue containing the inguinal and femoral triangle nodes is shown. The greater saphenous vein is identified by blunt and sharp dissection at the inferior portion of the groin dissection and at that point is doubly clamped, divided, and suture-ligated. The dissection is then directed in a cephalad manner, taking care to preserve the fascia over the adductor muscles. All tributary vessels are doubly clamped, divided, and ligated.

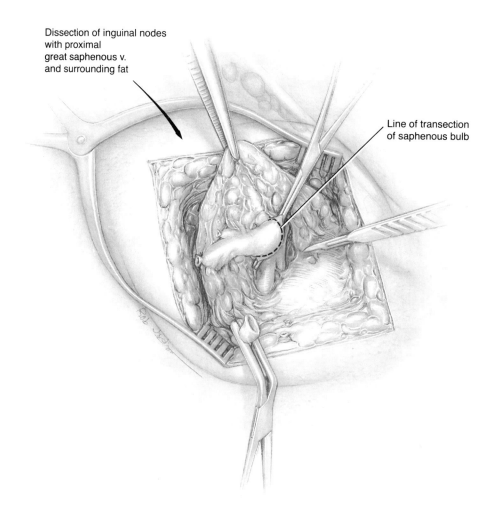

Dissection of inguinal nodes
with proximal
great saphenous v.
and surrounding fat

Line of transection
of saphenous bulb

FIGURE 121–3. The nodal tissue is carefully dissected away from the fascia of the quadriceps and sartorius muscles. Superiorly, Poupart's ligament is identified, and the node-bearing tissue is carefully dissected away by blunt and sharp dissection, with all vascular structures being carefully identified, clamped, and ligated. The saphenous bulb is identified and is doubly clamped, divided, and suture-ligated. The lymph nodes and lymphatic channels in the femoral canal are retracted inferiorly, permitting clamping and careful ligation. This permits removal of the superficial groin nodes. Meticulous hemostasis and lymphostasis are accomplished with ligatures and electrocoagulation.

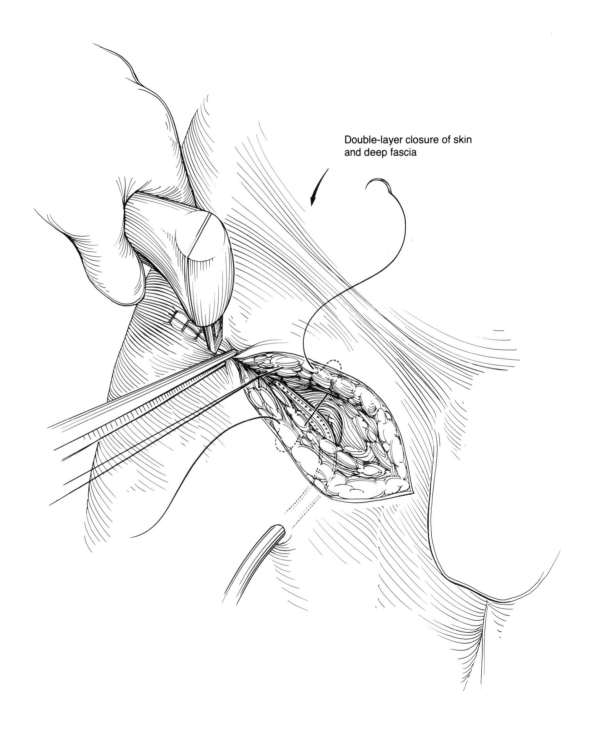

Double-layer closure of skin
and deep fascia

FIGURE 121–4. The wound is drained with a closed drainage system brought through the skin by a separate stab wound. The drain is fixed at the level of the skin with a suture ligature. The flaps are approximated with an absorbable suture in the subcutaneous tissue, and the skin is approximated with either skin staples or sutures.

122

Suture of Nerve

RICHARD D. GOLDNER, M.D.

Proper lighting and magnification by loupes are mandatory to adequately resect damaged nerve tissue adjacent to a laceration. Careful analysis of the cross-sectional architecture of the nerve is essential to achieve proper alignment of the motor and sensory segments. The nerve is inspected for vessels on the surface that are helpful in proper orientation and alignment of the cut nerve ends. Intraoperative nerve stimulation of motor fibers and histochemical staining may be helpful in achieving proper rotational alignment. Neurorrhaphy must be accomplished without tension on the repaired nerve.

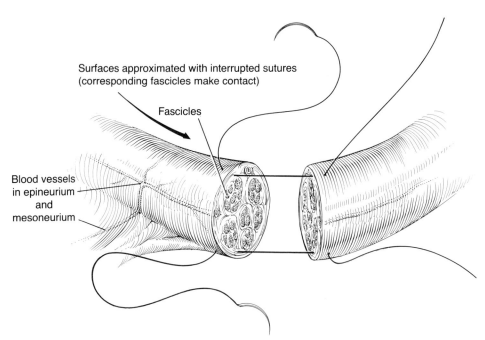

FIGURE 122–1. Larger nerves such as the median or ulnar are repaired with 8-0 nylon sutures, and smaller nerves such as those in the digits are repaired with 9-0 or 10-0 nylon sutures, using the operating microscope. Epineural repair of a nerve such as the median begins by passing 8-0 nylon suture through the epineurium of the adjacent proximal and distal ends of the severed nerve.

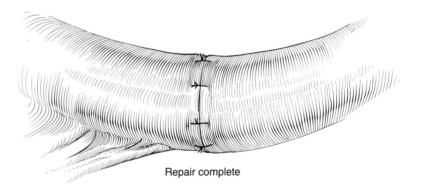

Repair complete

FIGURE 122–2. A second suture is placed opposite the first. Additional sutures are inserted midway between the previous ones, and the nerve is rotated for repair of the opposite side. The epineurium should not be closed so tightly that fascicular ends become infolded and mismatched. No fascicles should extrude between the suture lines. Microscopic repair of individual fascicles or groups of fascicles is appropriate under certain circumstances.

123

Suture of Tendon

RICHARD D. GOLDNER, M.D.

Because a tendon is composed of multiple longitudinal strands of collagen, repair of tendons with only simple sutures does not provide adequate strength. Suture techniques necessitating multiple passes through the tendon decrease vascular perfusion. The grasping techniques of Tajima and Kessler provide sufficient strength without producing ischemia.

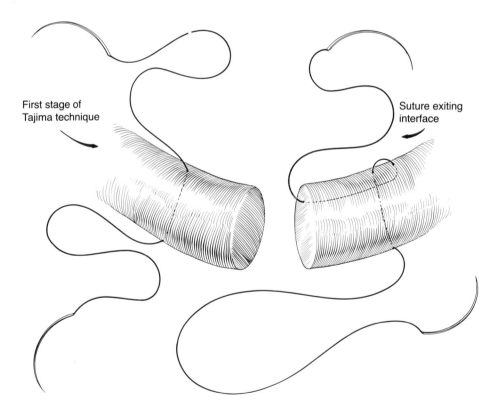

First stage of Tajima technique

Suture exiting interface

FIGURE 123–1. To repair a sharply lacerated tendon at the wrist, a suture of 3-0 braided polyester can be used. One of the needles is passed transversely across the tendon.

FIGURE 123–2. The needle is then inserted proximal to the point of exit of the transverse limb of suture and is directed within the body of the tendon, toward and out the cut surface of the tendon.

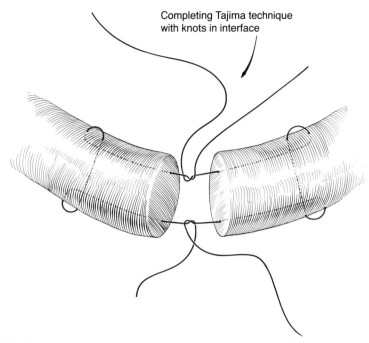

FIGURE 123–3. Similar suture placement is performed with the opposite end of the double-armed needle so that both ends of the suture exit the cut surface of the tendon. With the same technique, another double-armed suture is placed in the opposing cut tendon beginning with the transverse component, and, subsequently, each needle is passed from within the tendon out the cut interface. The surgeon and the assistant each tie one of the pairs of knots. This technique allows the knot to be buried within the cut ends of the tendon.

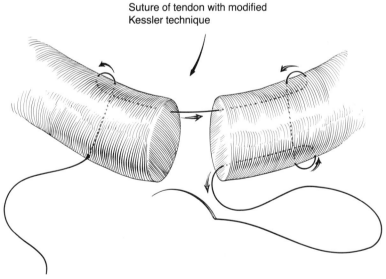

FIGURE 123–4. Suture of a tendon with a modified Kessler technique necessitates only one suture. Initially, the needle is passed transversely from one side of the tendon to the other. It is then inserted slightly proximally and is passed longitudinally within the tendon and out the cut surface. The needle is passed into the cut surface of the adjacent tendon end and exits along the side of the tendon. The two tendon segments are then properly positioned, as the subsequent transverse pass of the needle locks the suture and stabilizes the position of the tendon. The needle is inserted slightly proximally and passed longitudinally to exit the cut end of the tendon.

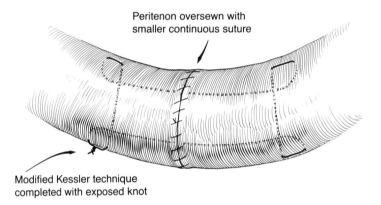

Peritenon oversewn with
smaller continuous suture

Modified Kessler technique
completed with exposed knot

FIGURE 123–5. The needle is then passed into the cut end of the opposing tendon and exists along the side where the knot is tied. In order to improve the strength and to smooth the edges of the tendon, a smaller continuous suture is placed in the peritenon.

124

Drainage of Hand Infections

RICHARD D. GOLDNER, M.D.

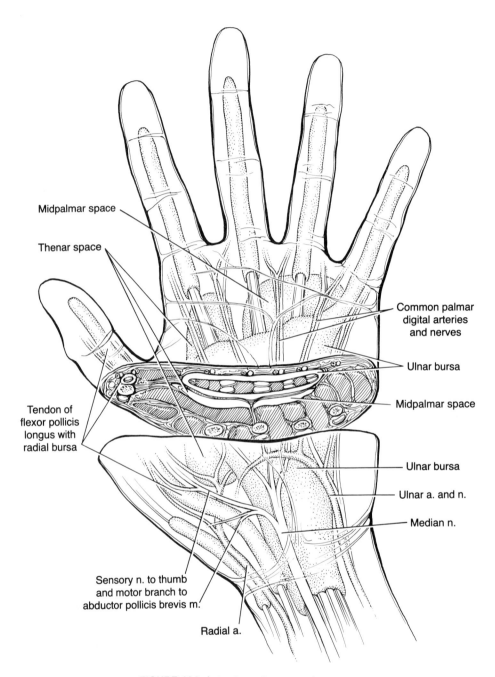

FIGURE 124–1 *See legend on opposite page*

FIGURE 124-1. The deep palmar space lies between the dorsal surface of the flexor tendons and the palmar surface of the interossei and adductor pollicis muscles. This potential space is subdivided by a septum that extends from the connective tissue surrounding the flexor tendons to the palmar surface of the long finger metacarpal. This septum divides the deep palmar space into two components: thenar and midpalmar. Causes of deep palmar space infection include purulent flexor tenosynovitis of the fingers, distal palmar abscesses extending proximally through the lumbrical canal, and penetrating injuries.

Infection along the flexor pollicis longus tendon involves the radial bursa, and infection in the small finger flexor sheath can extend to the ulnar bursa. Spread of infection between the radial and the ulnar bursae is termed a *horseshoe* abscess and involves Parona's space, which is bordered dorsally by the pronator quadratus muscle, radially by the flexor pollicis longus tendon, ulnarly by the flexor carpi ulnaris tendon, and on the palmar aspect by the flexor tendons.

When a palmar incision is made, several structures must be avoided: the superficial palmar vascular arch, which is a continuation of the ulnar artery and traverses the midpalm; the common and proper digital arteries, which arise from the superficial arch; the median nerve and its motor branch to the thenar muscles, in addition to common and proper digital nerves to the thumb, index finger, long finger, and radial aspect of the ring finger; and the ulnar nerve with branches to the ulnar intrinsic muscles and sensory branches to the ulnar aspect of the ring finger and to the small finger.

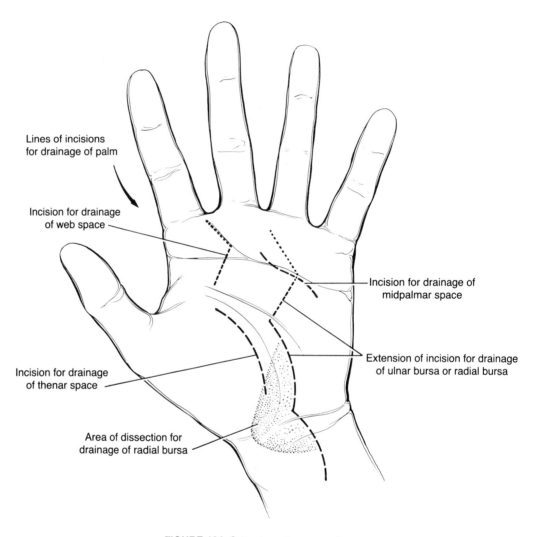

Lines of incisions
for drainage of palm

Incision for drainage
of web space

Incision for drainage of
midpalmar space

Extension of incision for drainage
of ulnar bursa or radial bursa

Incision for drainage
of thenar space

Area of dissection for
drainage of radial bursa

FIGURE 124–2 *See legend on opposite page*

FIGURE 124–2. Drainage of the midpalmar space can be accomplished through one of several incisions. A slightly curved incision can be made just proximal to the distal palmar crease overlying the long finger and ring finger metacarpals. The palmar fascia is carefully divided, and the digital nerves and arteries are identified and protected. Blunt dissection radial and deep to the ring finger flexor tendon produces drainage.

The thenar space (anterior adductor space) can be drained by a curvilinear incision in the palm, parallel and slightly radial to the midpalmar crease at the base of the thenar eminence. The palmar fascia is spread gently in line with the incision, and the digital nerves and flexor tendons to the index finger are identified. The spaces dorsal to the flexor tendons are entered by blunt dissection, taking extreme care to avoid the superficial and deep palmar arches and the motor branch of the median nerve.

The ulnar bursa and Parona's space are drained by an incision beginning obliquely at the flexion crease of the wrist and extending proximally in line with the ring finger metacarpal. The skin and subcutaneous tissue are divided, and the median nerve is identified radial to the incision. The ulnar nerve and artery are identified dorsal to the flexor carpi ulnaris tendon, which is ulnar to the incision. The flexor tendons are identified and retracted radially in order to enter Parona's space palmar to the pronator quadratus muscle. The flexor pollicis longus tendon, which lies within the radial bursa, is identified by elevating the skin and subcutaneous tissue and avoiding the median nerve and its palmar cutaneous branch, which lies radial to it and, by deeper dissection, adjacent to the finger flexors.

In more extensive hand infections, an incision adjacent to the midpalmar crease can be extended distally in a zigzag manner to cross the transverse skin creases obliquely. The incision can be extended proximally by transversing the flexion crease of the wrist obliquely and then extended further proximally in line with the ring finger metacarpal. If the volar carpal ligament is divided, the median nerve is seen. Flexor tendons dorsal to it and both the thenar and the midpalmar spaces can be reached. The proximal extension of this incision to expose the radial and ulnar bursa is described above. Distal extension of the incision allows access to the flexor tendon sheaths and lumbrical muscles. Digital nerves and arteries must be protected.

Infection at the web space usually begins on the palmar surface and extends dorsally through or around the transverse metacarpal ligament. A *collar button abscess* is a dorsal and palmar abscess connected by a thin stalk in the webs between the digits. Although swelling is often most prominent dorsally, the palmar component of the infection should not be overlooked.

Drainage of a web space infection is accomplished by a zigzag incision in the palm, just proximal to the web. The skin is divided, and the subcutaneous tissue is spread. Digital arteries and nerves are identified and protected, and the superficial transverse intermetacarpal ligament and palmar fascia are divided. Deeper tissues are spread with a clamp to drain the abscess. If a collar button abscess is present, a second incision is made on the dorsum.

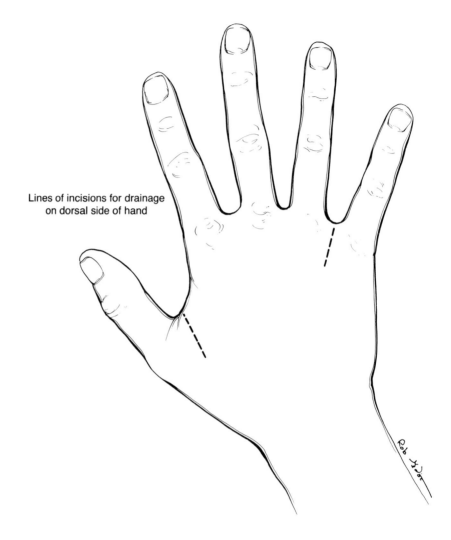

Lines of incisions for drainage
on dorsal side of hand

FIGURE 124–3. The dorsal incision begins just proximal to the web at the level of the metacarpophalangeal joints and extends 1 to 2 cm. proximally. After the skin is incised, the tissue is spread with a hemostat to drain the abscess.

Infection in the posterior adductor space is drained by a dorsal longitudinal incision between the index finger and the thumb that begins just proximal to the thumb-index web in order to avoid scar contracture. The skin and subcutaneous tissue are divided, the fascia is incised, the first dorsal interosseous muscle is retracted ulnarly, and the extensor pollicis longus tendon is retracted radially. The tissue beneath the fascia is spread with care to avoid the digital nerves and arteries and to open the abscess.

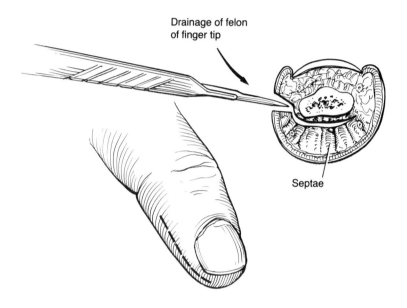

FIGURE 124-4. A *felon* is a subcutaneous abscess of the distal pulp of a digit and is associated with severe pain and swelling. The abscess involves the multiple vertical fibrous septae that divide the pulp into several small compartments. Therefore, infection in the distal digital pulp is a series of small, closed space infections, each requiring drainage. The abscess can extend into the distal phalanx and produce osteomyelitis, and, in severe cases, the pressure from the abscess can cause occlusion of digital vessels and necrosis of distal tissue.

After a metacarpal block for anesthesia (xylocaine without epinephrine), a lateral incision is made on the ulnar aspect of the index, long, or ring fingers and on the radial aspect of the thumb or small finger. The incision begins approximately 0.5 cm. distal to the distal interphalangeal joint flexion crease and extends distally in a straight line approximately 0.5 cm. from the edge of the nail plate and slightly distal to the nail matrix. The incision should be sufficiently dorsal that it does not damage the digital nerves and arteries and sufficiently distal to the flexor tendon sheath that it does not produce an iatrogenic tenosynovitis. The scalpel is inserted just palmar to the cortex of the distal phalanx. The tissue is separated from the periosteum of the distal phalanx, and the fibrous septae are divided to allow drainage. A gauze wick is inserted for 24 to 48 hours, and warm soaks are begun.

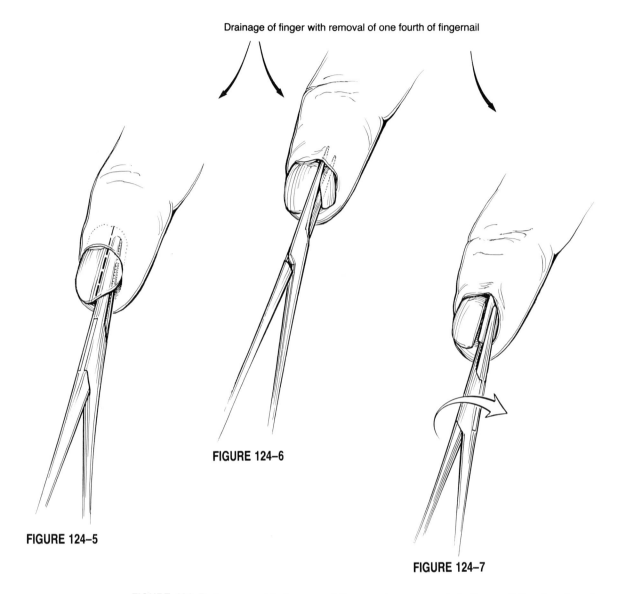

Drainage of finger with removal of one fourth of fingernail

FIGURE 124–6

FIGURE 124–5

FIGURE 124–7

FIGURE 124–5. A *paronychia* is one of the most common infections of the hand and involves the soft tissues around the fingernail. The cause is usually *Staphylococcus aureus* introduced into the paronychia by a hangnail or by nail biting or other trauma.

After a metacarpal block (xylocaine without epinephrine), a small, blunt hemostat is used to separate the deep surface of the nail plate from the underlying nail matrix and to separate the superficial surface of the nail plate from the overlying nail fold and eponychium.

FIGURE 124–6. Approximately one fourth of the nail plate, on the same side as the paronychia, is incised longitudinally with a pair of sharp small scissors. The incision extends from the distal nail plate, proximally beneath the nail fold and eponychium, to the base of the entire nail plate. Care should be taken to avoid incising the nail matrix, which could subsequently produce scarring and a ridge in the nail.

FIGURE 124–7. The detached segment of nail is grasped with a hemostat, gently manipulated counterclockwise and clockwise to detach any remaining soft tissue connections, and extracted. A gauze wick is inserted beneath the nail fold for 24 to 48 hours, and warm soaks are begun.

125

Surgical Procedures for Morbid Obesity

JOHN P. GRANT, M.D.

VERTICAL BANDED GASTROPLASTY

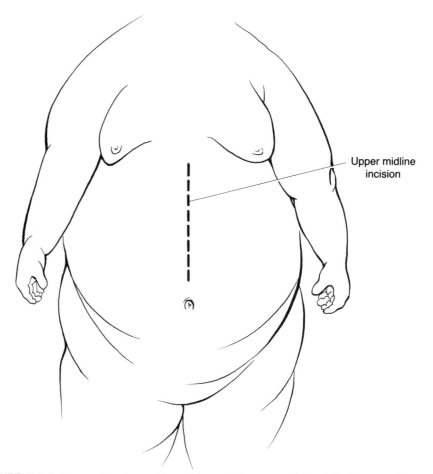

Upper midline incision

FIGURE 125–1. The patient is positioned in a slight reverse Trendelenburg position and placed under general anesthesia. A midline incision is extended from the xiphoid to the umbilicus.

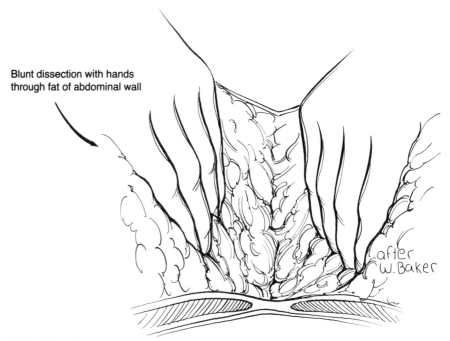

Blunt dissection with hands through fat of abdominal wall

after W. Baker

FIGURE 125–2. The subcutaneous tissues are separated by blunt dissection.

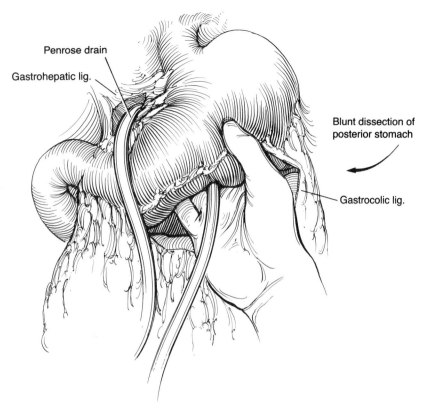

FIGURE 125–3. After abdominal exploration, an 8- to 10-cm. opening is made in the gastrocolic ligament, and the posterior wall of the stomach is freed from all attachments up to the gastroesophageal junction. An opening is made in the gastrohepatic ligament, and a Penrose drain is passed around the stomach for retraction.

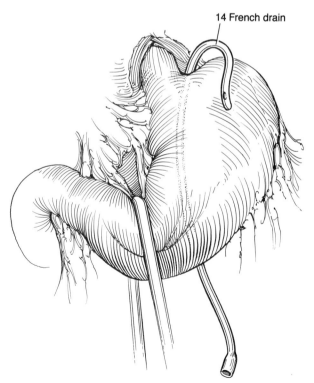

FIGURE 125–4. The peritoneum is opened overlying the distal esophagus, with care being taken not to injure the vagus nerve. A finger is passed posteriorly into the lesser sac just at the angle of His. A 14 French chest tube is inserted through this opening into the lesser sac, drawn caudally, and exited through the opening in the gastrocolic ligament.

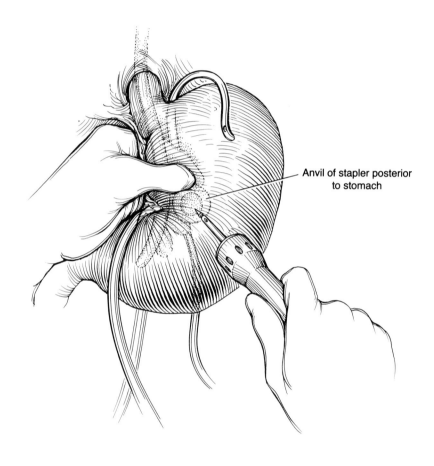

Anvil of stapler posterior
to stomach

FIGURE 125–5. A 24 French Maloney dilator is passed orally into the stomach and positioned along the lesser curvature. A 15-mm. EEA stapler is passed through the anterior and posterior walls of the stomach, with the anvil positioned along the lesser curvature against the Maloney dilator. The EEA stapler is fired and removed.

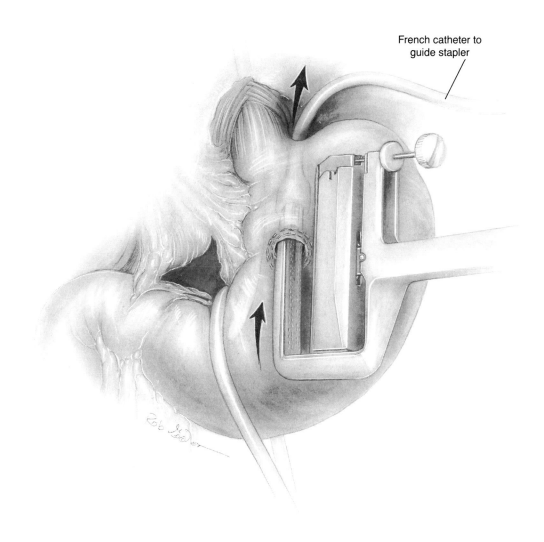

French catheter to
guide stapler

FIGURE 125–6. The 14 French chest tube is drawn through the EEA stapler hole and attached to the anvil of a TA-9OB stapler* or a V. Mueller PI-90 stapler† with 4.8-mm staples. The chest tube is carefully withdrawn, manipulating the anvil of the stapler along the posterior stomach wall and out at the angle of His.

*AutoSuture, U.S. Surgical Corporation, Norwalk, CT.
†3M Company, St. Paul, MN.

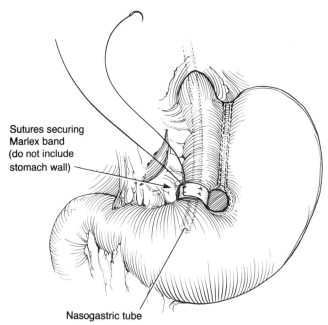

Sutures securing
Marlex band
(do not include
stomach wall)

Nasogastric tube

FIGURE 125–7. The stapler is positioned against the lesser curvature along the Maloney dilator and fired, placing four rows of staples and creating a 10- to 15-ml. gastric pouch. The mesentery along the lesser curvature at the opening for the EEA is carefully dissected bluntly, and a 1.5 × 6 cm. Marlex mesh strip is then wrapped around the lesser curvature through the EEA opening. The mesh is secured with 2-0 nylon sutures in two rows to create a 45- to 47-mm.-circumference ring. The sutures should not incorporate any stomach wall. Adjacent omentum is laid over the Marlex mesh and sutured in position.

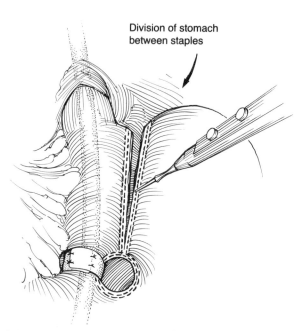

Division of stomach
between staples

FIGURE 125–8. If the Mueller stapler is used, the tissue is divided between the staple lines and each line is oversewn. The Maloney tube is removed, and a nasogastric tube is passed so that the tip is in the distal stomach just beyond the Marlex ring. The midline fascia is closed, and hemostasis is achieved in the subcutaneous fatty tissue. The skin is closed with staples, and a sterile dressing is applied. The nasogastric tube can usually be removed on the second postoperative day, and feedings can be initiated.

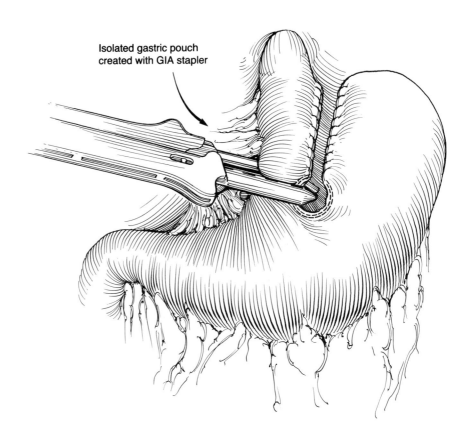

Isolated gastric pouch
created with GIA stapler

FIGURE 125–9. The operative procedure is that of the vertical banded gastroplasty with the PI-90 stapler and dividing between staple lines. The gastric pouch is then separated from the remainder of the stomach with a GIA stapler.

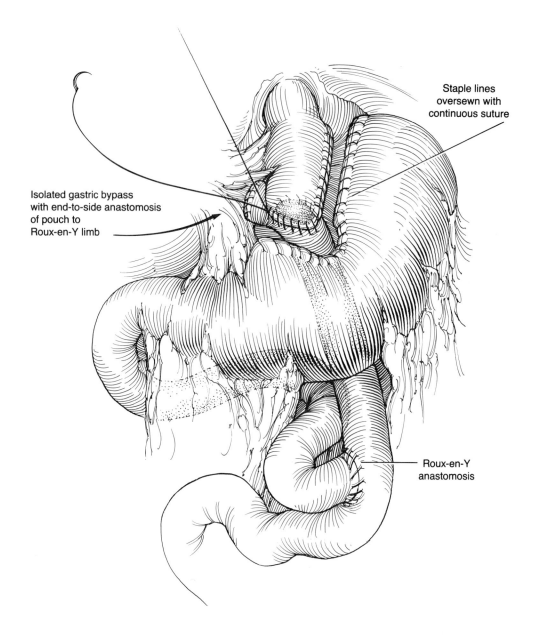

Staple lines
oversewn with
continuous suture

Isolated gastric bypass
with end-to-side anastomosis
of pouch to
Roux-en-Y limb

Roux-en-Y
anastomosis

FIGURE 125–10. The jejunum is divided and brought through the transverse mesocolon behind the stomach to the gastric pouch. An end-to-side anastomosis is made approximately 10 to 15 mm. in diameter with a single-layer suture of 3-0 Prolene or PDS. Staple lines are oversewn, and a nasogastric tube is passed with the tip just beyond the anastomosis. Some surgeons place a Stamm gastrostomy tube in the distal stomach for decompression, which is removed after 4 to 6 weeks. The proximal jejunal segment is sutured end-to-side into the distal jejunum 40 to 45 cm. beyond the jejunogastric anastomosis, and the abdomen is closed.

GASTRIC BYPASS (GREENVILLE ROUX-EN-Y PROCEDURE)

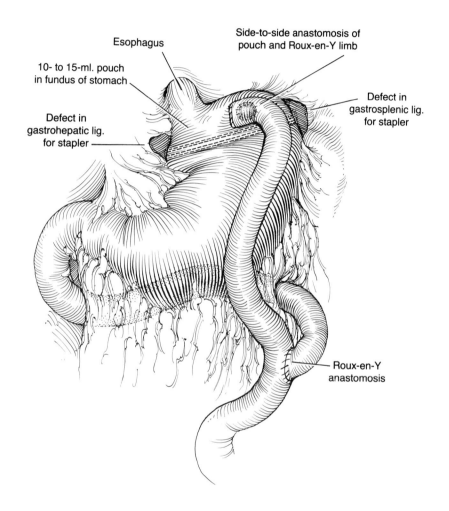

FIGURE 125–11. After entry into the abdomen and exploration, a defect is made in the gastrohepatic ligament 2 cm. beyond the gastroesophageal junction. Care is taken not to injure the vagus nerves. A second defect is made in the gastrosplenic mesentery just above the short gastric vessels. The loose fibrinous attachments posteriorly are freed between the two openings, and a TA-9OB or PI-90 stapler is passed. The stapler is fired, creating a 10- to 15-ml. gastric pouch.

The jejunum is divided with a GIA stapler 30 to 45 cm. distal to the ligament of Treitz, and the distal arm is brought up to the gastric pouch. A 15-mm. opening is made in both the gastric pouch and the jejunum, and a side-to-side single-layer anastomosis is constructed with continuous 3-0 Prolene or PDS sutures. A nasogastric tube is passed through the anastomosis, with the tip positioned just within the jejunum. The proximal jejunal segment is sutured end-to-side into the distal jejunum 40 to 45 cm. beyond the jejunogastric anastomosis. The abdomen is then closed.

INDEX